Fifth edition

Jones' Clinical Paediatric Surgery

Diagnosis and management

By the staff of the Royal Children's Hospital, Melbourne

Edited by:

John M Hutson
BS MD(Monash) MD(Melb) FRACS
Professor of Paediatric Surgery, Department of Paediatrics
Director, Department of General Surgery
Royal Children's Hospital

Alan A Woodward
MBBS, FRCS, FRACS
Head of Urology Service
Deputy Director, Department of General Surgery
Royal Children's Hospital

Spencer W Beasley
MbChB(Otago) MS (Melb) FRACS
Professor of Paediatric Surgery
Christchurch Hospital

b

Blackwell
Science
Asia

© 1999 by Blackwell Science Asia Pty Ltd

Published by Blackwell Science Asia Pty Ltd

First printed 1999

EDITORIAL OFFICES:

54 University Street, Carlton South,
Victoria 3053, Australia
Osney Mead. Oxford OX2 OEL, UK
25 John Street, London WC 1N 2BL, UK
23 Ainslie Place, Edinburgh EH3 6AJ, UK
350 Main Street, Malden,
MA 02148-5018, USA

OTHER EDITORIAL OFFICES:

Blackwell Wissenschafts-Verlag GmbH
Kurfilrstendamm 57
10707 Berlin, Germany
Zehemergasse 6
1140 Wien, Austria

Design by Design and Print Centre
Typeset by Graphicraft, Hong Kong
Printed by Brown Prior Anderson, Australia

DISTRIBUTORS

Blackwell Science Pty Ltd
54 University Street,
Carlton South, Victoria 3053, Australia

Orders Tel: 03 9347 0300
Fax: 03 9349 3016
E-mail: info@blacksci-asia.com.au
Internet: www.blackwell-science-asia.com.au

NORTH AMERICA

Blackwell Science, Inc.
Commerce Place, 350 Main Street,
Malden, MA 02148-5018

Orders Tel: 617388 8250
              800759 6102
Fax: 617388 8255

CANADA

Copp Clark Professional
200 Adelaide Street, West, 3rd Floor,
Toronto, Ontario M5H IW7

Orders Tel: 416597 1616
              800 8159417
Fax: 416 597 1616

UNITED KINGDOM

Marston Book Services Ltd
PO Box 87
Oxford, OX2 ODT

Orders Tel: 01865 791155
Fax: 01865 791927
Telex: 837515

CATALOGUING-IN-PUBLICATION DATA

5th ed.
Includes index.
ISBN 0 86793 012 8

1. Children - Diseases - Treatment. 2. Children - Surgery. 3. Pediatrics. I. Jones, Peter G. II. Hutson, John M. III. Beasley, Spencer W. IV Woodward, Alan A. (Alan Arthur). V. Royal Children's Hospital. VI. Title : Clinical paeditric surgery.

617.98:21

Contents

Abdomen

Urinary Tract

Trauma

Orthopaedics

Chest

Skin/Soft Tissues

Index

Contributors

A.W. Auldist, FRACS

Chairman, Division of Surgery
General Surgeon

S.W. Beasley MS, FRACS

Professor of Paediatric Surgery, University of
Otago, Christchurch Hospital, New Zealand
Previously General Surgeon
Senior Lecturer, University of Melbourne

R. Berkowitz, MD, FRACS

Director, Department of Otolaryngology
Otolaryngologist

A. Briedahl, FRACS

Craniofacial Surgeon

P.A. Dewan, MS, MD, FRCS, FRACS

Associate Professor, University of Melbourne
General and Urological Surgeon

J.E. Elder, FRACO, FRACS

Director, Department of Ophthalmology
Ophthalmologist

K. Graham, MD, FRCS (Ed), FRACS

Professor of Orthopaedic Surgery, University of
Melbourne
Director, Department of Orthopaedics

J.M. Hutson, MD, MD, FRACS

Professor of Paediatric Surgery, University of
Melbourne
Director, Department of General Surgery

B.R. Johnstone, FRACS

Plastic Surgeon

E.J. Keogh, FRCS, FRACS

Burns Surgeon

J Rosenfeld, MS, FRACS, FRCS, FACS,
FACTHM

Associate Professor of Neurosurgery, University
of Melbourne
Director, Department of Neurosurgery

K.B. Stokes, FRACS

General Surgeon

R.G. Taylor, FRACS

General and Burns Surgeon

A.A. Woodward, FRCS, FRACS

Deputy Director, Department of General Surgery
General and Urological Surgeon

Foreword to the First Edition

The progressive increase in the body of information relative to the surgical specialties has come to present a vexing problem in the instruction of medical students. There is not time in the medical curriculum to present everything about everything to them and in textbook material one is reduced either to synoptic sections in textbooks of surgery, or to complete and authoritative textbooks in the specialty too detailed for the student or the non-specialist.

There has long been a need for a book of modest size dealing with paediatric surgery in a way suited to the requirements of the medical student, general practitioner and paediatrician. Peter G. Jones and his associates from the distinguished and productive group at the Royal Children's Hospital in Melbourne have succeeded brilliantly in meeting this need. The book could have been entitled 'Surgical Conditions in Infancy and Childhood', for it deals with the child and his afflictions, their symptoms, diagnosis and treatment rather than the surgery as such. The reader is told when and how urgently an operation is required, and enough about the nature of the procedure to understand its risks and appreciate its results. This is what students need to know and what paediatricians and general practitioners need to be refreshed on.

Many of the chapters are novel, in that they deal not with categorical diseases but with the conditions which give rise to a specific symptom; thus: Vomiting in the First Month of Life, The Jaundiced Newborn Baby, Surgical Causes of Failure to Thrive. The chapter on genetic counselling is a model of information and good sense.

The book is systematic and thorough. A clean style, logical sequential discussions and avoidance of esoterica allow the presentation of substantial information over the entire field of paediatric surgery in this comfortable-sized volume with well chosen illustrations and carefully selected bibliography. Many charts and tables, original in conception, enhance the clear presentation.

No other book so satisfactorily meets the needs of the student for broad and authoritative coverage in a modest compass. The paediatric house officer (in whose hospital more than 50 per cent of the patients are, after all, surgical) will be serviced equally well. Paediatric surgeons will find between these covers an account of the attitudes, practices and results of one of the world's great paediatric surgical centres. The book comes as a fitting tribute to the 100th Anniversary of the Royal Children's Hospital.

MARK M. RAVITCH

PROFESSOR OF PEDIATRIC SURGERY
UNIVERSITY OF PENNSYLVANIA

Tribute to Mr Peter Jones

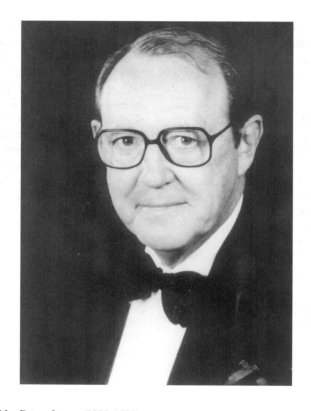

Mr Peter Jones (1922–1995) MB, MS, FRCS, FRACS, FACS, FAAP. The first Australian surgeon to obtain the FRACS in paediatric surgery, and member of RACS Council (1987–95), Vice-President of the Medical Defence Association of Victoria (1974–1988) and President of the Australian Association of Surgeons (1983–1986). He was legendary as a medical historian and in heraldry, as a great raconteur, but primarily as a great student teacher.

Preface to the Fifth Edition

The objective of the first edition of this book was to bring together information on surgical conditions in infancy and childhood for use by medical students and resident medical officers. It is a great satisfaction to our contributors that the book has fulfilled this aim successfully, and that a fifth edition is now required. Family doctors, paediatricians and many other people concerned with the welfare of children have also, it seems, found the book useful.

A knowledgeable medical publisher once commented to Peter Jones that this is not a book about surgery but about paediatrics, and that is what it should be, given the omission of almost all details of operative surgery.

The plan for the fourth edition has been retained, although each chapter now begins with clinical histories and some key questions, allowing students to focus on the problems. Many of the contributors to this edition are new members of the surgical staff, and bring to the fifth edition a fresh outlook and state-of-the-art ideas. We have maintained the previously successful style, while including many new photographs and drawings.

Mr Peter Jones died in 1995 and this edition is dedicated to him. Peter was a great teacher and it remains a daunting task for those who follow in his footsteps. We hope this new edition will continue to honour the memory of a great paediatric surgeon who understood what students need to know.

John M. Hutson

Alan A. Woodward

Spencer W. Beasley

MAY 1999

Acknowledgements

Many members of the Royal Children's Hospital community have made valuable contributions to this fifth edition. We thank the staff of the Education and Resource Centre for the quality of their photography, which continues to be at a very high standard. The secretarial staff of the Department of Surgery, and particularly Mrs Elizabeth Vorrath, are thanked sincerely for their untiring effort. Rowena and Iain Hutson are thanked for helping to sort the illustrations. Finally, we express our gratitude to Shirley Green of Blackwell Science Asia for bringing this edition to fruition.

—1—

Antenatal Diagnosis —
Surgical Aspects

CASE 1

At 18 weeks' gestation, right fetal hydronephrosis is diagnosed on ultrasonography.

Q. 1.1   *Discuss the further management during pregnancy.*

Q. 1.2   *Does the antenatal diagnosis improve the postnatal outlook for this condition?*

CASE 2

An exomphalos is diagnosed at the 18-week ultrasonographic examination.

Q. 2.1   *What further evaluation is required at that stage?*

Q. 2.2   *Does this anomaly influence the timing and mode of delivery?*

Antenatal diagnosis is one of the most rapidly developing fields in medical practice. While the genetic and biochemical evaluation of the developing fetus provides the key to many medical diagnoses, the development of accurate ultrasonography has provided the impetus to the diagnosis of surgical fetal anomalies. At first, it was expected that the antenatal diagnosis of fetal problems would lead to better treatment and an improved outcome. In some cases this has been true. Antenatally diagnosed fetuses with gastroschisis have been delivered in a tertiary level obstetric hospital with neonatal intensive care in order to prevent hypothermia, and the results of treatment have improved. In other cases, such as diaphragmatic hernia, these expectations have not been fulfilled because antenatal diagnosis has opened a Pandora's box of complex and lethal anomalies, which in the past never survived the pregnancy, and were recorded in the statistics of fetal death *in utero* and stillbirth.

INDICATIONS AND TIMING FOR ANTENATAL ULTRASONOGRAPHY

All pregnancies are now assessed with mid-trimester ultrasonography usually performed at 17 to 18 weeks' gestation. The main purpose of this examination is to assess the obstetric parameters of the pregnancy, but the increasingly important secondary role of this study is to screen the fetus for anomalies (Fig. 1.1). Most anomalies are detectable at 18 weeks but some only become apparent later in the pregnancy. Earlier ultrasonography examinations may be performed with transvaginal scanning in special circumstances, such as a previous pregnancy with a neural tube defect, and increasingly to detect early signs of aneuploidy.

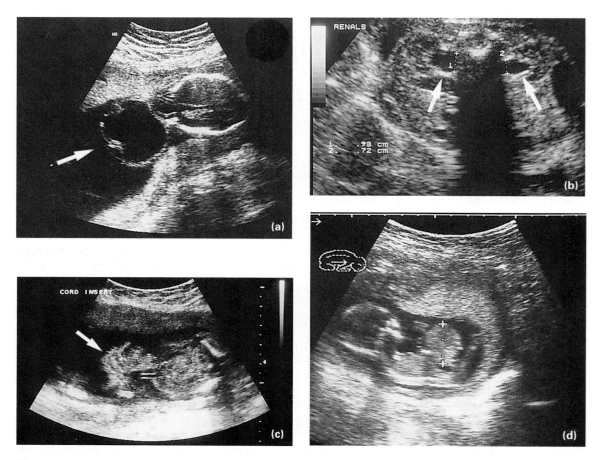

Fig. 1.1 (a) Encephalocele shown in a cross-section of the fetal head. The sac protruding through the posterior skull defect is arrowed. (b) Bilateral hydronephrosis shown in an upper abdominal section. The dilated renal pelvis containing clear fluid is marked. (c) The irregular outline of the free-floating bowel in the amniotic cavity of a term baby with gastroschisis. (d) A longitudinal section through a 14-week fetus showing a large exomphalos. The head is seen to the left of the picture. The large sac (marked) is seen between blurred (moving) images of the arms and legs.

NATURAL HISTORY OF FETAL ANOMALIES

Before the advent of ultrasonography, paediatric surgeons saw only a selected group of infants with congenital anomalies. These babies had survived the pregnancy and lived long enough after birth to reach surgical attention. Thus the babies coming to surgical treatment were already a selected group, mostly with a good prognosis.

Antenatal diagnosis has brought surgeons into contact with a new group of conditions with a poor prognosis, and at last the full spectrum of pathology is coming to surgical attention. For example, posterior urethral valves causing obstruction of the urinary tract were thought to

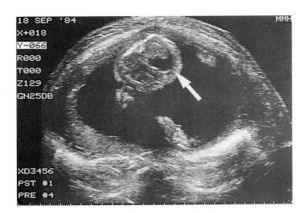

Fig. 1.2 Cross-section of a uterus with marked polyhydramnios. The fetal chest is seen in cross-section within the uterus. The fluid-filled cavity within the left side of the chest is the stomach protruding through a diaphragmatic hernia (arrow).

be rare, with an incidence of 1 : 5000 male births; most cases did well with postnatal valve resection. It is now known that the true incidence of urethral valves is 1 : 2500 male births and these additional cases did not come to surgical attention because they were severe examples of intrauterine renal failure with either death *in utero* or early neonatal death from respiratory problems of Potter's syndrome. It was thought that antenatal diagnosis would improve the outcome of such congenital anomalies, but the overall results have appeared to become worse with these severe 'new' cases being included.

There are similar problems with the antenatal diagnosis of diaphragmatic hernia (Fig. 1.2). Congenital diaphragmatic was not associated with multiple congenital anomalies when cases presented after birth. Now antenatal diagnosis of diaphragmatic hernia has uncovered a more severe subgroup with associated chromosomal and multiple developmental anomalies. It would seem that the earlier the diaphragmatic hernia is diagnosed, the worse is the outcome.

Despite these problems, there are many advantages in antenatal diagnosis. The outcome of many conditions is improved by the prior knowledge of these 'congenital' anomalies.

MANAGEMENT FOLLOWING ANTENATAL DIAGNOSIS

Fetal management

Cases diagnosed antenatally may be classified into three groups:

Good prognosis

In some cases, such as a unilateral hydronephrosis, there is no place for active management, and the main task is to track the progress of the problem through pregnancy with serial ultrasonography. The detailed diagnosis is made with the more sophisticated range of tests available after birth, and UTIs are prevented with prophylactic antibiotics commenced at birth. Thus a child with severe vesico-ureteric reflux may go through the first year of life without any UTIs. If the parents receive counselling by a surgeon experienced in the care of the particular problem, they have time to understand the condition. Thus, in the case of cleft lip seen on fetal ultrasonography, the parents will have time to understand the nature of the problem by seeing photographs of the condition before and after surgery, and will have the chance to meet other families with this condition. With such preparation, the family can cope better with the birth of a malformed baby.

The paediatric surgeon also has an important role to play in advising the obstetrician on the prognosis of a particular condition. Some cases of exomphalos are easy to repair, whereas in others, the defect may be so large that primary repair will be difficult. Moreover, in some fetuses there may be major chromosomal and cardiac anomalies associated with the exomphalos that may alter the outcome. In exomphalos, therefore, the prognosis varies from good to poor. In other conditions, the outlook for a congenital defect may change as treatment improves. Gastroschisis was a lethal condition before 1970, but now management has changed and there is a 95 per cent survival rate. In those cases with a good prognosis, fetal intervention is not indicated and the pregnancy should be allowed to run its course. The mode of delivery will usually be determined on obstetric grounds. Babies with exomphalos may be delivered by vaginal delivery if the birth process is easy. There is evidence that spina bifida fetuses undergo further nerve damage at vaginal delivery, and caesarian section may be preferred in this circumstance. If urgent neonatal surgery is required, for example, for gastroschisis, the baby should be delivered at a tertiary obstetric unit with a neonatal intensive care unit and neonatal surgical service. In other cases, for example, cleft lip and palate, where urgent surgery is not required but good family and nursing support is important, delivery close to the family's home may be more appropriate. Antenatal planning and family counselling give us the opportunity to make the appropriate arrangements for the birth. A baby born with gastroschisis in the middle of winter in a bush nursing hospital in the mountains, many hours away from surgical care, will have a very different outlook from a baby with the same condition born at a major neonatal centre.

Poor prognosis

Anencephaly, diaphragmatic hernia with major chromosomal anomalies, or urethral valves with early intrauterine renal failure, are examples of conditions with a poor prognosis. These are lethal conditions, and the outcome is predetermined before the diagnosis is made.

Late deterioration

Initial assessment of the fetal anomaly indicates a good prognosis with no reason for interference, but later in gestation, the fetus deteriorates and some action must be undertaken to prevent a lethal outcome. An example would be the lower urinary tract obstruction seen in posterior urethral valves. Loss of liquor with oligohydramnios is a sign of intrauterine renal failure. There are several ways to treat this problem. If the gestation is at a viable stage, for example, 36 weeks, labour could be induced and the urethral valves treated at birth. If the risks of premature delivery are higher, for example, at 28 weeks' gestation, temporary relief may be obtained by using percutaneous transuterine techniques to place a shunt catheter from the fetal bladder into the amniotic cavity. These catheters tend to become dislodged by fetal activity. A more definitive approach to drain the urinary tract is intrauterine surgery to perform a vesicostomy and allow the pregnancy to continue. This procedure has been performed with success in a few cases of posterior urethral valves. These patients are highly selected and there are very few centres in the world performing intrauterine surgery. At present this surgery is regarded as experimental, and reserved for rare situations.

Antenatal ultrasonography has become the most important means of diagnosing fetal anomalies and has given us a valuable means of understanding the natural history of developmental abnormalities.

SURGICAL COUNSELLING

When a child is born with unanticipated birth defects there is inevitably shock and confusion for the family until the diagnosis is clarified and they can assimilate and accept the information given to them, and make plans for the future. Important treatment decisions will have to be made urgently while the new parents are often still too stunned to play any sensible part in the ongoing care of their baby. Antenatal diagnosis has changed this situation. New parents may now have many weeks to understand and come to terms with their baby's problem. With suitable preparation they can play an active role in the postnatal diagnosis and treatment choices for their newborn baby.

The paediatric surgical specialist who treats the particular problem uncovered by antenatal diagnosis is in the best position to advise the parents on the prognosis and further treatment of the baby. Detailed information on the management after birth with photographs before and after corrective surgery allows the parents to understand and come to terms with the surgical procedures. The opportunity to meet other families with a child treated for the same condition gives time for the pregnant woman and her husband to understand the problem before the birth. Handling and nurturing the baby immediately after birth is an important part of bonding. Parents and nursing staff suddenly confronted with a newborn baby with the unexpected finding of a gross anomaly, such as sacro-coccygeal teratoma, may be afraid to handle the baby who is then taken away to another hospital for complex surgery. Parents in this situation may take many months to relate to the new baby and understand the nature of the problem. However, when prepared by antenatal diagnosis the nursing staff and parents will quickly realise that they can handle and nurture the baby. Parents will understand the nature of the surgery and bond with the baby. Thus, instead of being stunned by the birth of a malformed baby, the new parents can play an active part in postnatal surgical management and provide better informed consent for surgery.

FURTHER READING

Gibbs D.L., Piecuch R.E. Graf J.L., Leonard C.H., Farrell J.A. & Harrison M.R. (1998) Neurodevelopmental outcome after open fetal surgery. *J. Pediatr. Surg.* **33**: 1254–6.

Harrison M.R. (1998) The fetus as a patient. In: O'Neill J.A., Rowe M.I., Grosfeld J.L., Fonkalsrud E.W. & Coran A.G. (eds), *Pediatric Surgery*, 5th edn, Mosby, St. Louis, pp. 33–42.

Kimble R.M., Harding J.E. & Kolbe A. (1998) Does gut atresia cause polyhydramnios? *Pediatr. Surg. Int.* **13**: 115–17.

Lewis D.A., Rickert C., Bowerman R. & Hirschl R.B. (1997) Prenatal ultrasonography frequently fails to diagnose diaphragmatic hernia. *J. Pediatr. Surg.* **32**: 352–6.

Najmaldin A.S., Burge D.M. & Atwell J.D. (1990) Antenatally-diagnosed urological abnormalities: where do we stand? *Pediatr. Surg. Int.* **5**: 195–7.

Nielson O.H. (1996) The paediatric surgeon and prenatal diagnosis. Editorial. *Pediatr. Surg. Int.* **11**: 1–3.

Nielson O.H., Kvist N. & Brocks V. (1996) Abdominal wall defects in the era of prenatal diagnosis. *Pediatr. Surg. Int.* **11**: 4–7.

Scott J.E.S. & Renwick M. (1990) Northern region fetal abnormality survey results 1987. *J. Pediatr. Surg.* **25**: 394–7.

Thorup J., Leng K., Rabol A., Passalides A. & Nielson O.H. (1996) Follow-up of prenatally diagnosed unilateral hydronephrosis. *Pediatr. Surg. Int.* **11**: 18–21.

Zachai E.H. & Robin N.H. (1998) Clinical genetics. In: O'Neill J.A., Rowe M.I., Grosfeld J.L. Fonkalsrud E.W. & Coran A.G. (eds) *Pediatric Surgery*, 5th edn, Mosby, St. Louis, vol. 1, pp. 19–32.

— 2 —

The Care and Transport of the Newborn

CASE

A 30-week gestation infant is born with gastroschisis.

Q. 1.1   *What advice would you give the referring institution about the management of this infant prior to transport to a tertiary institution?*

The newborn infant with a major surgical condition should be transported and treated in a neonatal unit with paediatric surgical facilities. It is only in such a unit that the specialised surgical, anaesthetic and nursing expertise necessary for neonatal surgery will be found.

A detailed pre-operative assessment is necessary to detect associated or coexistent developmental anomalies. Vital disturbances should be corrected before operation, and predictable complications of the abnormalities should be anticipated and recognised early.

RESPIRATORY CARE

The aims of respiratory care are: (i) to maintain a clear airway; (ii) to prevent abdominal distension; (iii) to avoid aspiration of gastric contents; and (iv) to provide supplementary oxygen if necessary. Assessment of gestational age and weight will identify the premature infant who is susceptible to hyaline membrane disease and apnoeic episodes. Small-for-dates babies are more likely to suffer asphyxia at birth, meconium aspiration and pneumothorax. An emergency tray with appropriately sized oral airways, face mask and bag, laryngoscope, endotracheal and suction tubes should be readily available.

Placing the baby in the prone position improves the airways and reduces gastro-oesophageal reflux and the likelihood of aspiration of gastric contents.

Suction of the pharyngeal secretions maintains a clear airway, especially in the premature infant with poorly developed laryngeal reflexes, and in the infant with oesophageal atresia.

A nasogastric tube, size 8 french, will prevent life-threatening aspiration of vomitus, provided the tube is kept patent and allowed to drain freely with additional aspiration at frequent intervals. It will also reduce abdominal distension and improve pulmonary ventilation in patients with intestinal obstruction or congenital diaphragmatic hernia.

Oxygen therapy, endotracheal intubation and ventilation will be required in the pre-operative resuscitation of some neonates with conditions such as congenital diaphragmatic hernia.

CIRCULATING BLOOD VOLUME

Conditions that diminish the circulating volume include neonatal bowel obstruction and gastroschisis. The fluid is lost from vomiting, ileus and evaporation.

Blood loss in the neonatal period may be due to birth trauma, haemorrhagic disease from Vitamin K deficiency or clotting defects associated with sepsis. The blood volume of a full-term infant is 80 mL/kg. Blood loss of only 30 mL in a neonate is equivalent to losing 500 mL in an adult.

Fresh whole blood is cross-matched for major operations in the neonatal period. Blood loss during surgery is kept to a minimum and measured by weighing all swabs and packs used. The haemoglobin concentration in the first few days of life is about 19 g/dL and the haematocrit 50 to 70 per cent. Blood viscosity is relatively high, and blood loss in this circumstance may be replaced in part with blood and in part with a crystalloid solution, which lowers the viscosity of the blood.

Diminished blood volume in a sick neonate with a bowel obstruction will lead to poor peripheral circulation. The baby will be lethargic and pale, with cool limbs, venoconstriction and cyanosis. Acidosis becomes a complicating factor. In this situation a 'bolus infusion' of a crystalloid solution such as Hartmann's solution over 15 minutes at 10 mL/kg is used for resuscitation. When this is effective, the peripheral circulation will improve dramatically. If this initial infusion is not adequate, further bolus infusions of crystalloid at 10 mL/kg may be given and the clinical response monitored.

CONTROL OF BODY TEMPERATURE

The sick neonate with a surgical condition is prone to hypothermia, defined as a core body temperature of less than 36°C. In hypothermia, heat production is stimulated above normal metabolic requirements and may be boosted by thermogenesis from increased metabolism of brown fat deposits. However, if heat loss exceeds heat production, the body temperature will continue to fall, leading to acidosis and the depression of respiratory, cardiac and nervous functions.

All metabolic functions are altered by hypothermia. Newborn infants, especially the premature, are at risk of excessive heat loss because of the relatively large surface area to volume ratio and the lack of subcutaneous insulating fat.

Heat loss occurs from the body surface to the environment by radiation, conduction, convection and the evaporation of water. Excessive heat loss during transport, assessment and operation must be avoided, particularly in conditions such as gastroschisis where the eviscerated bowel provides a very large surface area for evaporation. Heat loss is controlled once the bowel is wrapped in domestic clear plastic wrap to prevent evaporation, and the baby is placed in the warm environment of a humidicrib.

Radiant overhead heaters are of particular value during procedures such as intravenous cannulation or the induction of anaesthesia because they allow unimpeded access to the infant. Wet packs should never be applied to a neonate as they will accelerate evaporative and conductive heat losses.

FLUIDS, ELECTROLYTES AND NUTRITION

Many infants with a surgical condition cannot be fed in the perioperative period. Intravenous fluids provide daily maintenance requirements and prevent dehydration. The total volume of fluid given must supply maintenance requirements, restore fluid and electrolyte deficits and replace ongoing losses.
- Maintenance water requirements are:
  60–80 mL/kg on day 1 of life
  80–100 mL/kg on day 2
  100–150 mL/kg on day 3 and thereafter.
- Maintenance electrolyte requirements are:
  Sodium: 3 mmol/kg per day
  Chloride: 3 mmol/kg/day
  Potassium: 2 mmol/kg per day.

- Maintenance joule requirements are: 100–140 kJ/kg per day.

These maintenance requirements can be provided in the first week by a solution made up of 5 per cent dextrose in 0.225 per cent sodium chloride (sodium: 35 mmol/L) with the addition of potassium chloride at 20 mmol/L. However, this solution is inadequate for long-term maintenance of body functions as it has many deficiencies, especially in kJ.

Replacement of fluid and electrolyte deficiencies may be necessary in surgical patients, such as those with neonatal bowel obstruction. Before birth, the placenta maintains fluid and electrolyte balance. At birth, electrolyte levels are normal despite long-standing bowel obstruction, and extracellular water levels are relatively high. Persistent vomiting after birth soon causes dehydration and electrolyte imbalance. The degree of dehydration can be measured by the clinical parameters of tissue turgor, the state of peripheral circulation, depression of the fontanelle, dryness of the mouth and urine output. Body weight loss also gives an approximation of water loss.

The rule of thumb for estimating water loss is that dehydration of 5 per cent or less of body mass has few clinical manifestations: 5 to 8 per cent shows moderate clinical signs of dehydration; 10 per cent shows severe signs and poor peripheral circulation. Thus a 3000-gram infant who has been vomiting and has a diminished urine output, but shows no overt signs of dehydration, may have lost approximately 5 per cent of body mass and will require 3000 × 5 per cent mL = 150 mL fluid replacement to correct the deficit. Maintenance fluid requirements must be administered also.

Electrolyte estimations are most useful for identifying a deficiency of electrolytes that are distributed mainly in the extracellular fluid, for example, sodium, but will not be as reliable for electrolytes that are found mainly in the intracellular space, for example, potassium. Fluid and electrolyte deficiency due to vomiting will need to be replaced with a crystalloid solution that contains adequate levels of sodium, for example, 0.9 per cent sodium chloride (sodium: 150 mmol/L).

Continuing losses of fluid and electrolytes need to be measured and replaced. Losses may arise from nasogastric tube aspirates in bowel obstruction, diarrhoea from an ileostomy, and the excessive urinary losses that may occur after the relief of urinary obstruction; for example, after the resection of posterior urethral valves. When the losses are high they are best measured and replaced with an intravenous infusion of electrolytes equivalent to those of the fluid being lost.

Intravenous nutrition will be required when the period of starvation extends beyond 4 to 5 days. Common indications for intravenous nutrition in the neonatal period include necrotising enterocolitis, extensive gut resection and gastroschisis. The aim of intravenous nutrition is to provide all substances necessary for normal growth and development. Intravenous nutrition may be maintained for weeks or months as required. Complications of prolonged nutrition include sepsis and jaundice.

Oral nutrition is preferred where possible and breastfeeding is best. Surgery to the alimentary tract may make oral feeding impossible for a variable period: gut enzyme function may be poor and various substrates in the feeds may not be absorbed. Lactose intolerance is seen commonly and leads to diarrhoea with the passage of acidic fluid stools. Other malabsorptive problems relate to sugars, protein, fat and the osmolarity of the feeds. These can be handled by altering the conformation of the feeds or, in severe cases, by a period of intravenous nutrition to allow the gut enzymes time to recover.

BIOCHEMICAL ABNORMALITIES

Important problems include metabolic acidosis, hypoglycaemia and hypocalcaemia. These are corrected before operation because they may adversely influence the infant's response to anaesthetic agents.

Metabolic acidosis

Metabolic acidosis, which may result from hypovolaemia, dehydration, cold stress, renal failure or hypoxia, increases pulmonary vascular resistance and impairs cardiac output. Acidosis is corrected by giving a dose of sodium bicarbonate, which is calculated from the estimated base deficit, using the formula: Base deficit $\times$ weight (kg) $\times$ 0.3 = dose of sodium bicarbonate (mmol).

Hypoglycaemia

Hypoglycaemia occurs in the sick newborn, especially if premature. Liver stores of glycogen are small, as are fat stores. Starvation and stress will use up liver glycogen rapidly, and there will be a switch to fatty acid metabolism to maintain blood glucose levels, with consequent ketoacidosis. Gluconeogenesis from amino acids or pyruvate is slow to develop in the newborn, due to the relative inactivity of liver enzymes. A point is soon reached when blood glucose levels cannot be maintained and severe hypoglycaemia will result, causing apnoea, convulsions and cerebral damage. These complications of hypoglycaemia may be prevented by intravenous dextrose infusions. Young babies should not be starved for longer than 4 hours before surgery.

Hypocalcaemia

Hypocalcaemia may occur in infants with respiratory distress. The ionized calcium level in the blood maintains cell membrane activity. Hypocalcaemia may cause twitching and convulsions, and can be corrected by slow infusion of calcium gluconate.

PREVENTION OF INFECTION

The poorly developed immune defences of the newborn infant predispose to infection with Gram positive and Gram negative organisms. Infection may spread rapidly and result in septicaemia.

Signs of systemic infection in the neonate include hypothermia, pallor and lethargy.

Early recognition and treatment of infection is aided by bacteriological cultures from the infant's nose, throat, umbilicus and rectum, both on admission to hospital and subsequently on a regular basis. This is important in picking up 'marker organisms' such as multiple antibiotic-resistant *Staphylococcus aureus*. When infection is suspected, a 'septic work-up' is performed, taking specimens of CSF, urine and blood for culture and starting appropriate intravenous antibiotics immediately.

Infants undergoing surgery are at special risk of infection, and care must be taken not to introduce pathogenic organisms: this applies particularly to cross-infection in the neonatal ward. Prophylactic antibiotics may be used to cover major surgery.

PARENTS

An important part of the care for neonates undergoing surgery is the reassurance and support of the infant's anxious parents. The mother may be confined in a maternity hospital while her baby is separated from her and undergoing major surgery in another institution. Close communication is important in this situation, and the mother and baby should be brought together as soon as possible. The parents should handle and fondle the baby to facilitate bonding and for the infant's general welfare. With goodwill, gentle contact between infant and mother can be achieved, even in difficult circumstances.

GENERAL PRINCIPLES OF NEONATAL TRANSPORT

The transport of a critically ill neonate is a precarious undertaking, and the following principles should be followed:
(1) The infant's condition should be stabilised before embarkation.

(2) The most experienced/qualified personnel available should accompany the patient.

(3) Specialised neonatal 'retrieval' services should be used.

(4) Transport should be as rapid as possible, but without causing further deterioration or incurring unnecessary risks to the patient or transporting personnel.

(5) Transport should be undertaken early rather than late.

(6) All equipment should be checked before setting out.

(7) The receiving institution should be notified early so that additional staff and equipment can be prepared for arrival.

TRANSPORT OF NEONATAL EMERGENCIES

A list of the more common emergencies is given in Table 2.1. Most infants with these conditions

Table 2.1 Neonatal surgical conditions requiring transportation

Obvious malformations	Exomphalos/gastroschisis
	Myelomeningocele/ encephalocele
	Imperforate anus
Respiratory distress	
Upper airways obstruction	Choanal atresia
	Pierre–Robin syndrome
Lung compression	Congenital lobar emphysema
	Pulmonary cyst(s)
	Pneumothorax (should have chest drain inserted)
	Congenital diaphragmatic hernia
Congenital heart disease	
Acute alimentary or abdominal emergencies	Oesophageal atresia
	Intestinal obstruction
	Necrotising enterocolitis
	Haematemesis and/or melaena
Ambiguous genitalia	

should have transport arranged as soon as the diagnosis is apparent or suspected.

Some developmental anomalies do not require transportation, and specialist consultation at the hospital of birth may suffice (for example, cleft lip and palate, orthopaedic deformities). Where doubt exists concerning the appropriateness or timing of transportation, specialist advice should be sought.

Choice of vehicle

The choice between road ambulance, helicopter or fixed-wing aircraft will depend on distance, availability of vehicle, time of day, traffic conditions, airport facilities and weather conditions. In general, fixed-wing aircraft offer no time advantages for transfers of under 160 km (100 miles).

Patients with entrapped gas (for example, pneumothorax or significant abdominal distension) are better not to travel by air. If air travel is necessary, the aircraft should fly at low levels if it is unpressurised, otherwise expansion of the trapped gases with a decrease in the ambient atmospheric pressure may make ventilation difficult.

Communication

Good communication between the referring and receiving institutions can be crucial to survival and expedites treatment prior to transportation. Any change in the patient's condition should be reported to the receiving unit in advance of arrival. Detailed documentation of the history and written permission for treatment, including surgery, should be sent with the infant. In addition, neonates require 10 mL of maternal blood to accompany them, as well as cord blood and the placenta, if available.

Details of stabilisation procedures can be discussed with the headquarters of the transport team if difficulties arise while awaiting their arrival.

Written permission for transport is required. A full explanation of what has been arranged and why, and an accurate prognosis should be given to the parents. They should be allowed as much

Table 2.2 Oxygen cylinders

Size	Volume (L)	Duration of supply (h)		
		2 L/min	5 L/min	10 L/min
B	220	1.75	0.75	0.33
C	440	3.25	1.5	0.75
D	1500	12.25	5.0	2.5

access to the infant or child prior to transport as is possible. The parents can be given a 'Polaroid' photograph of the infant, taken before departure or at admission to hospital, if they are to be separated from their infant.

Equipment required

If a specialised retrieval team is not available, the following basic equipment is required.

Newborn infants require a portable incubator that operates from the ambulance battery or a self-contained source. A thermometer or temperature probe is used to monitor temperature; protection against cold stress can be aided by the use of plain plastic wrap or baby blankets.

An adequate supply of oxygen must be taken; cylinders must be immobilised carefully in the transporting vehicle, and the volume of oxygen required is calculated from the flow rate and the estimated time of transport (+50 per cent for unexpected delays) (Table 2.2).

Suction for clearing secretions is required. Low suction pressures should be used in neonates, so care is needed if suction provided for adult transport in ambulance vehicles is to be used. Controlled suction can be provided by the use of an oral mucus extractor.

A bag and mask of suitable size for emergency hand ventilation should be carried for any patient at even remote risk of respiratory failure.

A battery-operated infusion pump is required for a patient who has an intravenous infusion line. In the absence of a mechanical pump, controlled rates can be provided by the use of a three-way tap and syringe to give an intermittent bolus at 1 minute intervals. Restraining devices immobilize the stretcher, incubator and other equipment, and secure the patient safely. Drugs vary with the requirements of the individual patient, but may include analgesics, vasopressors and hydrocortisone.

STABILISATION OF NEONATES PRIOR TO TRANSFER

Temperature control

An incubator or radiant warmer is used to keep the infant warm. Recommended incubator temperatures are shown in Table 2.3. The infant should be covered except for parts required for observation or access. Axillary or rectal temperatures should be taken half-hourly, or quarter-hourly if under a radiant warmer.

Respiratory distress

Oxygen requirements

Enough oxygen should be given to abolish cyanosis and ensure adequate saturation. If

> **Box 2.1 Neonatal medical conditions requiring stabilisation before transport**
>
> (1) Prematurity
>
> (2) Temperature control problems
>
> (3) Respiratory distress causing hypoxia and/or respiratory failure
>
> (4) Metabolic derangements
> — hypoglycaemia
> — metabolic acidosis
> — hypocalcaemia
>
> (5) Shock
>
> (6) Convulsions

Table 2.3 Incubator temperature

Baby's weight (g)	Incubator temperature (°C)
< 1000	35–37
1000–1500	34–36
1500–2000	33–35
2000–2500	32–34
< 2500	31–33

measurements of blood gases are available, an arterial P_{O_2} of 50 to 80 mmHg is desirable. Although an excessively high P_{O_2} is liable to initiate retinopathy of prematurity, a short period of hyperoxia is less likely to be detrimental than a similarly short period of hypoxia.

Respiratory failure

Infants in severe respiratory failure (on clinical grounds or $P_{CO_2} > 70$ mmHg), or those with apnoea, may require endotracheal intubation and intermittent positive pressure ventilation.

Metabolic derangements

Hypoglycaemia should be corrected by intravenous infusion of glucose. Monitoring of babies at risk should be done with Dextrostix. Intravenous infusion may be by the umbilical, or a peripheral, route.

An infusion of blood or plasma expander at 10 to 20 mL/kg, i.v. over 0.5 to 1 hour may be required to correct shock.

Acid-base balance should be estimated if facilities are available. Otherwise, a small volume of sodium bicarbonate (3 mmol/kg, slowly i.v.) may be given to an infant who has been asphyxiated severely, has had recurrent hypoxia, or shows signs of poor peripheral circulation.

Convulsions should be controlled with phenobarbitone (10 to 15 mg/kg i.v. or orally) or diphenylhydantoin (15 mg, i.v. or orally).

Specialist advice regarding management of specific conditions should be sought from the transporting agency. For example, in gastroschisis and exomphalos the exposed viscera should be wrapped in clean plastic wrap to prevent heat-loss; moist packs or gauze should never be used. A nasogastric tube with continuous drainage is required for patients with diaphragmatic hernia (Chapter 5), bowel obstruction (Chapter 7) or exomphalos (Chapter 9). In oesophageal atresia, frequent aspiration of the blind upper oesophageal pouch, at 10 to 15 minute intervals, is essential to avoid aspiration (Chapter 6).

FURTHER READING

James A.G. (1993) Resuscitation, stabilisation and transport in perinatology. *Curr. Opin. Pediatr.* **5**: 150–5.

Strafford M.A. (1998) Cardiovascular physiology and care. In: O'Neill J.A., Rowe M.I., Grosfeld J.L., Fonkalsrud E.W. & Coran A.G. (eds), *Pediatric Surgery*, 5th edn, Mosby, St. Louis, pp. 103–34.

Teitelbaum D.H. & Coran A.G. (1998) Nutrition. In: O'Neill J.A., Rowe M.I., Grosfeld J.L. Fonkalsrud E.W. & Coran A.G. (eds), *Pediatric Surgery*, 5th edn, Mosby, St. Louis, pp. 171–96.

— 3 —

The Child in Hospital

CASE 1

Erin is seen in the surgical clinic because of an inguinal hernia. During the explanation prior to filling out the consent form, the surgeon describes the use of 'invisible stitches', a waterproof dressing and local anaesthetic.

> Q. 1.1   *Should the operation be done under local anaesthetic?*
>
> Q. 1.2   *Why are 'invisible stitches' important?*

CASE 2

Jacob attends the surgical clinic very reluctantly because he is apprehensive about an upcoming orchidopexy.

> Q. 2.1   *What are his major fears likely to be?*

Great effort should be made to minimize psychological disturbances in children undergoing surgery. The important factors to consider are the age and temperament of the child; the site, nature and extent of the surgical procedure; the degree and duration of discomfort after operation; and the time spent in hospital.

Children between 1 and 3 years of age are the most vulnerable, and procedures should be carried out in the first year of life, or postponed until 4 to 6 years of age when the child can comprehend and co-operate better.

The temperament and ability of children to cope with stress are infinitely variable; the trust that children are prepared to grant those who care for them is a measure of the confidence they have in their own family circle. Major disturbances within the family may affect the patient's equanimity and the ability of the parents to give them support, and for these reasons elective surgery may be deferred until after the birth of a sibling or the death of a close relative.

PREPARATION FOR ADMISSION

Preparation for elective admission is important for children over 4 or 5 years of age and, whether assisted by a booklet (see Further Reading) or advice, it is largely in the hands of the mother, whose acceptance of the situation is its endorsement in the child's eyes.

The child needs a brief and simple description of the operation, and if something is to be removed, it should be made clear that it is dispensable. Children should also be told that they will be asleep while the operation is performed, that it will be over when they wake, that they will be 'stiff' and a little 'sore' for a day or so, and when they will be able to go home. It is pointless to say that it will not hurt at all, for honesty is essential to preserve trust.

How the child's questions are handled is just as important as the factual content of the answers; possible sources of fear should be dealt with and the pleasant aspects suitably emphasized. The amount of information must be adjusted to the child's age and particular needs; more detail will be expected by older children.

EFFECT OF SITE OF SURGERY

Operations on the genitalia or the body's orifices, including circumcision after the age of 2 years, are more likely to cause emotional upset than other operations of the same magnitude. One or both parents should stay with the patient and suitable occupational or play therapy is of considerable value.

Anal and oesophageal surgery should be completed shortly after birth, and subsequent dilatations performed under anaesthesia wherever possible. Many boys who have experienced both operations would prefer, in retrospect, bilateral orchidopexy to tonsillectomy by even the gentlest hands.

DAY SURGERY

Time spent in hospital should be as short as possible. 'Day Surgery', with admission, operation and discharge on the same day, is cost-effective, convenient and suitable for at least 80 per cent of elective paediatric surgery.

The greatest advantage is minimizing the psychological impact on the child, which is magnified by sleeping away from home for even one night. There are many other obvious advantages, including minimal disturbances of breastfeeding and reduced travelling by parents.

Although surgical technique is important (haemostasis, secure dressings), day surgery has been made safer and more acceptable by improved anaesthetic techniques; timing and choice of premedication and anaesthetic agents, minimal trauma during intubation (particularly the use of the laryngeal mask rather than tracheal intubation), quick recovery, and long-acting local anaesthetic blocks or caudal analgesia in lieu of the usual postoperative injections of narcotics.

In the most vulnerable 1 to 3 year age group, day surgery has reduced the likelihood of behavioural disturbances. Suitable operations for day surgery depend on parental attitudes, logistics and careful selection of individual patients.

WARD ATMOSPHERE AND PROCEDURES

Unlimited visiting by parents, living-in quarters for mothers and a more understanding approach by all who care for children have led to a less formal and more friendly atmosphere in hospital.

The procedures necessary for investigation, or in preparation for the operation, should be scrutinized carefully to see whether they are necessary. Blood tests or X-rays are rarely required for elective day surgery.

The induction of anaesthesia may be a source of fear and distress. Effective premedication, skilful intravenous induction and the prompt administration of hypnotics and analgesics after the operation keep discomfort to the absolute minimum.

Even after major abdominal surgery some toddlers will be walking within 24 hours. They might just as well be playing on the floor or sitting at a table, and today that is where they are, with no subsequent ill-effects. The playroom is not required for most postoperative patients, since once they can walk to the toilet and playroom, they can be discharged home. The children usually set the pace of convalescence, and as a general rule they will show no desire to move when they should rest; for example, during a period of paralytic ileus.

Play materials, a day room, television and bright surroundings act as constant stimuli to those who are well enough to be 'up and doing'.

A single, absorbable subcuticular stitch can be used to close almost all incisions; this avoids the anxiety and time spent in removing sutures.

PARENTAL SUPPORT

The parents always require consideration, especially when a first-born baby is transferred to a children's hospital on the first day of life. The baby may stay there for several weeks, at precisely the time when the mother's emotions are in turmoil and she would normally be establishing a new and unique relationship. Feelings of guilt at producing an infant with a congenital abnormality, or inadequacy following removal of the infant from her care and the lack of close physical contact, may lead her to reject the baby and exaggerate the usual puerperal emotional forms of instability. To help overcome this when separation is unavoidable, the mother should be given a Polaroid photograph of her baby, she should see the baby again as soon as possible, and care for it as much as the illness permits (Chapter 2).

RESPONSE OF THE CHILD

The average child's natural optimism, freedom from unfounded anxiety, remarkable powers of recuperation and apparent short memory for unpleasant experiences can make even major surgery a relatively short and simple matter; most patients are out of bed in 2 to 3 days and active for much of the day or already at home by 3 to 6 days.

Even when minor surgery has been uneventfully concluded the child may show some disturbances up to 2 months after leaving hospital, and the parents should be made aware of this possibility. Signs of insecurity, increased dependency and disturbed sleep are not uncommon but fortunately are of short duration when met with warm affection, reassurance and understanding by the parents.

The undesirable psychological effects of surgery must be put in proper perspective by mentioning the beneficial effects that so often follow the operation; for example, the well-being after removal of an uncomfortable hernia, the freely expressed satisfaction at the excision of an unsightly lump or blemish.

Finally, in older children there is, not infrequently, a detectable increase in confidence and poise that comes from facing, and coping adequately with, an operation. This is often the first occasion that the child has been away from home, and metaphorically at least, standing on his or her own two feet.

THE TIMING OF SURGICAL PROCEDURES

Surgical conditions in infancy and childhood can be classified according to the degree of urgency with which treatment should be carried out. Three categories can be distinguished:
(1) The immediate group — where conditions require immediate investigation and/or a definitive operation.
(2) The intermediate group — where treatment is not urgent but should be undertaken without undue delay.
(3) The elective group — where operation is performed at an optimum age determined by one or more factors that affect the patient's best interests.

The immediate group

Trauma, acute infections, abdominal emergencies and acute scrotal conditions naturally fall into this category.

A particularly important subgroup is neonatal emergencies. Most of these are the result of developmental abnormalities causing disorders of function that threaten life. The best prognosis depends on early diagnosis, speedy transport to a hospital where appropriate skills and equipment are available, and effective surgical management (see Chapters 4 to 11).

The intermediate group

Inguinal hernias are prone to strangulation, especially in the first year of life. For this reason, herniotomy should be performed within a few days of diagnosis in those less than 1 year of age. The '6–2 rule' may be useful here: a baby less than 6/52 needs herniotomy within 2 days, less than 6/12 within 2 weeks, and less than 6 years within 2 months.

Investigation of swellings or masses suspected to be malignant should be undertaken within a day or two of their discovery.

The elective group

Factors favouring deferment of operation

Factors that favour the deferment of an operation, and hence may determine an optimum age, include:

(1) The possibility of spontaneous correction or cure. In infants, scrotal hydroceles, encysted hydroceles of the cord, true umbilical hernias and sternomastoid tumours all show a strong tendency to spontaneous resolution.

(2) Strawberry naevi (intracutaneous capillary haemangiomas), although they may progress and enlarge in the first year of life, usually involute and fade spontaneously in the ensuing 2 to 4 years (Chapter 50). In general, they should be left alone for this to occur, for surgical measures are required rarely.

(3) The difficulties posed by minute and delicate structures can be avoided by postponing the operation until the patients are more robust, although this is seldom the sole reason for deferring an operation; for example, an undescended testis can be repaired more easily in a 6- to 12-month-old boy than shortly after birth.

(4) The supposedly greater capacity of older children to tolerate major operations, which is now much less important. With modern methods of anaesthesia and adequate resuscitation, including immediate replacement of blood loss, major operations are often performed on very young infants.

(5) The greater ability of the patient to co-operate and comprehend with age. Voluntary exercises are important after some operations and it may be desirable to defer surgery until the necessary degree of co-operation is forthcoming.

(6) The importance of growth. Chest wall deformities are corrected at adolescence, once chest wall growth is almost complete.

(7) Coexistent anomalies and intercurrent diseases; for example, infections will affect the timing of operations. The situation in each patient should be assessed to establish the order of priorities when there are multiple abnormalities, and to determine whether the treatment of non-urgent conditions should be deferred temporarily.

Factors favouring early operation

Factors that favour early operation rather than deferred treatment include the capacity for healing and adaptation in the very young. For example, a fracture of a long bone at birth causes such an exuberant growth of callus that clinical union occurs in 7 to 10 days, and the subsequent moulding will remove any residual bony deformities.

(1) Stimulation of development by early treatment occurs in infants with a congenital dislocation of the hip. When splinting is commenced in the first week of life, this will prevent the secondary dysplasia of the acetabulum and femur, which in the past was thought to be the primary cause of the dislocation.

(2) Malleability of infantile tissues is an advantage; for example, in talipes, in which the best results are obtained when treatment is commenced in the first few days after birth.

(3) Avoidance of undesirable psychological effects. Often these can be prevented by completing treatment, including repetitive painful procedures, before the memory of things past is established or before the child

goes to school, where obvious deformities or disabilities are likely to attract attention.

(4) Effect on the parents. The family as a whole should be considered and when it is not disadvantageous to the child, early operation may resolve parental anxiety and prevent rejection of the child.

FURTHER READING

Bar-Maor J.A, Tadmore C.S., Birkhan J. & Shoshany G. (1989) Effective psychological and/or 'pharmacological' preparation for elective pediatric surgery can reduce stress. *Pediatr. Surg. Int.* **4**: 273–6.

Ludman L., Spitz L. & Lansdown R. (1990) Developmental progress of newborns undergoing neonatal surgery. *J. Pediatr. Surg.* **25**: 469–71.

Ramanujam T.M., Uma G., Usha V., Ramanathan S. & Sryaritha R. (1998) Advantages and limitations of day surgery in children in a developing country. *Pediatr. Surg. Int.* **13**: 512–14.

Suruga K., Miyazawa R., Kimura K. & Miyano T. (1990) A study on more than 20 years of postoperative follow-up in pediatric surgical cases. *J. Pediatr. Surg.* **25**: 731–6.

— 4 —

Respiratory Distress in the Newborn

CASE 1

Antenatal ultrasonography has revealed a large solid lesion occupying most of the right chest. At birth, respiratory distress develops rapidly: a chest X-ray shows a partly cystic and solid lesion in the right lower zone.

> Q. 1.1   *What is the differential diagnosis?*
>
> Q. 1.2   *What treatment is needed?*

CASE 2

After a breech delivery, acute cyanosis and respiratory distress develops in a term infant. Breath sounds are diminished over the left chest.

> Q. 2.1   *What is the likely problem?*
>
> Q. 2.2   *What emergency treatment may be needed?*

When a newborn baby breathes more rapidly than normal, respiratory distress is present. The degree of distress may be slight initially, but progressive deterioration may culminate in irreversible respiratory failure.

Neonatal respiratory distress is not normally the province of the paediatric surgeon, but it may occur in a specific group of neonatal patients in whom the causes are amenable to surgical correction. Respiratory failure may have developed already when the baby presents, and prompt action can save life and regain the opportunity for corrective surgery. Those concerned with the care of the newborn must be able to recognize respiratory distress and the paediatric surgeon must be familiar with its causes and the principles of management.

In only a few cases can a firm diagnosis be made solely on clinical grounds, and X-rays of the thorax and abdomen should be obtained as soon as possible.

RECOGNITION OF RESPIRATORY DISTRESS

The most important clinical feature is a raised respiratory rate. Tachycardia is almost invariably present as well, and if the rate is more than 200/min the situation is serious. Bradycardia also is a dangerous sign and often portends imminent respiratory failure.

Other cardiovascular signs, such as the presence of apparent 'dextrocardia', and the nature of the peripheral pulses, will provide further clues.

The abdomen may be scaphoid in babies with a diaphragmatic hernia, but it can be distended when there is a pulmonary cause for the respiratory distress. Intestinal obstruction and neonatal peritonitis also can cause abdominal distension and respiratory embarrassment.

The mechanics of respiration should be assessed; respiration may be 'laboured' or associated with deformity of the chest wall or may exhibit inspiratory (sternal) retraction indicative of obstruction of the airways.

A surgical cause is present in a minority of babies with respiratory distress, and the surgeon must be familiar with other conditions that enter into the differential diagnosis; for example, hyaline membrane disease and cerebral birth injuries (Table 4.1). The clinical evidence

Table 4.1 Causes of neonatal respiratory distress

Type of obstruction	Examples
Nasal	Choanal atresia
Pharyngeal	Pierre–Robin syndrome
	Hamartoma of tongue
Laryngeal	'Infantile larynx'
	Vocal cord palsy
	Subglottic haemangioma
	Laryngeal web/cyst
Tracheal	Tracheomalacia
	Massive cystic hygroma
	Vascular ring
Lower airways	Meconium aspiration
	Aspiration of gastric contents
	Lobar emphysema
Alveolar disease	Hyaline membrane disease
	Pneumonia
	Congenital heart disease
	Pulmonary oedema
	Diaphragmatic hernia
Pulmonary compression	Pneumothorax
	Diaphragmatic hernia
	Repaired exomphalos or gastroschisis
	Congenital lobar emphysema
	Congenital lung cysts
	Duplication cysts
	Abdominal distension
Neurological disease	Birth asphyxia
	Apnoea of prematurity
	Intracranial haemorrhage
	Convulsions

including the obstetrical details and any abnormal physical signs will help determine the cause of tachypnoea. For example, a baby who is pale and cyanosed and improves following the administration of oxygen may have a diaphragmatic hernia (Chapter 5). A scaphoid abdomen and barrelled chest with the heart sounds best heard on the right are supportive physical signs and a chest X-ray will confirm the diagnosis. By contrast, an infant with cyanosis and respiratory distress that is relieved by crying may have choanal atresia (Chapter 14).

THE PRINCIPLES OF MANAGEMENT

When respiratory failure is present already, urgent treatment is required, regardless of the underlying cause.

An accurate diagnosis of the cause is made on the clinical signs and the results of investigation, usually radiology. The degree of respiratory or metabolic acidosis must be determined as a guide to the resuscitation required.

Where applicable, surgery is undertaken to correct the cause, usually after correction of the physiological disturbances.

SPECIFIC CONDITIONS

One of the important aspects of neonatal respiratory distress is that many of the causes have a wide clinical spectrum; for example, one diaphragmatic hernia may produce a direct threat to life within minutes of birth, while another may cause no distress in the neonatal period and give rise to symptoms only after several weeks (Chapter 5). Congenital cysticadenomatoid malformations and pulmonary sequestration often are diagnosed on antenatal ultrasonography.

Choanal atresia is discussed in Chapter 14 and oesophageal atresia in Chapter 6.

Pulmonary dysplasia

Malformations of part or all of one lung causing respiratory distress in the newborn are: congenital lobar emphysema and congenital cysts of the lung, either solitary or multiple. The physical signs are never diagnostic and X-rays are required to make the diagnosis. Again there are considerable variations in the clinical picture, and when there is obvious respiratory distress, surgery is indicated. Resection of the affected segment of the lung not only removes functionless pulmonary tissue in which there is little or no gaseous exchange, but also it allows expansion of the normal areas that have been compressed by the overdistended segment, lobe or lobes.

Congenital lobar emphysema

The underlying abnormality is bronchomalacia from congenital deficiency of the cartilage. It results in expiratory obstruction and the trapping of air in the affected lobe, leading to massive distension of a pulmonary lobe.

The cardinal symptom is tachypnoea, most noticeable when the baby is being fed. Not infrequently there is a dry cough and stridor. Cyanosis is usually an indication for urgent treatment. The mediastinum is displaced and the chest wall over the affected area is prominent and relatively immobile; breath sounds are diminished and the percussion note typically is hyper-resonant.

X-rays show an area of increased radiolucency in which there are some bronchovascular markings. There is also a downward displacement of the diaphragm on the affected side, and the overdistended lung may herniate across the midline (Fig. 4.1).

The lobes most commonly affected are the left upper lobe or the right middle lobe and the treatment is lobectomy.

Congenital cystic lung

The clinical features are similar to those of lobar emphysema: respiratory distress occurs early,

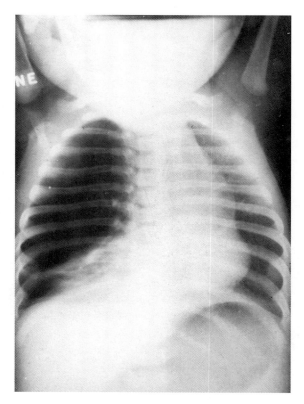

Fig. 4.1 Congenital lobar emphysema of the right upper lobe that is overdistended and herniating across the midline.

but usually it is more urgent and severe. X-rays show a large cyst with a sharply defined border (Fig. 4.2) or an extensive multicystic area; the findings are otherwise similar to those of lobar emphysema; namely, compression and collapse of unaffected areas of the lungs and displacement of the mediastinum.

The aim of surgery is to remove the portion of the lung that is not only functionless but also interfering with the function of the remainder. The distribution of disease determines the area to be removed, and segmental resection, lobectomy, or even pneumonectomy, may be required.

Pulmonary sequestration

Pulmonary sequestration is an uncommon malformation in which there is non-functioning

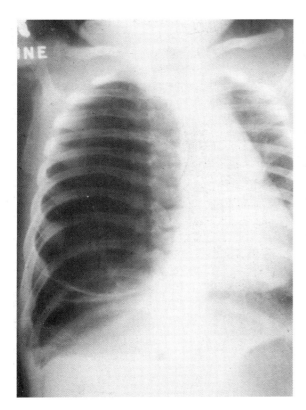

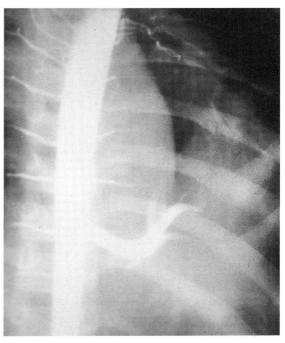

Fig. 4.3 Anomalous blood supply from the aorta to a left pulmonary sequestration.

Fig. 4.2 Congenital cystic lung. A giant cyst replaces the right lower lobe, compresses the remainder of the right lung and herniates across the midline to displace the heart and compress the left lung.

lung tissue that has no connection with the normal bronchial tree, and a blood supply that arises from an anomalous systemic artery, often the aorta (Fig. 4.3) (Chapter 49). It usually occurs on the left side and may be either intralobar or extralobar, depending on whether it shares visceral pleura with the normal lung. It may present as a pulmonary infection, because of its space-occupying effect, or be found incidentally on a chest X-ray.

Congenital cystic adenomatoid malformation

Congenital cystic adenomatoid malformations (CCAMs) include a range of localised abnormalities in which the bronchiolar tissue is abnormal, with communicating cysts and a relative paucity of cartilage. They may be diagnosed on antenatal ultrasonography as a cystic or solid mass in one part of the lung. Maternal polyhydramnios and mediastinal shift are common. CCAM presents postnatally in 3 ways: (i) respiratory distress (60 per cent); (ii) infectious complications, for example, recurrent pneumonia (20 per cent); and (iii) as an incidental finding on a chest X-ray (20 per cent). Many CCAMS observed on antenatal ultrasonography regress and have resolved by term. CCAMS identified postnatally are resected.

Mediastinal conditions

Very rarely, large cystic teratomas and duplication cysts cause respiratory distress and should be removed. In the neonate, oesophageal duplication cysts present with increasing respiratory distress.

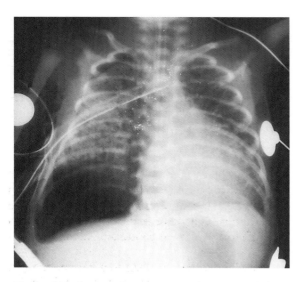

Fig. 4.4 Severe pulmonary interstitial emphysema.

Pulmonary interstitial emphysema

This is an acquired condition of extreme prematurity seen in infants where assisted ventilation is required for severe hyaline membrane disease. High ventilatory pressures force air into the lung interstitium, which tracks along peribronchial spaces, producing interstitial cysts that have a characteristic appearance on X-ray (Fig. 4.4). Treatment is directed at reducing the ventilatory pressures. In severe and progressive cases, thoracotomy may be required to deflate the cysts. Refinements in neonatology have resulted in a significant decrease in the incidence of this condition.

PLEURAL CONDITIONS

Neonatal pneumothorax

Pneumothorax may occur as a complication of diffuse pulmonary disease or of a localized abnormality such as a subpleural emphysematous bleb. The pneumothorax may be suspected on clinical grounds by sudden deterioration in condition, displacement of the trachea or apex beat, and a hyper-resonant percussion note, but X-rays are required to confirm the diagnosis.

In neonates, the severity of the symptoms frequently is out of proportion to the size of the pneumothorax. Even a small pneumothorax may be associated with severe respiratory distress when there is pre-existing parenchymatous lung disease. Intercostal drainage is urgent.

Empyema

Empyema occasionally occurs in the early days of life and is usually staphylococcal, but also may be caused by a Gram-negative organism. Early diagnostic paracentesis is helpful to identify the organism and to determine its sensitivities. Drainage of the pleural cavity by an intercostal catheter may be effective in the early stages of the disease process, but once pus is thick or loculated, open thoracotomy for drainage may be required.

Haemothorax

Haemothorax is an infrequent complication of haemorrhagic disease of the newborn and may produce an alarming clinical picture; this is due to mechanical factors that interfere with respiration and to the reduction of the circulating blood volume. Pleural paracentesis and blood transfusion are required.

THE MEDICAL MANAGEMENT OF ACUTE RESPIRATORY FAILURE

Acute respiratory failure occurs when oxygenation and/or ventilation are impaired sufficiently to be an immediate threat to life.

Cause of respiratory failure

Acute respiratory failure in neonates is usually the result of asphyxia due to:
(1) Birth asphyxia.

Table 4.2 Factors predisposing infants to respiratory failure

Factor	Comment
Metabolic rate	Metabolism per kg is twice that of adults
Respiratory rate	Lung surface area per kg is about the same as for an adult; so the infant has much less respiratory reserve
Compliance	The chest wall of the infant is less able to adjust to a reduction in lung compliance or an increase in airways resistance
Airways calibre	Relatively larger total airways resistance than in older children or adults
Airways obstruction	The narrow airways are more prone to obstruction by oedema and secretions
Temperature control	Temperature regulation is poor in the newborn, especially in the premature. In a cold environment, oxygen consumption may increase two- or three-fold. With limited respiratory reserve, respiratory failure can occur rapidly

(2) Injuries sustained during birth.
(3) Developmental anomalies, including congenital heart disease.
(4) Immaturity of the pulmonary system (part of prematurity).
(5) Increased susceptibility to infection. The factors in infants that predispose to respiratory failure are summarized in Table 4.2.

Signs of respiratory failure

In the neonate, especially the premature, acute hypoxia causes pallor, apnoea, bradycardia, hypotension and lethargy. The clinical signs of hypercapnia — sweating, tachycardia and hypertension — are seen rarely, but pulmonary haemorrhage, cerebral haemorrhage, severe hyperkalaemia and hypoglycaemia all may occur as the result of hypoxia.

Treatment

General management of respiratory failure is directed by the clinical features, supported by serial estimations of the blood gases.

Nursing care

An infant with incipient respiratory failure requires close observation at all times. Neonates should be nursed in an isolette or under a radiant heater so that the temperature is controlled and observation unimpeded.

Handling should be kept to a minimum, for it can increase oxygen consumption dramatically.

The position most favourable in nursing neonates is prone, with hips and knees flexed, and the head turned regularly and frequently from one side to the other. This reduces apnoeic episodes, shortens gastric emptying time and reduces the risk of regurgitation and aspiration. The supine position is preferred if bag and mask ventilation or resuscitation are needed.

Oxygen

The method of delivery of oxygen depends on the age of the infant and oxygen concentration required; for example, isolette, head box, mask, nasal catheter(s) oxygen cot and tent. The concentration required depends on the disease process.

All patients having prolonged oxygen therapy should have arterial blood gas estimations and adjustment of inspired oxygen concentrations to ensure adequate arterial saturation. Premature infants receiving oxygen therapy are at risk of retinopathy of prematurity and frequent blood gases are necessary to maintain the arterial P_{O_2} in the range of 6.6 to 10.6 kPa (50 to 80 mmHg). Dependence on hypoxia for 'ventilatory drive' is extremely rare in children and so is pulmonary oxygen toxicity; neither should be considered as reasons for restricting oxygen therapy.

Fluids and feeding

Oral feeding should be suspended in children with severe dyspnoea and nasogastric feeding should be substituted. If abdominal distension occurs, feeding must be discontinued to avoid regurgitation and aspiration, and to prevent restriction of descent of the diaphragm: these are all potential causes of additional respiratory embarrassment.

Nasogastric feeding can be recommenced once artificial (mechanical) ventilation has been instituted.

Intravenous fluids are required to prevent dehydration and to supply parenteral nutrition, but fluids may need to be restricted in some patients with pulmonary disease.

Sodium bicarbonate may be required to correct metabolic acidosis (Chapter 2). Regular biochemical monitoring and an accurate fluid balance are the key to fluid management.

Temperature control

Seriously ill neonates are particularly vulnerable to cold stress, and the maintenance of body temperature is of vital importance before, during and after operation (Chapter 2).

The neonate has a narrow 'thermoneutral' range in which oxygen consumption is minimal and optimal: abdominal wall skin temperature is optimal between 36° and 36.5°C. Exposure to an environmental temperature of 20° to 25°C increases oxygen consumption threefold and may precipitate cardiorespiratory failure.

For reasons of access, critically ill neonates should be nursed in open cots with servo-controlled radiant heat. Insensible water loss may be increased, particularly in infants of very low birth weight, but this can be taken into account when planning fluid requirements.

Respiratory physiotherapy

In the newborn, gentle suction is performed at intervals to remove pooled secretions and to stimulate coughing. However, pharyngeal and endotracheal suction may cause a sudden fall in Pa_{O_2} that necessitates an increase in the concentration of oxygen in the inspired gases.

Monitoring

Respiratory and cardiovascular signs should be monitored, along with the oxygen concentration in the inspired air. Blood for gas analysis is obtained by percutaneous puncture or, more accurately, in samples from an indwelling catheter in a peripheral artery, which also can be used for a continuous record of the arterial pressure. Continuous transcutaneous monitoring of oxygen and carbon dioxide levels is used widely.

Ventilatory support

In neonates, nasotracheal intubation is the preferred type of artificial airway (Table 4.3). Tubes of appropriate size and composition can be left *in situ* for long periods with minimal adverse effects or complications.

Table 4.3 Use of nasotracheal tube in neonates

Advantages	Disadvantages
Protects or ensures uninterrupted airway	Narrows the upper airways
Overcomes upper airway obstruction	Bypasses natural humidification, heating and filtering of inspired gases
Allows precise tracheo-bronchial toilet and suction	Prevents coughing and expectoration of secretions
Facilitates continuous positive airway pressure	May cause subglottic irritation and stenosis: a risk that can be minimized by using a tube of the correct size allowing a small air leak during positive pressure ventilation
Enables mechanical ventilation	

Humidification of dry inspired gases is necessary to avoid viscid and retained sputum, atelectasis, blockage of the endotracheal tube with inspissated secretions, and to preserve mucociliary function.

Inspired gases should be delivered to the trachea at 37°C, fully saturated with water vapour, using a safe, servocontrolled humidifier. This is an important contribution to the maintenance of body temperature and to reduce insensible fluid losses from the airways.

Suction of the trachea is necessary to stimulate coughing and to remove accumulated secretions, usually once an hour, but in some cases more frequently. Suction can cause hypoxia and atelectasis and may introduce infection, and techniques are used to avoid these risks. Gentle 'bagging' with an oxygen-rich mixture is used before and after suction to reduce hypoxia and re-expand the lung. In infants at risk of retinopathy of prematurity, the oxygen concentration in the 'bag' should not be more than 10 per cent higher than the mixture used for ventilation. In older children, 100 per cent oxygen can be used.

Continuous positive airways pressure

This is a technique that employs a distending pressure (5 to 10 cm H_2O) applied to the airways of a patient who is breathing spontaneously. It is used in pulmonary conditions causing hypoxaemia due to atelectasis, alveolar instability and intrapulmonary shunting. Continuous positive airways pressure (CPAP) increases functional residual capacity and compliance, re-expands areas of atelectasis, decreases intrapulmonary shunting and increases arterial P_{O_2}. In premature infants, CPAP often will improve the regularity of respiratory movements and decrease apnoeic episodes. The technique requires careful control to avoid reduced cardiac output, retention of fluids, rupture of alveoli and pneumothorax.

Intermittent positive pressure ventilation

Intermittent positive pressure ventilation (IPPV)

is used to correct hypoventilation, and sometimes (for example, raised intracranial pressure, pulmonary hypertension) to produce hyperventilation and to lower Pa_{CO_2}. Mechanical ventilators have been designed specifically for neonatal and paediatric use. IPPV is often combined with positive end-expiratory pressure (PEEP). PEEP is used for the same reasons as CPAP; that is, as a means of improving oxygenation. The hazards of IPPV are greater than those of CPAP and related directly to the level of pressure applied. Barotrauma to immature lungs may result in a chronic lung disease in neonates known as bronchopulmonary dysplasia.

Intermittent mandatory ventilation (IMV) is a technique of mechanical ventilation in which a predetermined minute volume is guaranteed, while, in addition, the patient breathes independently from the ventilator. With infant ventilators, a constant flow is provided during the expiratory phase from which the infant can breathe. It is a technique useful for weaning from mechanical ventilation and as a means of mimimizing barotrauma.

Controlled ventilation involves the use of relaxants and sedatives that paralyse respiratory movements, to completely abolish the work of breathing and improve gas exchange. The technique is useful in critically ill neonates and those with difficult ventilatory problems, but it should only be employed where expert surveillance and sophisticated monitoring are available. Inappropriate pressure settings can cause a pneumothorax with sudden deterioration, and inadvertent disconnection rapidly results in potentially fatal hypoxia.

FURTHER READING

Resuscitation of the Newborn. In: *Advanced Paediatric Life Support: the Practical Approach*, 2nd edn, BMJ Publishing Group (1997) pp. 55–61.

Kellnar S. & Trammer A. (1990) Therapy of neonatal chylothorax. *Pediatr. Surg. Int.* **5**: 216–17.

Wensley D.F., Goh T.H., Menahem S., Edis B., Venables A.W. & Robertson C.F. (1989) Management of pulmonary sequestration and scimitar syndrome presenting in infancy. *Pediatr. Surg. Int.* 4: 381–415.

Wilson J.M. & DiFiore J.W. (1998) Respiratory Physiology and Care. In: O'Neill J.A., Rowe M.I., Grosfeld J.L., Fonkalsrud E.W. & Coran A.G. (eds) *Pediatric Surgery*, 5th edn, Mosby, St. Louis, pp. 71–88.

— 5 —

Diaphragmatic Hernia

CASE 1

Within minutes of birth, a full-term infant boy develops increasing respiratory distress and becomes cyanosed. He fails to improve with upper airway suctioning. The pregnancy was uneventful. He looks barrel-chested and his abdomen is scaphoid.

Q. 1.1   *What is the diagnosis?*

Q. 1.2   *What investigation will confirm the diagnosis?*

Q. 1.3   *What factors determine the outcome in these situations?*

CASE 2

A newborn infant with a recently diagnosed left-sided congenital diaphragmatic hernia is about to be transferred to a paediatric surgical institution by air. He is currently being ventilated through an endotracheal tube and he is just maintaining adequate blood gas levels.

Q. 2.1   *Should his ventilation be increased during transport?*

Q. 2.2   *Should any other manoeuvre be performed to reduce the likelihood of problems during transport?*

Q. 2.3   *If he suddenly deteriorates what complication may have happened?*

DEFINITIONS

The diaphragm develops largely from three structures: (i) the pleuroperitoneal membrane; (ii) the septum transversum; (iii) marginal growths from the muscles of the body wall.

Congenital diaphragmatic hernia results from failure of formation or fusion of the components of the diaphragm that allows abdominal contents to move through the defect into the chest. Failure of muscularisation may produce a thin, weak diaphragm, referred to as an eventration of the diaphragm.

The Bochdalek type of diaphragmatic hernia is the most common type of congenital diaphragmatic hernia (1 in 5000 live births) and results from a defect in the postero-lateral part of the diaphragm. During intra-uterine development, the small bowel, stomach, spleen and left lobe of the liver pass through the defect into the chest, limiting the space available for the developing lung. This causes lung hypoplasia, which in many infants is severe enough to produce severe respiratory distress within minutes of birth, and may not be compatible with life.

The Morgagni type of diaphragmatic hernia is rare, and results from a defect close to the anterior midline, between the costal and sternal attachments of the diaphragm (Fig. 5.1). It usually

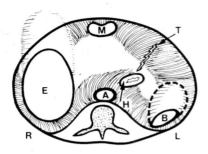

Fig. 5.1 Diaphragmatic hernias. Diaphragm as seen from below, showing: (B) Bochdalek left posterolateral defect; (M) anterior or Morgagni type; (H) hiatus for oesophageal and hiatus hernia; (E) large eventration in the tendinous portion of the right cupola; (T) a tear that causes a post-traumatic hernia; (A) aorta.

contains part of the colon or small bowel, and less commonly, part of the liver.

Occasionally, a hernia may occur through the apex of the cupola or at the periphery adjacent to the costal margin. Oesophageal hiatal hernias also occur and usually produce symptoms caused by gastro-oesophageal reflux.

CLINICAL FEATURES

Most congenital diaphragmatic hernias become symptomatic at or shortly after birth. Where pulmonary hypoplasia is severe, the infant becomes cyanosed with severe respiratory distress within minutes of birth. In other patients there is tachypnoea, increased respiratory effort, hyperinflated chest, scaphoid abdomen and heart sounds are on the right side. This is because 85 per cent of postero-lateral hernias involve the left hemidiaphragm. The remainder are right-sided (12 per cent) or bilateral (3 per cent).

Unlike postero-lateral hernias, most anterior hernias are symptomless unless strangulation occurs; that is, except in the rare event that the hernia protrudes into the pericardial cavity rather than into the inferior mediastinum and causes cardiac tamponade, presenting as cardiorespiratory distress in the neonatal period.

Diaphragmatic hernias are being diagnosed on antenatal ultrasonography with increasing frequency. This allows their transfer to a tertiary paediatric surgical centre before birth.

INVESTIGATION

Diagnosis of a postero-lateral hernia is confirmed by a chest X-ray (Fig. 5.2). Loops of bowel can be seen in the left chest. The heart is deviated to the contralateral side, usually to the right. Little room is left for the lungs, particularly the left lung. It may be difficult to distinguish in a diaphragmatic hernia from basal lung cysts: in this case a repeat chest X-ray is performed after a nasogastric tube has been inserted, the tip of which can be seen in the chest. Alternatively, a barium study will show the bowel within the thoracic cavity when a hernia is present.

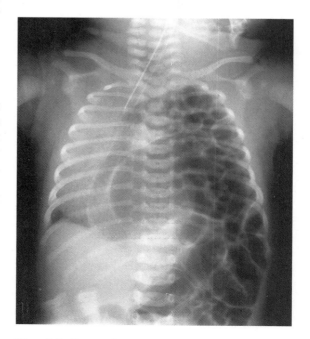

Fig. 5.2 X-ray of congenital diaphragmatic hernia (Bochdalek type). Multiple bowel loops fill the left pleural cavity and the heart is displaced to the right.

TREATMENT

Postero-lateral (Bochdalek) hernias

Where antenatal ultrasonography examination has identified a diaphragmatic hernia, the best outcome is achieved if the child is transferred to a tertiary paediatric surgical centre prior to birth. This is because the rapid development of severe pulmonary distress postnatally makes subsequent transfer difficult and potentially dangerous.

Initial treatment involves intensive cardiorespiratory support and decompression of the bowel by insertion of a nasogastric tube to prevent bowel dilatation within the chest. Care must be taken to avoid hyperinflation and barotrauma of the small hypoplastic lungs. Ventilation with a face mask ('bagging') should be avoided as this forces air into the stomach, increasing its volume at the expense of the already compromised lungs. Vigorous endotracheal ventilation should also be avoided because of the risk of causing a tension pneumothorax, which can lead to the rapid demise of the infant.

Sudden deterioration of the infant's condition during initial resuscitation or during transport suggests the development of a tension pneumothorax, and this may require prompt drainage by needle aspiration or intercostal intubation. The infant should be transferred to a tertiary neonatal intensive care unit.

Surgery to return the bowel to the abdominal cavity and to repair the defect in the abdomen is performed when the infant's condition is stable. This may be anywhere between 12 hours and 7 or more days after birth. In left-sided defects, a left transverse or subcostal abdominal incision is used. The management of the infant with severe hypoplastic lungs is difficult and may involve extracorporeal membrane oxygenation or even, in the future, heart-lung transplantation. The major cause of death remains pulmonary hypoplasia and pulmonary hypertension. The combined lung weight in infants dying with this condition is often less than 1/3 of normal.

Anterior diaphragmatic hernia

Anterior diaphragmatic (Morgagni) hernias are often diagnosed on an incidental X-ray of the chest in a symptomless patient, but repair is still advisable because of the risk of strangulation.

FURTHER READING

Greenholz S.K. (1996) Congenital diaphragmatic hernia: an overview. *Seminars in Pediatr. Surg.* **5**: 216–23

Harrison M.R., Adzick S.N. & Flake A.W. (1993) Correction of congenital diaphragmatic hernia *in utero* VI: Hard-earned lessons. *J. Pediatr. Surg.* **28**: 1411.

Puri P. (1994) Congenital diaphragmatic hernia. *Current Problems in Surgery*, pp. 794–836.

Stolar C.J.H. (1997) Congenital diaphragmatic hernia. In: Oldham K.T., Colombani P.M. & Foglia R.P. (eds). *Surgery of infants and children: scientific principles and practice*. Lippincott-Raven, Philadelphia, pp. 883–95.

Stolar C.J.H. & Dillon P.W. (1998) Congenital diaphragmatic hernia and eventration. In: O'Neill J.A., Rowe M.I., Grosfeld J.L., Fonkalsrud E.W. & Coran A.G. (eds). *Pediatric Surgery*, 5th edn, Mosby, St. Louis, pp. 819–37.

Langer J.C. & Harrison M.R. (1996) Congenital diaphragmatic hernia and eventration of the diaphragm. In: Puri P. (ed) *Newborn Surgery*, Butterworth-Heinemann, Oxford, pp. 209–15.

— 6 —

Oesophageal Atresia and Tracheo-oesophageal Fistula

CASE 1

Mrs W has been admitted to a district hospital where she has delivered a baby boy at 38 weeks' gestation who, despite initial suctioning, appears to be salivating excessively and is very 'mucousy'. He has mild tachypnoea, but is pink.

Q. 1.1   What manoeuvre must be undertaken to establish the cause of his excessive drooling?

Q. 1.2   Are there any other abnormalities likely to be present?

Q. 1.3   What needs to be done before and during transfer to a paediatric surgical institution?

CASE 2

Annabel R, aged 38, had difficulty conceiving but now has an infant girl. The baby looks dysmorphic and has a deformed forearm and thumb abnormalities, and an anorectal abnormality. An orogastric tube could not be passed into the stomach.

Q. 2.1   What other abnormalities are likely and how would they be detected?

Q. 2.2   What would you do before proceeding to surgery?

Oesophageal atresia is a congenital anomaly in which there is complete interruption of the lumen of the oesophagus in the form of a blind upper pouch, and a lower oesophageal segment that usually communicates with the trachea via a distal tracheo-oesophageal fistula. Less common variations of the abnormality occur also (Fig. 6.1).

PATHOPHYSIOLOGY

The effect of oesophageal atresia on the infant is that saliva, or milk if the infant has been fed, accumulates in the upper oesophageal pouch and spills over into the trachea, causing choking and cyanosis, and soiling of the lungs. Gastric contents may be aspirated through the distal tracheo-oesophageal fistula into the bronchial tree. Pulmonary complications follow, initially atelectasis, and then pneumonia. Abdominal distension from air passing down the fistula into the stomach may elevate and splint the diaphragm, adversely affecting the infant's ability to ventilate adequately.

EARLY DIAGNOSIS

Oesophageal atresia should be recognised as soon

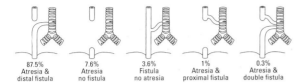

| 87.5% | 7.6% | 3.6% | 1% | 0.3% |
| Atresia & distal fistula | Atresia no fistula | Fistula no atresia | Atresia & proximal fistula | Atresia & double fistula |

Fig. 6.1 The anatomical variants of oesophageal atresia and/or tracheo-oesophageal fistula. The percentage frequency of each variant is shown.

after birth as possible, for delay leads to progressive pulmonary complications. The diagnosis is made when a catheter cannot be passed through the oesophagus into the stomach (see below).

Maternal polyhydramnios

The association with polyhydramnios is sufficiently common that in <u>every baby born to a mother with polyhydramnios, a firm 10 gauge catheter should be introduced through the mouth and passed carefully down the oesophagus;</u> if it becomes arrested at about 10 cm from the gums, the diagnosis of oesophageal atresia has been established. A small catheter will curl up in the upper oesophagus and give a false impression of oesophageal continuity (Fig. 6.2).

Symptoms soon after birth

Oesophageal atresia should be suspected when a newborn infant appears to be drooling excessively or has been resuscitated at birth by adequate aspiration of mucus with a catheter, and then within minutes or hours, develops rattling respirations, tachypnoea or fine frothy white bubbles of mucus in the nostrils or on the lips.

Diagnosis before feeding

Oesophageal atresia should be diagnosed before the infant is fed because feeding causes an acute episode of spluttering, coughing and cyanosis, with aspiration of milk into the lungs.

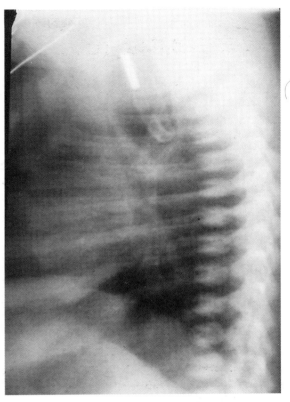

Fig. 6.2 A small catheter will curl up in the upper oesophageal pouch and give a false impression of oesophageal continuity. Therefore, a wide-bore catheter, for example, No. 10 gauge, should be used.

PRE-OPERATIVE INVESTIGATION

X-ray

An X-ray of the thorax and abdomen is taken to demonstrate the presence of air in the stomach and small bowel, which indicates that there is a fistula between the trachea and the lower segment of the oesophagus (Fig. 6.3). The X-ray also provides information on the state of the lungs and the presence of vertebral and rib anomalies. It may show evidence of a right-sided aortic arch.

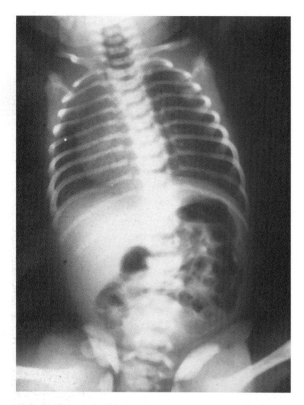

Fig. 6.3 Plain X-ray of the chest and abdomen shows air in the oesophageal pouch stomach and small bowel, indicating that there is a distal tracheo-oesophageal fistula.

Table 6.1 Multiple malformation associations seen with oesophageal atresia

VATER	CHARGE
Vertebral	Coloboma
Ano-rectal	Heart disease
Tracheo-oesophageal	Atresia choanae
Radial/Renal	Retarded growth
	Genital hypoplasia
	Ear anomolies

Renal ultrasonography

If the infant has not passed urine, a renal ultrasonography must be performed to exclude bilateral renal agenesis. If the infant has no kidneys or has severely dysplastic kidneys, as occurs in 3 per cent of infants, no surgery is justified.

Genetic consultation

If the infant has dysmorphic facies and other features suggestive of a major chromosomal abnormality, early genetic consultation is mandatory. There are a number of malformation clusters, such as VATER and CHARGE, that are well known to occur with oesophageal atresia (Table 6.1). In some cases, treatment may be delayed until after chromosomal analysis.

Echocardiography

Nearly 25 per cent of infants with oesophageal atresia have congenital heart disease. It is important to identify cardiac lesions pre-operatively because a prostaglandin E_1 infusion will need to be commenced before the repair of the oesophagus if the lesion is 'duct-dependent'. In most babies the cardiac defect does not delay the oesophageal surgery, and oesophageal repair takes precedence over surgery to the heart. An echocardiograph may identify a right aortic arch and influence the surgical approach to the oesophagus.

TREATMENT

The condition is treated by early complete correction. In preparation for surgery, the upper pouch should be kept empty by frequent suction. The infant should be placed in an incubator or under an overhead heater to avoid excessive heat loss. Vitamin K is given intramuscularly and intravenous fluids commenced. Antibiotics are given during surgery.

The operation is performed usually within 12 hours of admission to hospital. Through a right posterolateral extrapleural thoracotomy, the fistula is divided and closed, and a direct end-to-end anastomosis of the upper and lower segments of the oesophagus is constructed. Postoperatively, oral feeds can be commenced on days 3 or 4.

ANATOMICAL VARIATIONS

Oesophageal atresia without a fistula

In this situation the gap between the two segments of the oesophagus may be so great that a primary anastomosis is impossible at birth. On the initial X-ray these babies have no gas below the diaphragm (Fig. 6.4). A gastrostomy is fashioned to allow enteral feeding and the overflow of saliva from the upper pouch is controlled by frequent suction. At about 6 weeks an oesophageal anastomosis is performed. Occasionally this fails and oesophageal replacement is required.

'H' fistula

Sometimes the oesophagus is intact but there is a communication between the trachea and oesophagus, usually at the level of C7 or T1. These infants present in the first week or so of life with episodes of coughing, cyanosis during feeding and pulmonary complications. Sometimes they present later with a history of recurrent pulmonary infections or abdominal distension mimicking a bowel obstruction. The diagnosis is made by performing a barium swallow or mid-oesophageal contrast study, and observing the contrast passing through the fistula into the trachea. Treatment is by operative division of the fistula through a cervical approach.

SPECIAL PROBLEMS

Effect of prematurity

Prematurity is common in these infants. Provided facilities are available they should have their oesophageal atresia repaired early, before the

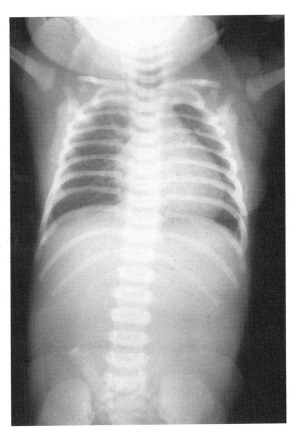

Fig. 6.4 In oesophageal atresia without a distal tracheo-oesophageal fistula there is air in the upper pouch, but none below the diaphragm. Most of these infants have no fistula, while a few have a proximal tracheo-oesophageal fistula.

expected respiratory distress of hyaline membrane disease becomes severe. Failure to divide the tracheo-oesophageal fistula early in these babies leads to severe problems with ventilation because air escapes preferentially through the fistula into the stomach and may even cause gastric perforation.

Gastro-oesophageal reflux

Gastro-oesophageal reflux is common with oesophageal atresia and may contribute to the development of an oesophageal stricture. If this occurs a fundoplication is required.

Tracheomalacia

Tracheomalacia is a structural weakness of the trachea and commonly occurs in association with oesophageal atresia. It is responsible for the 'seal bark' brassy cough characteristic of oesophageal atresia patients. It tends to improve with time but in the neonatal period may cause breathing difficulties. Occasionally, splinting of the trachea (tracheopexy, aortopexy) is required to prevent collapse of the trachea.

COMPLICATIONS OF SURGERY

There are three main complications: (i) leak from the oesophageal anastomosis; (ii) oesophageal stricture; and (iii) recurrent tracheo-oesophageal fistula. The majority of anastomotic leaks are minor and should be treated by antibiotics, total parenteral nutrition and withholding oral feeds. They usually seal spontaneously and surgery is required only if uncontrolled mediastinitis or empyema develops. Oesophageal stricture may present with dysphagia or choking on feeds. Gastro-oesophageal reflux is frequently a contributing factor and may need correction. Treatment involves fundoplication if gastro-oesophageal reflux is present, or oesophageal dilatation. A recurrent tracheo-oesophageal fistula rarely closes spontaneously and requires re-exploration and division.

PROGNOSIS

In the absence of associated congenital abnormalities or severe prematurity, survival in oesophageal atresia is virtually assured.

FURTHER READING

Beasley S.W., Chetchuti P.A.J. & Puntis J.W.L. (1998) Esophageal atresia. In: Stringer M.D., Mouriquand P.D.E., Oldham K.T. & Howard E.R. (eds) *Pediatric Surgery and Urology: Long-term Outcomes*, W.B. Saunders, London, pp. 166–88.

Beasley S.W., Hutson J.M. & Auldist A.W. (1996) Oesophageal atresia. In: *Essential Paediatric Surgery*, Arnold, London, pp. 3–6.

Beasley S.W., Myers N.A. & Auldist A.W. (1991) *Oesophageal Atresia*, Chapman & Hall, London.

Chetcuti P., Myers N.A. & Phelan P.D. et al. (1988) Adults who survive repair of congenital oesophageal atresia and tracheo-oesophageal fistula. *Br. Med. J.* **297**: 344–6.

Harmon C.M. & Coran A.G. (1998) Congenital anomalies of the esophagus. O'Neill J.A., Rowe M.I., Grosfeld J.L., Fonkalsrud E.W. & Coran A.G. (eds) *Pediatric Surgery*, 5th edn, Mosby, St. Louis, pp. 941–86.

— 7 —

Bowel Obstruction

CASE 1

A newborn baby develops abdominal distension with bile-stained vomiting and does not pass meconium.

Q. 1.1   *List three possible diagnoses.*

Q. 1.2   *How would you arrange transport to a neonatal surgical centre?*

Q. 1.3   *Discuss the principles of resuscitation in this circumstance.*

CASE 2

A diagnosis of Hirschsprung's disease is made on a newborn baby.

Q. 2.1   *What is the definitive diagnostic test for Hirschsprung's disease?*

Q. 2.2   *Discuss the surgical treatment.*

Q. 2.3   *Discuss the prognosis.*

CASE 3

A 1-day-old baby presents with bile-stained vomiting but no abdominal distension.

Q. 3.1   *List the causes of high-level neonatal bowel obstruction.*

Q. 3.2   *How do you distinguish between these on investigation?*

Q. 3.3   *Discuss the urgency of diagnosis and treatment.*

Neonatal bowel obstruction presents with the triad of bile-stained vomiting, abdominal distension and failure to pass meconium. A wide range of congenital anomalies of the gut can cause neonatal bowel obstruction, which in the neonatal period causes problems related to the special metabolism of the neonate.

ANTENATAL DIAGNOSIS

Dilated fluid-filled loops of gut may be seen on antenatal ultrasonography, indicating bowel obstruction. Sometimes the nature of the obstruction may be characteristic with the 'double bubble' of duodenal atresia, but more often the findings do not indicate a specific diagnosis. There is considerable variability in the normal appearance of the fetal gut and antenatal diagnosis of bowel obstruction should be reserved for those cases with gross gut dilatation. Polyhydramnios may be associated with intra-uterine bowel obstruction, particularly with the more proximal level of obstruction. Most pregnancies are now checked with ultrasonography at 17 to 18 weeks' gestation, but this may be too early to diagnose many cases of neonatal bowel obstruction. Intra-uterine segmental volvulus or intussusception in later pregnancy is the cause of many gut atresias and ultrasonography examination is not routinely performed in the later stages of pregnancy.

CLINICAL FINDINGS

Bile-stained vomiting in the neonatal period always is significant and must be evaluated carefully as it is indicative of bowel obstruction.

Adbominal distension is a less specific feature as gaseous distension may occur without bowel obstruction. Furthermore, some high bowel obstructions, for example, malrotation with volvulus or duodenal atresia, may not have abdominal distension.

The normal neonate passes meconium within 24 hours. Neonates with bowel obstruction do not pass meconium; however, there are three notable exceptions: (i) babies with Hirschsprung's disease may pass meconium, especially after rectal examination; (ii) some sticky meconium pellets may be passed in meconium ileus; (iii) the onset of symptoms in malrotation with volvulus may be delayed for some time after birth.

IMAGING

The plain X-ray (erect and supine) is the most important test and will show distension of the gut with fluid levels. The level of the obstruction may be related to the number of fluid levels; for example, a double bubble in duodenal atresia, three or four fluid levels in upper jejunal atresia and many fluid levels in ileal atresia or Hirschsprung's disease. Fine calcification indicates prenatal gut perforation with meconium peritonitis. Free gas in the peritoneal cavity is seen when perforation occurs after birth.

Contrast studies are useful in some patients.

Incomplete high obstructions are assessed with a barium meal, which will demonstrate a malrotation with volvulus or a duodenal web. A barium enema is a suitable test for low obstructions, such as Hirschsprung's disease or meconium ileus.

METABOLIC COMPLICATIONS

Neonatal bowel obstruction can lead to rapid and serious metabolic derangement. This is especially so if gut ischaemia occurs. Many of these metabolic problems are related to the neonatal period of development. These problems must be corrected before undertaking transport. Surgical correction cannot be contemplated until the baby has been fully resuscitated. The particular metabolic problems related to bowel obstruction are:

(1) Fluid losses from the lack of fluid intake, vomiting and sequestration of fluid in the gut and peritoneal cavity leads to diminished circulating fluid volume and poor tissue perfusion. This contributes to hypothermia and acidosis.

(2) Tissue glucose stores in the neonate are low. If oral intake is blocked and metabolism is stressed by bowel obstruction and poor tissue perfusion, glucose stores will be rapidly exhausted and the baby will switch to anaerobic metabolism with consequent acidosis. The acidosis has an adverse effect on cardiovascular activity exacerbating the problem.

(3) The sick neonate is particularly sensitive to hypothermia. Inadequate warming during examination, resuscitation and X-ray of the neonate compound the problems. Much of the preparation of the sick neonate for transport is spent correcting and maintaining body temperature.

(4) Respiratory distress is seen in many babies with bowel obstruction due to abdominal distension. Inhalation of vomitus may produce pneumonitis and atelectasis.

(5) Sepsis from gut organisms is due to transmigration of organisms through the

ischaemic or perforated gut wall, causing a rapid deterioration in all the other metabolic factors. Septicaemia with virulent gut organisms may lead to the rapid demise of the neonate.

GENERAL TREATMENT

Transport

The neonatal emergency transport service should be called to the sick neonate with a bowel obstruction. Sick neonates do not tolerate handling and movement; transport is a particularly stressful time and the metabolic problems should be corrected before transfer.

Nasogastric tube

The passage of a nasogastric tube to aspirate gut content relieves respiratory distress from abdominal distension and helps to measure the fluid losses. It is mandatory in all cases of bowel obstruction.

Resuscitation

Fluid replacement

An intravenous line is established while using an overhead heater to prevent heat loss. Rapid resuscitation with 10 mL/kg boluses of Hartmann's solution is given over 15 minutes for each bolus. The state of hydration of the baby is assessed in terms of peripheral circulation and urine output. Most babies would require 10 to 30 mL/kg of resuscitation fluid in a preparation for surgery.

Glucose replacement

Blood glucose levels should be monitored during resuscitation and a glucose solution should be given as well as Hartmann's solution. Lack of glucose exacerbates acidosis and can cause fitting.

Correction of acidosis

Acid-base measurement is an important part of neonatal resuscitation. Correction of hypothermia, fluid and glucose replacement will help to correct any acidosis, but sodium bicarbonate given intravenously may be needed.

Hypothermia

Hypothermia is a major risk to the sick neonate. A neonatal overhead heater with monitoring of the baby's temperature is used during resuscitation with the establishment of intravenous lines. X-ray imaging is another time of risk for hypothermia. Much of the expertise involved in neonatal transport services is directed to preventing hypothermia during transfer to a neonatal surgical centre.

Sepsis

There is a risk of sepsis with neonatal bowel obstruction, and intravenous antibiotics are commenced after cultures are taken.

HIRSCHSPRUNG'S DISEASE

In 1887, Hirschsprung described two infants who died with gross abdominal distension due to a massively dilated colon containing masses of faeces. Hirschsprung assumed that the disease affected the megacolon. However, the disease was later shown to be in the narrow distal bowel where there is a lack of ganglion cells in the submucosal and myenteric plexus, and where thickened abnormal cholinergic nerve fibres are found in the affected segment. The affected gut is in a constant state of spasm and will not relax. It is a functional obstruction.

Hirschsprung's disease occurs in 1 : 5000 births. Genetically there are two types:
(1) A larger group, in which males are affected five times as often as females, and there is a relatively short aganglionic segment, usually

involving the sigmoid colon, rectum and anal canal.

(2) A smaller group with a long aganglionic segment, equally common in boys and girls, with a higher degree of 'penetrance' and more likely to affect subsequent siblings.

Specific genetic abnormalities (for example, GDNF-ret oncogene; endothelin-endothelin B receptor system) are being described in Hirschsprung's disease and these genetic markers will become increasingly important in the understanding of the basis of this disease.

The affected segment begins at the anus and extends proximally for a variable distance — in most cases as far as the sigmoid colon, but sometimes as high as the ascending colon. In a few cases the affected segment extends into the small bowel, and in rare instances the entire alimentary canal is devoid of ganglia, excluding hope of survival.

The most common presentation is with complete bowel obstruction in the neonatal period. In some cases the baby may present at a few months of age with chronic constipation and failure to thrive. Paradoxically, these late-presenting cases may have long segment disease.

The three classic signs are: (i) delay in the passage of meconium; (ii) vomitus containing bile; (iii) abdominal distension.

Clinical features

Abdominal examination will reveal marked gaseous distension. Rectal stimulation with a probe may cause explosive decompression of meconium and faeces through the tight anal sphincters. A nasogastric tube will drain bile-stained fluid.

Investigation

Plain X-rays will show marked gaseous distension of the gut with air fluid levels. A contrast enema will show constriction of the segment of bowel affected by the Hirschsprung's disease tapering through a transition zone to a distended megacolon

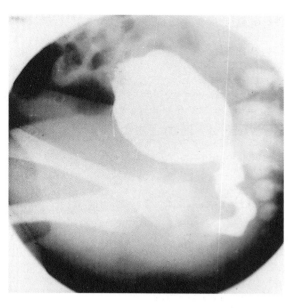

Fig. 7.1 Hirschsprung's disease transition zone between the dilated proximal colon and narrow distal bowel as seen on barium enema.

above the functional blockage of the affected segment (Fig. 7.1).

The diagnosis is made by rectal suction biopsy. The biopsy is processed to examine for ganglion cells by standard microscopy and histochemical preparations are made for acetylcholinesterase staining of cholinergic submucosal nerve fibres. The diagnosis of Hirschsprung's disease requires sophisticated paediatric pathological services.

Treatment

Following resuscitation, a laparotomy is performed and the surgeon works with the pathologist to take multiple biopsies from the bowel to identify the extent of the disease. A colostomy is then fashioned in the normally innervated bowel just above the transition zone.

The definitive pull-through operation is performed at the age of 3 to 6 months. The normally innervated bowel is brought down and sutured to the anus at the level of the anal valves.

Prognosis

The surgery for Hirschsprung's disease is life-saving, but there may be prolonged morbidity in some cases. Enterocolitis, either before or after surgery, can be life-threatening, with the outpouring of fluid stools causing rapid, severe electrolyte problems along with sepsis. Bowel and sphincter dysfunction with diarrhoea and soiling may be a long-term problem.

MECONIUM ILEUS

Cystic fibrosis causes a change in the physical properties of the meconium that fills the fetal gut. The meconium becomes excessively sticky and tenacious, causing a mechanical obstruction of the bowel. This phenomenon is called Meconium Ileus. In Western countries, cystic fibrosis is the usual underlying cause, and this can be diagnosed by genetic tests or by finding high sodium chloride levels in a sweat specimen. Occasionally, meconium ileus occurs as an isolated event and there is no underlying disease.

The sticky meconium impacts as a putty-like substance in the terminal ileum and the colon distal to this is a small unused 'microcolon'. The gut above the obstructed ileum is distended with sticky meconium.

Clinical findings

The baby presents with bile-stained vomiting, abdominal distension and failure to pass meconium. There may be a family history of cystic fibrosis. The loops of distended gut may be palpable as they are filled with meconium, rather than the gaseous distension in other forms of bowel obstruction. Rectal examination reveals no normal meconium, but pale mucus pellets.

Imaging studies

Plain X-rays show distended loops of gut filled

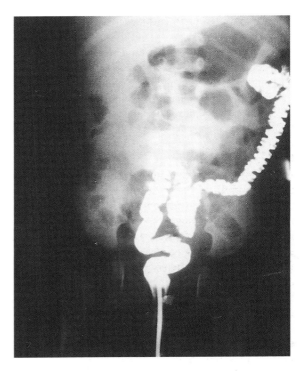

Fig. 7.2 'Microcolon'. The unexpanded but otherwise normal bowel distal to any complete intestinal obstruction *in utero*.

with a foamy substance. On the erect film there may be no air fluid levels as the meconium is too viscous to layer out with gravity. A contrast enema (Fig. 7.2) will show a microcolon with pellets in the terminal ileum. Contrast may then pass into the dilated small bowel above the obstructed ileum.

Treatment

Treatment is based on the assumption that these infants have cystic fibrosis. Antibiotics are commenced at once, and dehydration, which would make secretions even more tenacious, must be prevented.

Sometimes the obstructing meconium can be removed by a water soluble contrast enema under X-ray screening. If this non-invasive method fails, laparotomy is performed and a temporary enterostomy is performed to allow subsequent bowel wash outs to clear the meconium. The enterostomy is closed subsequently. The prognosis for meconium ileus depends on the nature of the underlying cystic fibrosis. Occasionally there is recurrent bowel obstruction due to faecal impaction in the terminal ileum. This is known as meconium ileus equivalent.

VOLVULUS NEONATORUM

The fetal alimentary canal returns from the extra-embryonic coelom into the abdomen at 8 to 10 weeks, and the bowel undergoes rotation and fixation at certain points by the attachment of its mesentery to the posterior abdominal wall.

When the process is incomplete or deviates from the normal plan, the result is malfixation or malrotation.

Commonly, the normal oblique attachment of the mesentery from the duodenojejunal flexure of the caecum is absent, and the small bowel is attached to the posterior abdominal wall by a narrow stalk based around the superior mesenteric vessels. The caecum is undescended; that is, situated in the right hypochondrium and abnormally fixed by peritoneal bands running laterally across the second part of the duodenum.

The poorly attached small bowel undergoes volvulus around the axis of the 'universal mesentery', which is twisted so that the flow of blood is cut off, producing a strangulating obstruction of the small bowel. This typically occurs in the newborn, hence the term 'volvulus neonatorum'. The terminal ileum and caecum are drawn into the volvulus and are wrapped around the stalk of the mesentery in two or three tight coils.

Clinical features

Bile-stained vomiting associated with a soft non-distended abdomen is the early feature of volvulus. The diagnosis should be made at this early stage before widespread ischaemic gut damage occurs.

No obstruction may occur in the first day or two after birth and meconium may be passed normally; then, with variable suddenness, bowel actions cease with the onset of obstruction.

The symptoms may be recurrent which is very suggestive of volvulus neonatorum.

The signs vary, depending on the degree of intestinal obstruction versus ischaemia. When strangulation occurs there are signs of shock, especially pallor, and a vague mass of congested bowel may be palpable in the centre of the abdomen. Blood or blood-tinged mucus may be passed rectally. Distension is variable and often absent or confined to the epigastrium when the duodenum is obstructed, for a large vomit can empty the stomach and proximal duodenum.

Investigations

A plain X-ray of the abdomen is not helpful in the early stage of volvulus. The most reliable radiological confirmation of malfixation is a barium meal with fluoroscopy, which will show that the duodenojejunal flexure is located at a lower level than (that is, caudal to) the pylorus. The contrast may show the spiral twist of the volvulus as well (Fig. 7.3).

Treatment

Laparotomy is urgently required, as ischaemia may lead to gangrene of the midgut. The volvulus is untwisted. The malfixation of the gut is then corrected by Ladd's operation. The narrow base of the mesentery is broadened by dissection that separates the caecum from the duodenum by dividing abnormal fascial bands. The small bowel is placed on the right side of the abdomen and the colon is placed on the left side, leaving the appendix in the left hypochondrium, and appendicectomy may be performed to prevent confusion. Sometimes the early diagnostic features of volvulus are missed and extensive gut ischaemia occurs. When the surgeon opens the abdomen, nearly all the gut is gangrenous. This situation poses a major problem for future

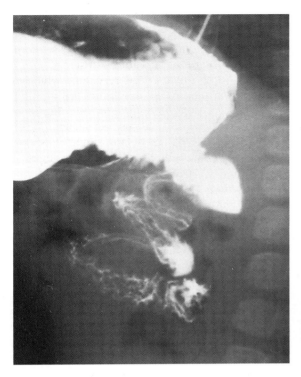

Fig. 7.3 Volvulus neonatorum. Barium meal shows a spiral twist of the bowel below the mid-duodenum.

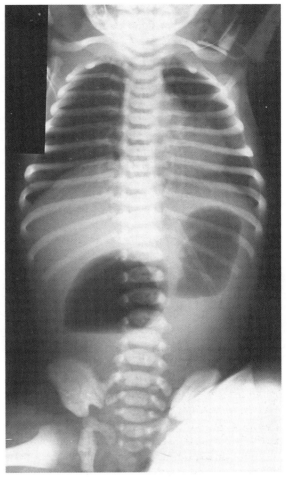

Fig. 7.4 Duodenal atresia. Plain X-ray shows a 'double bubble', one in the stomach and the other in the dilated proximal duodenum.

management. The gut is untwisted and a 'second look' laparotomy is performed 24 to 48 hours later to see if any viable gut can be saved.

DUODENAL OBSTRUCTION

Duodenal obstruction is caused by duodenal atresia, or by stenosis due to a septum or membrane with a small hole in it. Still less commonly, an annular pancreas may be wrapped around the duodenum, but usually this is accompanied by severe stenosis or atresia of the duodenum at the site of the envelopment.

Atresia of the duodenum occurs most commonly in the second part and is associated with Down syndrome in about 30 per cent of affected infants.

Acute obstruction develops in the neonatal period, but signs may be delayed for a day or so while the secretions accumulate in the distended stomach and proximal duodenum.

X-rays of the abdomen show a 'double bubble' pattern: two large loops each with a fluid level and no aeration of the more distal bowel (Fig. 7.4).

A duodenal septum with a hole in the centre may form an incomplete obstruction with episodic vomiting that may be bile-stained. These babies may present in the neonatal period or at a later age if the obstruction is not so severe. The diagnosis is made on a barium meal study.

Treatment

In atresia of the duodenum, with or without an annular pancreas, the obstruction is circumvented by duodenoduodenostomy. The surgical treatment for duodenal septum is duodenoplasty, but the bile ducts may pose a special problem because they open very close to or actually into the edge of the septum.

SMALL BOWEL ATRESIA

Atresia of the bowel can occur at any point (Fig. 7.5), most frequently in the distal ileum (Fig. 7.6), but this is rare in the colon. There is often only one atresia, although there may be several close together or widely scattered.

The cause may be interruption of the mesenteric arcades by a vascular accident *in utero*, a theory supported by experimental surgery on fetal animals.

The form of the atresia may be a very tight stenosis with no functional orifice, or a thick septum with the bowel in continuity or a missing segment with a gap of a centimetre or more between the closed ends. The adjacent vascular arcades are distorted and their terminal branches may be very small or absent. All the bowel distal to the atresia is collapsed. A barium enema may demonstrate a microcolon.

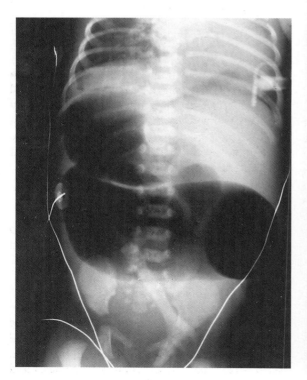

Fig. 7.5 Intestinal atresia. Plain X-ray shows obstruction of the jejunum. Infant also has *situs inversus*.

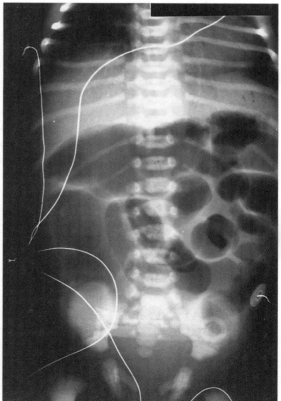

Fig. 7.6 Ileal atresia.

DUPLICATIONS OF THE ALIMENTARY TRACT

These are rare developmental anomalies in which a length of bowel is duplicated in such a way that the two segments share the same blood supply and a common wall, while the mucosal linings are separate. They can arise at any point from the mouth to the anus, and involve any length from 1 to 2 cm to the whole length of the large bowel. A duplication may or may not communicate with the main alimentary channel.

There are two basic types:

(1) Short closed cystic segments. The segment forms a cyst that bulges into the lumen or compresses and angulates the adjoining small bowel, causing obstruction. A small intraluminal cyst may cause obstruction in the neonatal period, but larger ones less intimately connected with the common wall usually cause progressive obstruction later in infancy or in early childhood. Occasionally a large tense cyst is palpable as a very mobile mass in a child without obstructive symptoms.

(2) Long tubular communicating duplications are much less common and more likely to be lined by ectopic (gastric) mucosa, which may cause a peptic ulcer (Chapter 23). If the diagnosis of a duplication containing ectopic gastric mucosa is suspected, it may be demonstrable by means of a technetium ^{99m} scan. The resection of a long duplication involves the removal of an equivalent length of bowel, and when this is unacceptable because of the inadequate length of bowel remaining, a practical alternative is to remove the lining alone.

NEONATAL NECROTIZING ENTEROCOLITIS

Necrotizing enterocolitis is a disease with combined ischaemia and infection of the bowel wall. Although not strictly a 'cause' of intestinal obstruction, it typically produces abdominal distension and bile-stained vomiting, resembling

---

Box 7.1 Predisposing factors and observed associations in neonatal necrotizing enterocolitis

Prematurity
Respiratory distress:
   Atelectasis
   Hyaline membrane disease
Birth asphyxia
Fetal distress during labour
Prolonged antepartum rupture of membranes
Twins
Caesarean section
Congenital heart disease
Jaundice
Catheterization of the umbilical vessels
Hyperosmolar feeds
Sepsis

---

obstruction, but distinguishable by features such as passage of blood and a characteristic radiological picture. A greater awareness of the entity may have contributed to the increased incidence in recent years, but there has been an absolute increase in the number of cases reported throughout the Western world.

Predisposing factors

Sick and premature neonates can develop necrotising enterocolitis as a further complication of the predisposing factors listed in Box 7.1.

Aetiology

The mechanism has not been elucidated fully. The most widely held theory to explain the intestinal ischaemia is that in a stressed, hypoxic state, blood is preferentially distributed to the heart and brain, at the expense of the splanchnic circulation, skin and muscle.

Local vascular changes have been implicated; for example, a catheter in the umbilical vein, if badly positioned, alters the portal haemodynamics. A catheter in the umbilical artery may have a similar effect on the arterial supply if advanced too far up the aorta, and also has the potential to produce emboli.

Certain bacteria appear to be important; *Klebsiella* species resistant to the commonly used antibiotics are found in a significant number of infants who develop necrotizing enterocolitis. Other enteropathogens (for example, *Escherichia coli*, *Clostridium difficile* and *Streptococcus faecalis*) and *Pseudomonas* species also have been isolated.

The type of feed and when it is commenced may have some relevance; for example, the disease appears to occur more frequently in infants who were fed early with artificial milk formulae. Breast milk may afford some protection against the disease in the 'at risk' infant, but this is not certain.

Pathology

Necrotizing enterocolitis may be generalized and involve most of the small and large intestine or be segmental in distribution, in which case the ileum and colon commonly are affected. There is histological evidence of impaired perfusion, resulting in tissue anoxia and necrosis. The mucosa is affected most, because of a shunting mechanism, but the process may involve the entire thickness of the bowel wall.

When the mucosa is damaged, production of mucus is impaired and bacteria normally present in the lumen can invade the intestinal wall, further damaging the bowel and entering the bloodstream to produce bacteraemia or septicaemia. The damaged mucosa bleeds into the lumen, and gas collects in the bowel wall (pneumatosis intestinalis) due to the activity of gas-forming organisms or by diffusion of intraluminal gas through breaches in the damaged mucosa.

The consequent pathological course varies: perforation with generalized peritonitis or local abscess formation follows transmural necrosis; healing with restoration of normal function occurs in the less-affected bowel; and fibrosis with the formation of a stricture may be the result of healing in a severely involved segment.

Clinical picture

The onset of symptoms is between 2 and 14 days after birth. The infant is ill, lethargic, febrile and not interested in feeds. Abdominal distension and bile-stained vomiting occur, and there may be passage of loose stools containing a variable amount of blood.

When complicated by peritonitis, the anterior abdominal wall becomes oedematous and red, with dilated veins, and palpation causes pain. A mass may be palpable if a localized intraperitoneal abscess has formed or if there is a persistently dilated loop of bowel.

Investigations

The radiological findings are typical. Plain films of the abdomen show dilated loops of bowel in which there are intramural bubbles of gas (pneumatosis intestinalis; Fig. 7.7). Gas outlining the portal vein and/or its radicles may be visible. Free gas in the peritoneal cavity, best seen under the diaphragm, is present if the intestine has perforated. Separation of adjacent loops of bowel suggests appreciable amounts of intraperitoneal exudate, an indication of peritonitis, with or without a perforation.

Bacteriological specimens, for example, blood culture and rectal swabs, should be taken before antibiotics are commenced or altered. The nose, throat and umbilicus also are swabbed.

Biochemistry, haematology, electrolytes, acid-base and bilirubin are monitored. The haemoglobin level may fall progressively as a result of sepsis and haemorrhage and serial measurements are required. The platelet and white cell counts are depressed in severe disease. The infants are acidotic.

Management

Initially this consists of stopping oral feeds,

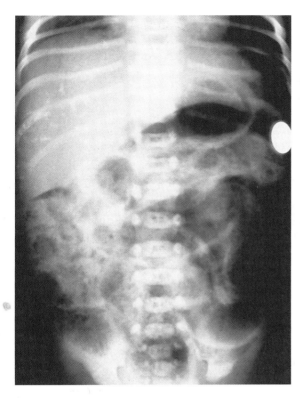

Fig. 7.7 Necrotizing enterocolitis. Intramural gas.

decompression of the intestine by suction via a wide bore nasogastric tube and parenteral administration of fluids and appropriate antibiotics.

Intensive measures listed in the section on the pre- and postoperative care of the neonate and adequate respiratory management also may be required. Acidosis is corrected.

Frequent clinical and radiological reassessment is essential, for it may show the need for surgery.

The indications for an operation are continued clinical deterioration despite intensive and appropriate resuscitation; or the development of a complication suggesting the presence of full-thickness bowel necrosis, such as perforation or intra-abdominal abscess. Features that are useful in determining the need for operation include free gas on X-ray, progressive signs of peritonitis (distended red and tender abdomen), persistent acidosis despite attempted correction, and a sudden and profound fall in the platelet count.

Operation is confined to the resection of perforated or necrotic bowel and drainage of any intraperitoneal abscesses. The mortality rate until recently was high, but with earlier diagnosis and more effective treatment this is diminishing.

FURTHER READING

Lister J. (1990) Intestinal atresia and stenosis, excluding the duodenum. In: Lister J. & Irving I.M. (eds) *Neonatal Surgery*, 3rd edn, Butterworths, London, pp. 453–72.

Lister J. (1990) Malrotation and volvulus of the intestine. In: Lister J., Irving I.M. (eds) *Neonatal Surgery*, 3rd edn, Butterworths, London, pp. 442–52.

Stauffer U.G. & Schwoebel M. (1998) Duodenal atresia and stenosis — annular pancreas. In: O'Neill J.A., Rowe M.I., Grosfeld J.L., Fonkalsrud E.W. & Coran A.G. (eds) *Pediatric Surgery*, 5th edn, Mosby, St. Louis, pp. 1133–44.

Teitelbaum D.H., Coran A.G., Weitzman J.J., Ziegler M.M. & Kene T. (1998) Hirschsprung's disease and related neuromuscular disorders of the intestine. In: O'Neill J.A., Rowe M.I., Grosfeld J.L., Fonkalsrud E.W. & Coran A.G. (eds) *Pediatric Surgery*, 5th edn, Mosby, St. Louis, pp. 1381–1424.

— 8 —

Abdominal Wall Defects

CASE 1

Mrs F. first realised there was a problem when ultrasonography at 18 weeks of gestation showed that her unborn baby had bowel loops within an expanded umbilical cord. Careful scan of the rest of the baby showed no other abnormality, although she was warned of the possibility. Amniocentesis and karyotyping failed to show trisomy 13 or 18, and it was elected to continue the pregnancy. A paediatric surgeon was consulted for advice about treatment at birth. The baby was delivered at the tertiary medical institution and the paediatric surgeon notified.

> Q. 1.1   *What is the abnormality?*
>
> Q. 1.2   *Why did it occur?*
>
> Q. 1.3   *What 'first aid' treatment is needed prior to transfer?*
>
> Q. 1.4   *What is the management and prognosis?*

CASE 2

Jody was 17, and did not want her parents to know she was pregnant. She presented in labour with no prior antenatal visits. A vigorous infant was soon delivered, but the midwife was horrified to see most of the small bowel hanging out through a small hole in the abdominal wall, just to the right of the umbilicus.

> Q. 2.1   *Will the baby live?*
>
> Q. 2.2   *Why is the baby's life at risk?*
>
> Q. 2.3   *Could there be other anomalies?*

CASE 3

Frank was born without trouble, at term. Antenatally, there had been some concern about no urine being visible in the bladder on ultrasonography. At birth the attachment of the cord was low, and adjacent to an ugly defect with wet, pouting mucosa. The penis was found to be bifid and one testis was undescended.

> Q. 3.1   *What is the embryological defect?*
>
> Q. 3.2   *Can this abnormality be treated?*
>
> Q. 3.3   *Why is the penis 'duplicated' and what is the outcome for sexual function and urinary control?*

EXOMPHALOS AND GASTROSCHISIS

These two developmental abnormalities in the region of the umbilicus are diagnosed on antenatal ultrasonography (Fig. 1.1) or present at birth as neonatal emergencies, and require urgent treatment.

The prevalence of exomphalos (omphalocele) and gastroschisis is relatively similar. The relatively high incidence of coexisting abnormalities in a fetus with exomphalos (35 per cent) has sometimes been accepted as grounds for termination, particularly if amniocentesis identifies a major chromosomal abnormality.

FIRST AID AT BIRTH

A baby with an anterior abdominal wall defect is at great risk of heat and water loss from evaporation because of the moist exposed viscera. For this reason, the baby should be placed in a humidicrib, with the entire torso wrapped, including the exposed viscera, in fresh plastic 'kitchen wrap' or aluminium foil. Care must be taken to ensure that the exposed bowel is not twisted at the level of the opening in the abdominal wall (Fig. 8.1). Do not use hot wet packs as these cool too quickly and chill the infant. The main objective is to prevent excessive fluid and heat loss during transfer to the receiving neonatal surgical unit.

Insert a nasogastric tube to keep the bowel empty and do not feed the baby: this facilitates operative reduction of the herniated bowel.

Commence an intravenous fluid infusion of 10 per cent dextrose + N/5 saline to prevent hypogylcaemia during transport, particularly if

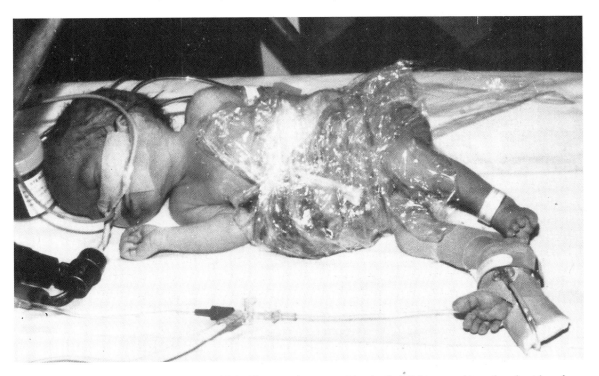

Fig. 8.1 First-aid management of gastroschisis. The torso is wrapped in plastic 'kitchen wrap' to reduce heat loss from evaporation. A nasogastric tube keeps the bowel decompressed, which facilitates operative reduction of the eviscerated bowel. An intravenous line has been inserted.

the baby has Beckwith's syndrome (organomegaly, exomphalos and hypoglycaemia secondary to excess fetal insulin-like growth factor production).

Transport

The infant with an abdominal wall defect should be referred to a fully equipped paediatric surgical centre without delay. Transport should be arranged via a specialised neonatal transport service, if available. If the diagnosis has been made on antenatal ultrasonography, the delivery should be undertaken in a centre with paediatric surgeons standing by.

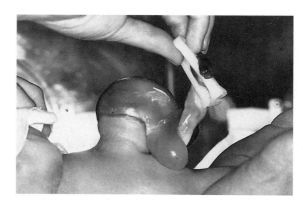

Fig. 8.2 Exomphalos.

EXOMPHALOS

This congenital hernia into the base of the umbilical cord is caused by incomplete folding of the embryonic disc and failure of the umbilical ring to form normally. The hernia is covered by fused amniotic membrane and peritoneum, which may rupture.

Very occasionally, the membrane ruptures before birth and the eviscerated bowel becomes matted and indurated with dense adhesions, so that the bowel appears to be shorter than normal. The inflammation is believed to be caused by chemical irritation from faeces in the amniotic fluid. Rupture may occur during delivery, in which case the bowel is normal.

The size of the defect in the abdominal wall and the size (capacity) of the sac are variable. An intact sac is shiny and translucent but lacks a blood supply and begins to dry out and deteriorate after birth. Within 12 hours it becomes opaque and yellowish; later, it becomes black, inelastic and dessicated.

The diagnosis is obvious (Fig. 8.2); the only difficulty may be in distinguishing a ruptured exomphalos from a gastroschisis. In the latter, there are no sac remnants and the defect is small and separate from the umbilical cord (see below).

Coexisting abnormalities are common in exomphalos, particularly cardiac and renal malformations. Malrotation occurs in 12 to 20 per cent of cases, but seldom causes volvulus, probably because of adhesions between loops and 'secondary' fixation to the parietes.

Beckwith–Wiedemann syndrome must be recognised early, because of the severe hypo-glycaemia that requires immediate correction. These babies produce excess insulin-like growth factor during gestation, which leads to organo-megaly, exomphalos and excess bodyweight. A large baby (for example, 4 kg) with exomphalos and macroglossia is suggestive of the diagnosis. The exomphalos appears to be secondary to the enlarged viscera, which cannot be accommodated inside the abdomen. Postnatal hypoglycaemia is transient but dangerous because of the risk of brain damage, which may occur if an immediate infusion of glucose is not provided.

Investigations

Chest X-ray and echocardiogram are required to exclude a cardiac lesion and intercurrent pulmonary conditions, such as atelectasis or meconium inhalation. The kidneys can be examined by ultrasonography. Careful physical examination may suggest other serious anomalies; for example, chromosomal aberrations, confirmation of which may modify or even preclude treatment.

Treatment

First aid and the method of transport to the tertiary centre are crucial for optimal outcomes, and are discussed earlier in this chapter. The aim of treatment is to reduce the contents of the exomphalos and repair the defect of the abdominal wall. The method of treatment depends on: (i) the general condition of the infant (size, birthweight, maturity, suitability for anaesthesia); (ii) presence of other anomalies; (iii) whether the sac is intact or ruptured; (iv) the size of the umbilical ring; (v) whether part of the liver has herniated into the sac.

Immediate operation and complete repair is the best course when the defect is less than 5 cm in diameter, the infant is fit for surgery and closure can be obtained.

Excision of the sac (or remnants, if ruptured), and construction of a cylindrical tube (a 'silo') can be used for larger defects. A sheet of silastic or teflon is sewn to the edge of the defect. Alternatively, Op Site can be attached to the skin around and over the defect, and used to serially reduce the volume of the exomphalos over 7 to 10 days by imbrication, so that the viscera are returned progressively to the abdomen. The prosthesis or Op Site is then removed and the defect repaired surgically. Use of a silo is indicated when the sac has ruptured with massive evisceration, but it is not without problems, such as infection around the sutures that anchor the prosthesis to the edge of the defect.

Non-operative management is best when anaesthesia is contra-indicated because of the poor condition of the infant (prematurity, cardiac anomaly, meconium inhalation) or when the defect is extremely large (> 5 cm in diameter) and contains herniated liver. The sac is painted with an astringent solution to make it a tough, dry eschar which separates when new skin has covered the area beneath it, after 8 to 12 weeks. Any substance applied to the exomphalos sac may be absorbed by the baby and care should be taken to use non-toxic substances sparingly.

Subsequent wound contraction reduces the hernia progressively over 4 to 8 months and makes the definitive repair easier. Once the eschar has formed, and normal feeding and stools are established, the infant can be managed safely at home, avoiding prolonged, costly and risky (because of cross-infection) hospitalisation. The appearance of the hernia and eschar may be intimidating to the parents, who need support and encouragement to achieve satisfactory bonding.

GASTROSCHISIS

Recent antenatal ultrasound observations suggest that gastroschisis may result from the rupture of a physiological hernia in the cord at 6 to 10 weeks' gestation. The fetus usually is normal genetically but has had an 'accident' affecting the umbilical cord. The defect in the abdominal wall is small (1 to 3 cm in diameter) and is nearly always to the right of the umbilicus.

The evisceration may involve almost all the small and large bowel, which become densely matted and adherent with amniotic (chemical) peritonitis and fibrin from defaecation *in utero* (Fig. 8.3), particularly during the last trimester.

It differs from a ruptured exomphalos in that there is:

(1) a greater risk of hypothermia;
(2) a smaller abdominal wall defect and no covering sac;
(3) lower incidence of serious coexisting malformations;
(4) a greater (but still small) incidence of a small bowel atresias, but these may be 'occult' or hidden by the matted fibrin surface of the exposed bowel.

Treatment

Only two methods are available; and (i) immediate operative reduction of the viscera and primary repair; and (ii) a prosthetic 'silo' as described above, reducing the viscera over 7 to 10 days, followed by

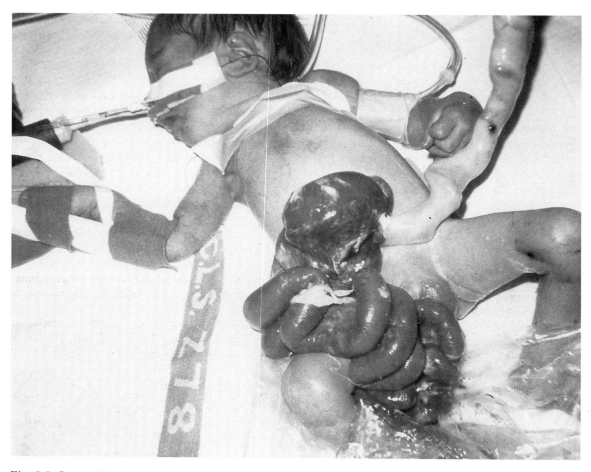

Fig. 8.3 Gastroschisis.

definitive ('secondary') repair. Immediate surgical repair is the method of choice, but success depends on a series of complementary adjuvant steps, and requires expert intensive care and nursing. The method involves:

(1) Correction of any physiological disturbances (temperature, hydration etc).

(2) Anorectal digital dilatation under anaesthesia to decompress the colon.

(3) Nasogastric suction to minimise bowel gas.

(4) Enlargement of the defect and intraperitoneal 'milking' of the bowel to evacuate as much meconium as possible through the anus.

(5) Stretching of the scaphoid anterior abdominal wall to enlarge the capacity of the abdomen.

(6) Postoperative mechanical ventilation to counteract splinting of the diaphragm caused by high intra-abdominal pressure when the viscera are 'reduced'.

(7) Total parenteral alimentation until effective peristalsis has been restored, sometimes after many weeks.

(8) Careful examination of the bowel at laparotomy to detect an 'occult' atresia.

When all these are applied effectively, closure should be achieved and almost all infants should survive.

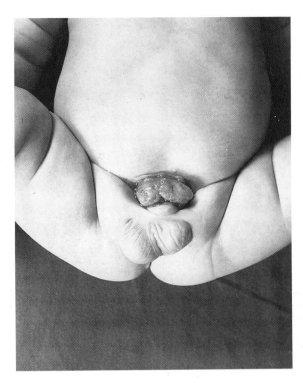

Fig. 8.4 Bladder exstrophy.

BLADDER EXSTROPHY (ECTOPIA VESICAE)

Failure of fusion of the lower abdominal wall during embryonic development leaves the bladder exposed as a flat plaque on the lower abdomen (Fig. 8.4). There is no covering muscle or skin. The pubic rami do not fuse in the midline. The ureters protrude from the exposed bladder and dribble urine. The urethra is exposed as a flat strip and the bladder outlet sphincters are not functional. Bladder exstrophy, also known as 'ectopia vesicae', is rare, with an incidence of 1 : 40 000 births. Reconstructive surgery to close the bladder and abdominal wall with restoration of bladder sphincters is one of the most difficult problems in paediatric surgery.

An even rarer variant of bladder exstrophy is known as cloacal exstrophy. In this condition, the right colon is fused on to the bladder exstrophy, and there may be an imperforate anus.

FURTHER READING

Beasley S.W. & Jones P.G. (1986) Use of mercurochrome in the management of the large exomphalos. *Aust. Paediatr. J.* **22**: 61–3.

Brock J.W., O'Neill J.A. (1998) Bladder exstrophy. In: O'Neill J.A., Rowe M.I., Grosfeld J.L., Fonkalsrud E.W. & Coran A.G. (eds). *Pediatric Surgery*, 5th edn, Mosby, St. Louis, pp. 1709–58.

Molenaar J.C. (1996) Exomphalos and gastroschisis. In: Puri P. (ed.) *Newborn Surgery*, Butterworth-Heinemann, Oxford, 1996, pp. 449–52.

Tracy T.F. (1997) Abdominal wall defects. In: Oldham K.T., Colombani P.M. & Foglia R.F. (eds) *Surgery of Infants and Children: Scientific Principles and Practice*. Lippincott-Raven, Philadelphia, pp. 1083–93.

Tunell W.P., Puffinbarger N.K. & Tuggle D.W. et al. (1995) Abdominal wall defects in infants. Survival and implications for adult life. *Ann. Surg.*, **221**: 525–8.

— 9 —

Spina Bifida

CASE 1

Jeannie was a regular drug-user and shared an apartment with several friends. She became pregnant at 18, avoided antenatal care and presented in labour. The baby had a red, ugly mass over the lumbar spine and no spontaneous leg movement.

> Q. 1.1   *What physical signs are important to note at birth?*
>
> Q. 1.2   *Will the baby have hydrocephalus?*
>
> Q. 1.3   *What is the prognosis for (a) intellect; (b) walking?*

CASE 2

Antenatal alphafetoprotein and mid-gestation ultrasonography did not reveal any fetal anomaly. At birth the infant had a small, skin-covered cystic mass over the sacrum. Leg movements were good but the bladder was palpable.

> Q. 2.1   *What are the urinary tract problems in spina bifida?*
>
> Q. 2.2   *How are urinary and faecal incontinence managed?*

Spina bifida is one of the most crippling congenital anomalies. The primary abnormality is incomplete fusion of the neural tube and overlying ectoderm leading to a defect between the vertebral arches. There is protrusion and dysplasia of the spinal cord and its membranes. The resulting nerve deficit may cause paraplegia, urinary and faecal incontinence and multiple orthopaedic deformities. Hydrocephalus is a frequent associated anomaly.

The severity of this anomaly has led to widespread antenatal screening with maternal alphafetoprotein levels and ultrasonography in mid-gestation. In many centres, termination of pregnancy is offered when screening reveals a myelomeningocele. Improved diet with correction of folic acid deficiency may also decrease the incidence of this anomaly. As a result of these two factors the incidence in Western countries of live-born infants with spina bifida has decreased dramatically in recent years.

EMBRYOLOGY

Spina bifida and anencephaly are neural tube defects. The fusion of the neural folds should be completed by the fourth week of embryonic development. The mesoderm around the neural tube forms the meninges, vertebral column and muscles. The less severe anomalies involve failure of vertebral arch fusion and protrusion of the meninges to form a meningocele. More severe anomalies involve the neuro-ectoderm with protrusion of the neural tube itself to form a myelomeningocele. Failure of fusion of the brain causes an encephalocele (see Chapter 12) or anencephaly.

AETIOLOGY AND ANTENATAL DIAGNOSIS

Spina bifida has been linked to folate deficiency in the maternal diet. There is a previous history of hydrocephalus, anencephaly or spina bifida in 6 to 8 per cent of cases: in these, the risk of spina bifida in subsequent pregnancies is 1 : 20. With two affected children, the risk is 1 : 8. Prenatal diagnosis in spina bifida is well established. Antenatal ultrasonography may detect the sac and the vertebral defect. The open sac weeps fetal cerebrospinal fluid (CSF) into the liquor and this can be detected by alpha-fetoprotein estimation of maternal blood or of amniotic fluid obtained by amniocentesis.

MYELOMENINGOCELE

This consists of a bifid spine with protrusion and dysplasia of the meninges and spinal cord. The dysplastic spinal cord is splayed over a meningeal sac filled with CSF and is associated with severe nerve deficits below the level of the lesion. This accounts for 94 per cent of neonates with spina bifida. There is a slight predominance of females. The incidence varies widely from one region to another and there are significant annual variations.

Clinical features

The sac is in the midline, usually in the lumbosacral region (Figs 9.1 and 9.2). The size of the sac is variable; there is an area of well-developed skin at the periphery but this is thin at the apex, which is covered by the delicate glistening arachnoid membrane with nervous tissue visible on the surface.

If left untreated the central area becomes ulcerated and infected, with a consequent risk of

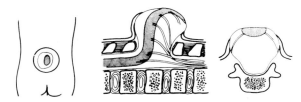

Fig. 9.1 Myelomeningocele. Tissue of the spinal cord forms part of the wall of the sac, as well as its contents.

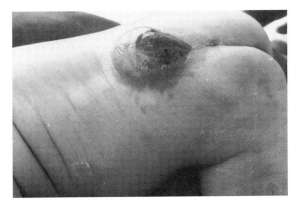

Fig. 9.2 Lumbar myelomeningocele. A moderately large sac with well-developed skin at its periphery. The glistening arachnoid membrane and nervous tissue is exposed on the apex of the sac.

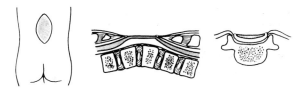

Fig. 9.3 Rachischisis. There is no sac and the central canal of the spinal cord lies wide open on the broad deficiency in the posterior vertebral laminae.

meningitis. Epithelialization occurs slowly, leaving a puckered scar covered with poor quality skin that is liable to ulceration. The coverings may rupture before, during or after birth, with escape of CSF. In rachischisis, the most severe form, the neural tube lies open, no sac is present and the spinal cord is a flattened, red, velvet-like ribbon down the centre of the back (Fig. 9.3).

Table 9.1 Assessment of level of paralysis

Level of lesion	Incidence (%)	Motor function
Cervical/upper thoracic	1	Paralysis of legs and trunk
Lower thoracic	27	Complete paraplegia, including psoas
Upper lumbar	23	Hip flexion and adduction present
Low lumbar/ upper sacral	45	Hip movements, knee extension, foot dorsiflexion
Lower sacral	4	All normal movement

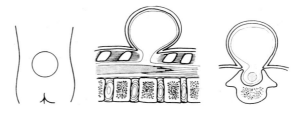

Fig. 9.4 Meningocele. The sac contains CSF only, and the spinal cord is normal.

Motor loss

There is a flaccid paralysis of the lower motor neurone type, the extent depending on the level of the neurological lesion. In some patients, upper motor neurone spastic paralysis is present also and is due to either isolated normal sections of the cord below the lesion, or to cerebral or spinal-cord damage from hydrocephalus or meningitis.

Children can be grouped according to the level of the lesion. The motor loss can be assessed by observing the infant's voluntary (not reflex) movements, and the determination of the level is helpful in assessing the probable extent of the eventual disability (Table 9.1).

Sensory loss

Sensory loss corresponds closely to the level of motor loss, although the lower level of normal sensation is usually about one segment higher than the lower level of normal motor power. Loss of sensation is most important in the feet, the buttocks and the perineum because of the risk of pressure sores in these areas.

MENINGOCELE

This is a simple meningeal sac lined by arachnoid membrane and dura, containing CSF and only occasionally nervous tissue (Fig. 9.4). It is relatively uncommon (6 per cent of cases of spina bifida cystica) and it may be associated with cutaneous lesions.

The sac may be of any size from a small bulge to an enormous protrusion. It may be tense, but more often is soft and fluctuant; some become tense when the baby cries or when pressure is applied to the fontanelle. The skin over the sac is generally intact but it may ulcerate occasionally, although this is more typical of myelomeningocele.

Hydrocephalus has been reported but it is rare. The mental state of the child is normal and there are no neurological abnormalities. Deaths are rare and are usually due to meningitis developing before or after operative repair.

Treatment consists of excision of the sac, and when the skin is sound there is no urgency; the repair can be done at any convenient time during infancy. If the sac is ulcerated it should be repaired immediately after birth, but if this opportunity is missed, epithelium should be allowed to cover the sac, which is then excised at a convenient time later in infancy.

VARIANTS OF SPINA BIFIDA

The vertebrae may be bifid without a meningocele or myelomeningocele sac. This may be a normal variant of spinal arch fusion or represent 'spina bifida occulta', which is more serious. Dysplasia of the skin over the spine is a sign of a potentially serious spina bifida: a hairy patch, pigmented naevus, haemangioma, lipoma or a sinus may be present. A dermal sinus over the spine may link with an intraspinal dermoid cyst. If this becomes infected, an intraspinal abscess may form with destruction of the adjacent spinal cord.

A spinal lipoma may be indicated by a bulge over the lumbosacral region. The lower lumbar and sacral nerves run through the fibrolipomatous tissue and progressive nerve damage may occur through spinal cord tethering. These lesions are best demonstrated on magnetic resonance imaging.

ASSOCIATED ANOMALIES AND SEQUELAE OF SPINA BIFIDA

Hydrocephalus

Hydrocephalus is the most important associated anomaly and it is present to some degree in almost all cases of myelomeningocele in early infancy. It needs investigation and treatment in about 70 per cent of affected infants. Hydrocephalus is relatively more common when the myelomeningocele is in the lower thoracic and upper lumbar areas, but it may occur with a myelomeningocele at any level.

The three most common causes of hydrocephalus are the Arnold–Chiari malformation, stricture of the aqueduct of Sylvius and failure of the subarachnoid space to open up at the level of the tentorium.

Hydrocephalus is an important factor that influences the child's survival and subsequent mental state.

Orthopaedic deformities

Orthopaedic deformities are common and greatly complicate management of the paraplegia. They include: kyphosis, lordosis, scoliosis, paralytic dislocation of the hips, flexion contractures of the hips and knees, and deformities of the feet. They are caused by inequality of muscular action and bony immobility leading to inadequate growth stimulus to the skeleton.

Urinary tract abnormalities

Ninety-five per cent of children with myelomeningocele have a neuropathic bladder. The kidneys are usually normal at birth, but there is a high incidence of progressive renal damage during the first few years of life if the problems of a high pressure, non-compliant bladder, vesicoureteric reflux and chronic pyelonephritis are not treated effectively.

Other anomalies

Many of the other anomalies that are associated with spina bifida are potentially lethal; for example, severe congenital heart disease and visceral malformations.

Complications

Meningitis

Meningitis accounts for approximately one-third of all deaths from spina bifida cystica; it arises either from infection of the ulcerated sac (especially if ruptured) or after surgical repair.

Mental retardation

Mental retardation is related to hydrocephalus, although separate cerebral deficiencies may occur also. Less than 10 per cent of children without clinical hydrocephalus are retarded, and with ventriculoperitoneal shunts. Sixty-six per cent have normal intelligence. Overall, children with myelomeningocele who survive to school-age have normal intelligence in approximately 77 per cent of cases; they are retarded but educable in special schools in 21 per cent of cases; and 2 per cent are grossly retarded.

Pressure sores

These may develop on the feet, sacrum and perineum; in the latter two sites the problem is accentuated by urinary and faecal soiling.

Prevention and treatment of pressure sores is of great importance. For deep, extensive sores in the buttock and sacral area, full-thickness skin grafts may be helpful to prevent recurrent breakdown.

Special senses

Paralytic squint (that is, sixth nerve palsy) is a common complication of hydrocephalus, and optic atrophy with blindness occasionally occurs from raised intracranial pressure, usually in older children. Deafness may also occur, apparently unrelated to the hydrocephalus.

Urinary infection

Stasis in the neurogenic bladder contributes to urinary tract infection and leads to chronic pyelonephritis that, if untreated, causes progressive renal scarring. Long-term low dose antibiotics and regular drainage of the bladder by intermittent catheterization may prevent or limit these problems.

Intermittent catheterization can be started shortly after birth. The parents pass a 'clean' catheter four to five times a day. In 80 per cent of cases the child wets a little between catheterization. In 20 per cent of cases there is marked wetting and the bladder storage capacity may be increased by using alpha-adrenergic or anticholinergic drugs.

In many children with spina bifida the neurogenic bladder pattern is that of retention leading to overflow incontinence; the rationale of 'clean intermittent catheterization' is to empty the bladder frequently, before overflow incontinence occurs. Paradoxically, catheterization usually lowers the incidence of urinary tract infections by removing stagnant residual urine. Some children on this regimen will also need daily low-dose antibiotics; for example, nitrofurantoin or Co-trimoxazole.

As children grow older, wetting becomes less acceptable. The main two causes of failure of intermittent catheterisation are: (i) poor urine storage due to deficiency in the function of the bladder outlet sphincter; and (ii) a small bladder capacity with a thick-walled, low compliance bladder. When these children reach school age, the bladder storage can be improved by the implantation of an artificial urinary sphincter around the bladder neck, and augmentation cystoplasty, after which intermittent catheterisation is still essential to empty the bladder.

Faecal incontinence

'Accidents' are common during early childhood; normal toilet training should be offered to these children, and the child is taught to evacuate the stool by contracting the abdominal muscles. Most children are constipated, and the aim is to produce a firm stool that is not soft enough to leak out, and not so hard that it will become impacted. This is achieved by diet, laxatives and bulking agents. After adolescence, most patients are clean and regular and evacuate a firm or hard stool. A few patients require a daily suppository or enema. Gross impaction with overflow is cleared by bowel wash outs. Biofeedback techniques are useful for some children.

PSYCHOLOGICAL AND SOCIAL MANAGEMENT

Many children show psychological disturbances as a result of their disabilities, especially in adolescence, although only a few are seriously disturbed. The disturbances are not directly proportional to the degree of disability or to the level of intellectual functioning; nor are they specific to children with spina bifida. Generally, counselling is sufficient, but some children require additional psychiatric treatment.

Many parents need help to enable them to accept their child's disability. This aspect presents few problems if they have been given a full picture of the condition soon after birth and they have been directly involved in the treatment; however, it can be difficult with parents with previous psychiatric or marital problems.

ASSESSMENT IN THE NEWBORN

Careful assessment by a specialist team is essential in the neonatal period. A treatment plan should be formulated as early as possible and the following points should be noted:

(1) The presence of other congenital abnormalities, especially those likely to lead to death in infancy or childhood.
(2) The type of spina bifida; that is, myelomeningocele or meningocele.
(3) The level, size and state of the sac.
(4) The presence of hydrocephalus and, in the older child, mental retardation.
(5) The presence of meningitis.
(6) The severity of the orthopaedic disability, recorded by charting muscle activity, especially that of the psoas major, quadriceps and the dorsiflexors and plantar flexors of the ankle.
(7) The presence of a neurogenic bladder and bowel, as shown by dribbling urine, a patulous anus, perineal anaesthesia and an expressible bladder.
(8) The presence of other urinary tract abnormalities, especially of the upper urinary tract, and of urinary tract infection.
(9) The dynamics of the family. Special problems exist with families who are unable to cope with the considerable strains imposed.

Most of the above points can be evaluated in the neonatal period, and the predicted disabilities should be fully discussed with the parents as soon as possible.

TREATMENT

The aim is to produce an ambulant patient, dry and free of the smell of urine and faeces, who is able to function at an optimal intellectual and physical level; and who is educable and capable of employment and independent living. The severity of the disease in some children precludes the attainment of all these objectives. Adverse factors that carry a high mortality or poor potential of

life include: high-level lesions associated with complete paraplegia (especially if associated with spinal kyphosis); hydrocephalus clinically present at birth; rapidly developing and progressive hydrocephalus; meningitis or ventriculitis; other severe congenital abnormalities; other life-threatening diseases; major renal impairment.

Initial examination and regular supervision in a special co-ordinated clinic are required for accurate assessment and optimal results.

The sac

Early operation reduces the incidence of meningitis and shortens the stay in hospital. It encourages acceptance of the child by the parents, but has no significance on the development of hydrocephalus. In some children the prognosis is so poor that the repair of the sac in these children may be best deferred.

The guidelines for treatment are as follows:

Treatment at birth

Caesarean section and immediate postnatal repair may preserve neurological function in some babies where antenatal ultrasonography demonstrates good leg movement. There is mounting evidence that trauma during delivery exacerbates the degree of neurological deficit. Immediate repair of the sac is indicated in all low lesions in the absence of the adverse factors listed above. Initial deferment of sac repair is appropriate in the presence of any of the adverse factors. If the sac is covered with sound skin there is no urgency for repair.

Hydrocephalus

A ventriculoperitoneal shunt is required for correction of hydrocephalus (Chapter 12), which commonly develops soon after sac closure.

Orthopaedic treatment

This is aimed at motor development, which should be as near normal as the degree of paralysis will allow. The child with extensive paralysis is given a supportive chair at the age of 3 or 4 months; physiotherapists and occupational therapists encourage activities appropriate to the child's age but which otherwise would be delayed by the paralysis. Standing and walking are encouraged as soon as the child is mature enough to co-operate; for the severely paralysed child this will be at a later age than normal. Few children fail to achieve walking, but many of those with high lesions will later cease walking because their mobility is greater in a wheelchair than with extensive orthoses and crutches. Children with low lesions walk well without orthoses. Children with high lesions (above L3) generally walk in long orthoses with extensions to the lower trunk and with elbow crutches. They tend to develop fixed flexion deformity of the hips and knees that may require surgical release.

The presence of an active quadriceps muscle enables the child to stand by extending the knee joint, so long callipers are not required. When the muscles acting on the feet are weak or inactive, plastic ankle-foot orthoses (AFO) are used to stabilize the feet.

In the common situation in which the dorsiflexors of the ankle are strong but the calf is paralysed, transfer of the tendon of the tibialis anterior posteriorly to the tendo Archilles and calcaneum will prevent progressive deformity.

No orthopaedic treatment is required for children with low sacral lesions.

Other deformities that may require treatment are kyphosis and scoliosis. Correction and fusion of paralytic spinal deformities in spina bifida require an operation on the vertebral bodies from in front and on the intact vertebral arches from behind. Internal fixation devices are inserted through both approaches.

Schooling and employment

Most children with spina bifida have a need for assistance at school. Difficulties with access, mobility and continence need to be overcome. Some children with shunted hydrocephalus have specific learning problems. Varying degrees of difficulty with concentration span, attention control and fine motor and perceptual functioning have been noted.

Almost all children with spina bifida cystica attend normal school, 5 to 10 per cent require special schools for the physically handicapped and a few attend special schools for the mentally handicapped. Because of the extensive assistance required, those children with the highest lesions may need to attend special school. During the early years in secondary school, vocational guidance is required to direct education and training towards suitable employment. Many professional, commercial, clerical and bench-type jobs are suitable for paraplegic patients.

PROGNOSIS

Until recently, the mortality of myelomeningocele had been 35 to 40 per cent. The causes of death were hydrocephalus (35 per cent), meningitis (51 per cent), with other congenital abnormalities and intercurrent infections contributing in 30 per cent of cases. Most deaths (83 per cent) occurred before the age of 1 year, 37 per cent between birth and 28 days, 46 per cent between 29 and 364 days, and 17 per cent at 12 months of age and over.

Deaths after 1 year of age are usually due to excessive intracranial pressure after failure of a shunt for hydrocephalus, or to urinary complications. Many children, even with severe disabilities, reach adult life.

The outlook for children with spina bifida has been transformed in recent decades and changes in approach and treatment are having a marked effect on the outcome.

FURTHER READING

Foster L.S., Kogan B.A., Cogen P.H. & Edwards M.S.B. (1990) Bladder function in patients with lipomyelomeningocele. *J. Urol.* **143**: 984–6.

Fuchs H.E. (1998) Pediatric neurosurgery: hydrocephalus and myelomeningocele. In: Stringer M.D., Mouriquand P.D.E., Oldham K.T. & Howard E.R. (eds) *Pediatric Surgery and Urology: Long-term Outcomes*, pp. 878–96, W.B. Saunders, London.

Hendren W.H. & Hendren R.B. (1990) Bladder augmentation: experience with 129 children and young adults. *J. Urol.* **144**: 445–53.

Hensle T.W., Connor J.P. & Burbige K.A. (1990) Continent: urinary diversion in childhood. *J. Urol.* **143**: 981–3.

Hutson J.M. & Beasley S.W. (1988) Spina bifida. *The Surgical Examination of Children*. Heinemann Medical, Oxford.

Peacock W.J. (1998) Management of spina bifida, hydrocephalus, central nervous system infections, and intractable epilepsy. In: O'Neill J.A., Rowe M.I., Grosfeld J.L., Fonkalsrud E.W. & Coran A.G. (eds) *Pediatric Surgery*, 5th edn, pp. 1849–58, Mosby, St. Louis.

Schulman S.L. & Duckett J.W. (1998) Disorders of bladder function. In: O'Neill J.A., Rowe M.I., Grosfeld J.L., Fonkalsrud E.W. & Coran A.G. (eds) *Pediatric Surgery*, 5th edn, pp. 1671–84, Mosby, St. Louis.

— 10 —

Ambiguous Sexual Development

CASE 1

After an uneventful second pregnancy, Mrs H. went into labour quickly. The baby was delivered by the midwife because the obstetrician was still on his way to the hospital. The midwife thought the baby was a boy, but when she arrived the obstetrician said it was probably a girl! Confusion in the labour ward staff was not resolved until a paediatrician confirmed ambiguous genitalia and arranged a transfer to the Children's Hospital. The parents were very upset and distraught.

Q. 1.1   *What are the criteria for diagnosis of ambiguous genitalia?*

Q. 1.2   *What should the parents be told?*

Q. 1.3   *Is this an emergency?*

Q. 1.4   *How is the gender of rearing decided?*

CASE 2

On routine genital examination the intern thought the newborn infant had a hypospadiac phallus and bifid scrotum, containing one testis.

Q. 2.1   *Can you be sure this baby is a boy?*

Q. 2.2   *What criteria discriminate intersex babies from those with hypospadias?*

No part of a newborn infant's anatomy arouses as much interest initially as the external genitalia. Throughout the pregnancy the parents have contemplated whether their child will be a boy or a girl. The announcement of the gender of the child triggers a set of socially predetermined and gender-related responses, gifts, congratulations and celebrations, giving the parents pride and pleasure.

It is a crisis, therefore, if the infant's genitalia are abnormal, so that the gender is in doubt (Fig. 10.1). The urgency of the situation is heightened by the fact that a genital malformation in the newborn may be the outward sign of a life-threatening internal disorder.

The responsibilities of the attending doctor are to minimize the distress of the parents and family, and to arrange for the immediate diagnosis and treatment of the underlying medical disorder that may accompany genital ambiguity.

DEFINITION

Genitalia are described as ambiguous when: (i) the phallus is too large for a clitoris and too small for a penis; (ii) the urethral opening is proximal, near the labioscrotal (genital) folds; (iii) the genital folds remain unfused, giving the

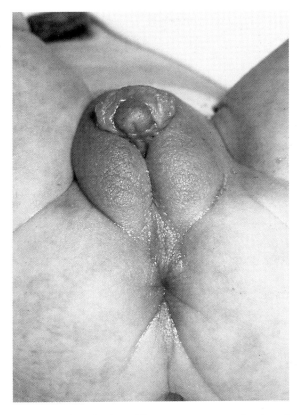

Fig. 10.1 Completely ambiguous appearance of external genitalia. Is it a boy or a girl?

appearance of labia or a cleft scrotum; (iv) the testes are either not descended or impalpable (Fig. 10.1).

THE CLINICAL PROBLEMS

In a newborn baby with ambiguous genitalia, the parents should be told as soon as possible that sexual development is incomplete, that the gender cannot be assigned and that consultation with the appropriate specialist will be arranged immediately. It will be the specialist's role to outline the steps required to obtain the necessary information to determine the sex of rearing. The investigations of this complex problem are

best carried out in the tertiary referral centre. Two specific entities are the principal source of ambiguity in the newborn: severe hypospadias with undescended testes and congenital adrenal hyperplasia.

Severe hypospadias with undescended testes

'Hypospadias with undescended testis' should be treated as intersex at birth, if the 'scrotum' is bifid or one or both testes are impalpable. A fused scrotum and two descended testes confirms normal androgenic function. In this situation a hypospadiac phallus can be treated as a local anatomical anomaly of penile development. Once intersex has been excluded, males with hypospadias and cryptorchidism can be treated by urethroplasty and orchidopexy at 6 to 12 months.

Congenital adrenal hyperplasia

This life-threatening condition occurs in 1 : 8000 live births and is the most important condition to be excluded in the management of ambiguous genitalia.

When congenital adrenal hyperplasia (CAH) occurs in females the appearance of the external genitalia may make the gender difficult to determine (Fig. 10.2). The ambiguous appearance results from an autosomal recessive defect causing a deficiency of adrenocortical enzymes, especially 21-hydroxylase. This enzyme is necessary for the biosynthesis of both cortisol and aldosterone. Cortisol levels are low, and this allows a marked increase in the secretion of pituitary adrenocorticotrophic hormone (ACTH), resulting in adrenal hyperplasia. Only androgens are produced and in a female these cause virilisation. Low aldosterone levels allow excessive sodium loss in the urine.

The degree of virilisation is often mild (Fig. 10.3). If the clitoral enlargement is only minor, the diagnosis may be overlooked — a potentially dangerous situation if the associated biochemical defect produces a 'salt-losing' situation.

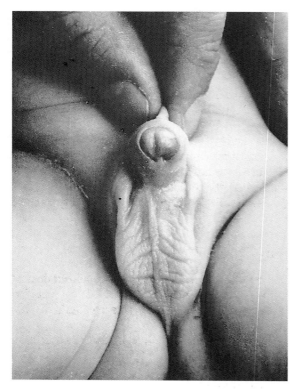

Fig. 10.2 Apparent hypospadias and impalpable testis (actually a female with CAH). (Reproduced with permission from Scheffer I.E., Hutson J.M., Warne G.L. & Ennis G. (1988) *Pediatr. Surg. Int.* **3**: 165–8.)

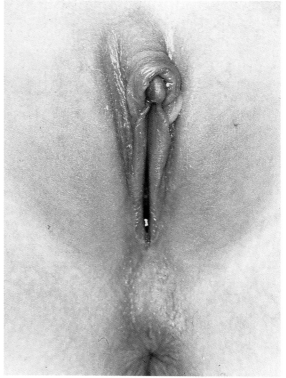

Fig. 10.3 An enlarged clitoris in a girl with CAH.

Investigations

(1) The serum electrolytes and blood glucose should be obtained with utmost urgency — within the hour. They are likely to reveal low sodium, high potassium and also hypoglycaemia.

(2) Serum 17 hydroxy-progesterone is estimated and the result obtained in 12 to 24 hours. This metabolite is high in all except rare forms of CAH.

(3) Chromosomal analysis is arranged but the result may take between 3 days and 3 weeks.

(4) A 24-hour urine specimen is collected for estimation of pregnanetriol and to obtain a gas-liquid chromatography steroid profile. The result is obtainable in 5 days.

(5) A urogenital sinugram shows a masculinized urethra but the presence of a vagina and cervix.

(6) A pelvic ultrasonography confirms the presence of a uterus and Fallopian tubes.

Treatment

(1) Intravenous rehydration, initially with 0.9 per cent saline.

(2) Hypoglycaemia is monitored and corrected with intravenous glucose–saline solution.

(3) Cortisone acetate or hydrocortisone are given as soon as blood and urine have been collected for examination.

The anatomy should be established as soon as the biochemical status is stabilized, but with less urgency. The anatomical information confirms the diagnosis but it is also required to enable the planning of subsequent surgical correction that involves clitoroplasty and vaginoplasty. It is important to realise, and to inform the parents, that females with CAH have normal reproductive potential.

Other types of ambiguity

This complex subject is beyond the scope of this chapter, but the background is summarized in the following sections.

Internal genitalia

Gonadal differentiation is determined by the karyotype with the Y chromosome being essential for testicular development. Other internal organs develop as persistent parts of the paired embronic ducts, the Wolffian and Mullerian ducts that are present initially in both males and females.

The testes *in utero* secrete two hormones: testosterone and Mullerian inhibitory substance (MIS). MIS is a protein that promotes regression of the Mullerian ducts. Absence of the Mullerian structures (uterus, Fallopian tubes and upper vagina) is evidence that MIS must have been secreted and that a testis must be present.

Development of Wolffian ducts requires local stimulation by testosterone, without which the Wolffian ducts atrophy, with a failure of the development of their derivatives (the epididymis, vas deferens and seminal vesicle).

Chromosomal regulation of sexual differentiation

The X, Y and autosomal chromosomes are responsible for sexual differentiation: the Y chromosome directs development of the testis via the SRY gene.

Normal development of the ovaries requires two X chromosomes, and the gene encoding for androgen receptors is also located in the X chromosome. The enzymes required for the synthesis of testosterone are regulated by autosomal genes, as is the enzyme 5 alpha-reductase.

PRACTICAL DECISIONS IN MANAGEMENT

Three aspects are important in the management of infants with ambiguous genitalia:
(1) The specific diagnosis.
(2) The sex of rearing.
(3) The explanation and counselling given to the parents.

Diagnosis

To reach a specific diagnosis the advice of a paediatric endocrinologist, and detailed biochemical and anatomical investigation, are required because:
(1) There may be genetic implications affecting counselling.
(2) The potential fertility of the infant should be established.
(3) Urgent medical treatment may be required, as in CAH.
(4) A plan for surgical management is necessary.
However, in many children no specific diagnosis is possible.

Sex of rearing

The sex of rearing is determined by (i) the underlying diagnosis (for example, CAH patients are normally raised as girls, despite virilisation); (ii) the size of the male vs female genitalia (for example, a child with a microphallus and large vagina may be better raised as a girl, despite XY chromosomes).

The appropriate sex of rearing maximises the patient's prospects of fertility and minimises the risk of psychological damage.

Fertility in the male depends on testes capable of spermatogenesis, a patent pathway and a penis with sufficient erectile tissue for erection and insemination. A good-sized phallus is rarely present in male infants with ambiguous genitalia, and fertility is usually impossible.

In the female, ovulation and a pathway to the uterus are required, but future developments in *in vitro* fertilization, using donor gametes and transplantation of an embryo, may permit pregnancy in a female with a uterus and vagina but no ovaries or Fallopian tubes. There are greater opportunities, therefore, for active participation in the reproductive process in those raised as females, provided a uterus is present.

Psychological damage is common to both sexes. In a patient raised unsuccessfully as a male, embarrassment due to a micro-phallus, inability to void standing and a phallus inadequate for intercourse all create major problems.

Counselling parents

Parents should be told frankly, when the gender is unclear, that tests will be carried out urgently, and how long it will take to fully understand the child's pathology.

The gender is the sex of rearing, and once decided it should be reinforced at every opportunity by referring to the infant as 'he' or 'she', and never 'it'. It is important to reassure parents that genital ambiguity and malformations do not lead to homosexuality, a fear many parents experience but few express. It is helpful to explain to parents that the genitalia go through an undifferentiated stage in both sexes, and that differentiation is extremely complex and not always complete at birth.

FURTHER READING

Donahoe P.K. & Schnitzer J.J. (1998) Ambiguous genitalia in the newborn. In: O'Neill J.A., Rowe M.I., Grosfeld J.L., Fonkalsrud E.W. & Coran A.G. (eds). *Pediatric Surgery*, 5th edn, Mosby, St. Louis, pp. 1819–33.

Grumbach M.M. & Conte F.A. (1992) Disorders of sexual differentiation. In: Wilson J.D. & Foster D.W. (eds) *Williams Textbook of Endocrinology*, 8th edn, W.B. Saunders, Philadelphia, p. 853.

Hutson J.M. (1995) Endocrine-related urological surgery. In: Brook C.G.D. (ed.) *Clinical Paediatric Endocrinology*, 3rd edn, pp. 371–82, Blackwell Science, Oxford.

Hutson J.M. & Beasley S.W. (1988) Ambiguous genitalia: is it a boy or girl? In: *The Surgical Examination of Children*, pp. 257–66, Heinemann Medical, Oxford.

Sharp R.J. (1996) Intersex. In: Puri P. (ed.) *Newborn Surgery,* Butterworth-Heinemann, Oxford, pp. 645–62.

Sheldon C.A. (1997) Intersex states. In: Oldham K.J., Colombani P.M. & Foglia R.P. (eds). *Surgery of Infants and Children: Scientific Principles and Practice*, Lippincott-Raven, Philadelphia, pp. 1577–616.

Warne G.L. & Hughes I.A. (1995) The clinical management of ambiguous genitalia. In: Brook C.G.D. (ed.) *Clinical Paediatric Endocrinology*, 3rd edn, pp. 53–68, Blackwell Science, Oxford.

— 11 —

Anorectal Anomalies

CASE 1

A baby boy is delivered in a country hospital. He is found to have an imperforate anus and has passed meconium per urethra.

Q. 1.1   *How would you arrange referral and transport?*

Q. 1.2   *What will you tell the parents about the management of imperforate anus in the first few weeks of life?*

Q. 1.3   *What is the long-term outlook for the baby?*

CASE 2

A child with a high imperforate anus has had an anorectal reconstruction, but at the age of 5 years he is soiling frequently and is about to start school.

Q. 2.1   *Which method of imaging would give the best visualisation of the relationship of the bowel to the anorectal sphincters?*

Q. 2.2   *If no fault is found with the reconstructive surgery how is this problem managed?*

Anorectal malformations are uncommon. Although 'imperforate anus' is the name given to this condition, in many cases there is a fistulous opening into the urinary tract in the male or the genital tract in the female. There are many different sub-types of anorectal anomalies and these anomalies are also associated with other syndromes such as the VATER association (*v*ertebral; *a*nal; *t*racheo-o*e*sophageal; *r*adial/renal). Surgical correction of these anomalies is difficult as the rectum and anus have lost their relationship to the sphincter muscles and these muscles may be abnormal in their development and nerve supply.

CLASSIFICATION

The number of variations seen in anorectal malformations makes the detailed diagnosis and treatment difficult. However, the key difference between the different types of anorectal malformation lies in the relationship of the terminal bowel to the pelvic floor muscles and the levator ani muscle in particular. The simple classification divides anorectal anomalies into high, intermediate and low lesions. High lesions have arrested development of the bowel above the pelvic floor muscles. This is a difficult problem to treat and the long-term prognosis for normal continence is not good. In low lesions the developing bowel passes down through the pelvic floor muscles and anal sphincters. The surgical correction is relatively easy and the long-term prognosis is good, but not always for normal continence. Intermediate lesions occur where the bowel passes down into the levator ani muscle

Table 11.1 'Wingspread' classification of anorectoral malformations (1984)

Male	Female
High	High
(1) Anorectal agenesis:	(1) Anorectal agenesis:
— with rectoprostatic/ urethral fistula	— with rectovaginal fistula
— without fistula	— without fistula
(2) Rectal atresia	(2) Rectal atresia
Intermediate	Intermediate
(1) Rectobulbar fistula	(1) Rectovestibular fistula
(2) Anal agenesis without fistula	(2) Rectovaginal fistula
	(3) Anal agenesis without fistula
Low	Low
(1) Anocutaneous fistula	(1) Anovestibular fistula
(2) Anal stenosis	(2) Anocutaneous fistula
	(3) Anal stenosis
Other	Other
Cloacal malformations	
Rare malformations	Rare malformations

but does not reach the anal canal sphincters. The prognosis for these intermediate lesions is a little better than the high lesions. The complexity of the complete classification is indicated by the 'Wingspread' classification (Table 11.1 and Fig. 11.1). The relationship of the bowel to the levator ani muscle and the nature of any fistula are the key features of this classification.

ASSOCIATED ANOMALIES

The mortality and morbidity of imperforate anus is influenced as much by the associated anomalies as the anorectal lesion itself. About 60 per cent of anorectal anomalies have a second abnormality. The commonest of these are genitourinary (30 per cent), vertebral (30 per cent), alimentary (10 per cent), or in the central nervous system (20 per cent). In the alimentary tract oesophageal atresia and duodenal atresia may be seen. Cardiac and major chromosomal abnormalities may be life-threatening. A wide range of urinary tract abnormalities including neuropathic bladder, vesicoureteric reflux, duplication of the ureter and ureterocele are commonly seen with imperforate anus and may increase the long-term morbidity. The vertebral anomalies may include sacral deficiency of the agenesis and pelvic nerves, compounding the problem with the anorectal sphincters.

INCIDENCE

Anorectal malformations occur in 1 : 5000 births with a slight preponderance in males. Males have high lesions more frequently whereas females tend to have low lesions. Most cases of imperforate anus are sporadic and the risk of this problem occurring in a future pregnancy is very small. There are, however, rare families with a very high incidence of anorectal anomalies, which follow an autosomal dominant inheritance pattern.

CLINICAL FEATURES

The newborn baby with a supralevator lesion presents with no visible anus and has intestinal obstruction (Fig. 11.2). However, in females the fistula to the genital tract is usually wide enough to decompress the bowel adequately. In males, a fistula to the urinary tract may lead to the appearance of meconium in the urine, an important diagnostic observation (Box 11.1).

A fistula opening on the perineal skin is easily visible when it is filled with meconium, but can be very minute and requires a careful search with good illumination (Fig. 11.3). The discovery of a fistula to the skin with even a tiny orifice is proof that it is a low anomaly, whereas a completely 'blind' perineum may be due to either a high or low anomaly, but usually the former.

In females, a detailed search of each perineal orifice is essential, and the internal anatomy can be predicted when the site of the external opening has been located. For example, faeces may be

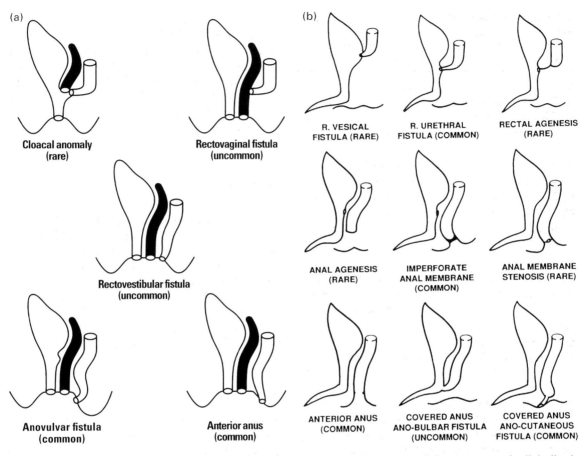

Fig. 11.1 Anorectal malformations. A schema showing the most common varieties encountered clinically in (a) females and (b) males.

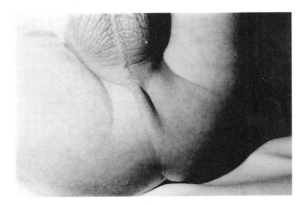

Fig. 11.2 The featureless perineum of a male body with a recto-urethral fistula.

described as coming from the vagina. However, rectovaginal fistulas are uncommon (Fig. 11.4), and more careful examination will reveal a small orifice tucked into the vestibule just outside the vaginal orifice. This may be the more common anovestibular fistula (covered anus), or a rectovestibular fistula.

The rarest anomaly seen in the female is the cloaca. There is one opening in the perineum; the urethra, vagina and bowel open at the vault of this cloacal channel. This is the most difficult of all the anorectal malformations to treat. A careful and complete physical examination of all babies with an imperforate anus must be conducted to

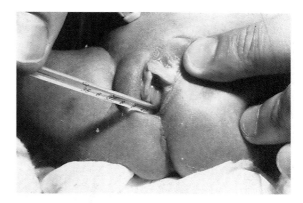

Fig. 11.4 High lesion in a female (rectovestibular fistula). The thermometer passes cranially up the fistula behind the vagina.

IMAGING

The newborn baby with an anorectal anomaly will have extensive imaging to determine the relationship of the rectum and anus to the sphincter muscles and also to demonstrate associated anomalies in the spine, urinary tract, cardiovascular and gastrointestinal systems.

(1) X-rays of the spine and chest will demonstrate any associated 'VATER' anomalies. Sacral agenesis is of particular importance as a loss of the pelvic nerves leaves a poor outlook for continence.

(2) The invertogram uses bowel gas as a contrast medium to measure the position of the terminal bowel against the bony landmarks, which indicate the position of the sphincter muscles. A line drawn from the pubic symphysis to the sacrococcygeal junction is called the PC line and shows the upper level of the pelvic floor muscles. If the bowel terminates above the PC line this is a high lesion. The lowermost part of the pelvic floor muscle is marked by the 'I point', which is the lowermost tip of the comma-shaped ischial bone. In low lesions the bowel gas extends beyond the 'I point' (Fig 11.5).

(3) Magnetic resonance imaging provides the best evaluation of the state of the sphincter

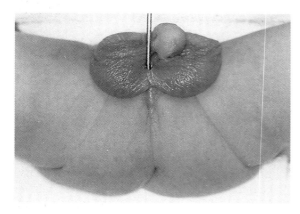

Fig. 11.3 Low lesion in a male with an anocutaneous fistula in the scrotal raphé (probe).

detect any associated spinal, gastrointestinal and cardiac anomalies. This should always include the passage of a stiff nasogastric tube to check for oesophageal atresia. Chromosomal abnormalities such as Down syndrome may also occur.

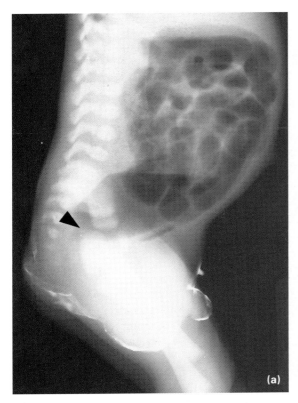 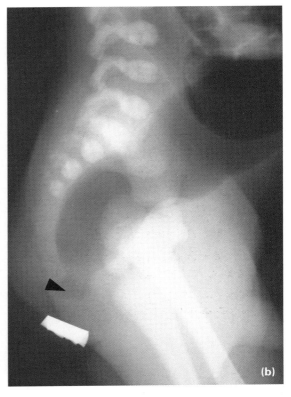

Fig. 11.5 'Invertogram'. Lateral X-ray of the pelvis with the baby inverted (pictures show an upright position for clarity): (a) a 'high' lesion; and (b) a low lesion; for example, imperforate anal membrane. The gas-filled bowel extends well below the PC line and the 'I point'.

muscles and their relationship with the rectum and anus.

(4) Ultrasonography in the first few weeks of life will image the state of the lower spinal cord and the urinary tract. Cardiac ultrasonography is also performed.

(5) A micturating cysto-urethrogram (Fig. 11.6) will show any fistula into the urinary tract and demonstrate other associated urinary tract problems; for example, vesico-ureteric reflux.

TREATMENT AND PROGNOSIS

Certain generalisations can be made:

- The identification of a fistulous opening in the perineum indicates that there is a low anomaly and the prognosis is good.
- Meconium in the urine indicates the need for a preliminary colostomy, for all recto-urinary communications are high anomalies.
- In females, a fistula should be expected and a thorough search made for it. Those with one or two orifices have a cloacal or rectal anomaly and a colostomy is required. In almost all those with three orifices, immediate local surgery is simple and the prognosis is good.
- An anterior anus is by definition normal except for its ectopic situation and requires no treatment.

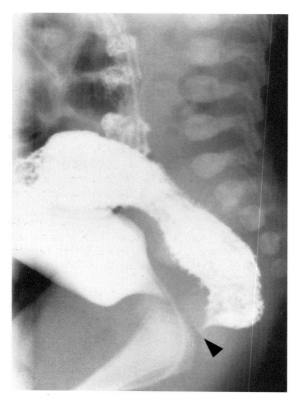

Fig. 11.6 A micturating cysto-urethrogram showing contrast in a recto-urethral fistula (arrow head).

- An expressible bladder with perineal anaesthesia and sacral agenesis indicates major nerve disruption to the bladder and anorectal sphincters. The prognosis for normal continence is poor.

Low lesions

The long-term outlook for continence is fair, apart from occasional smearing and staining of underwear, which usually is of little inconvenience.

An anocutaneous fistula in either sex, and anovestibular and anovulvar fistulas in females, require a cut-back along the fistula to display the covered anus. In females this may result in an anus contiguous with the posterior fourchette, but

this nearly always functions normally. However, if there is a cosmetic problem or if faeces enter the vagina during defaecation, the anus can be transplanted to the normal site by a sacroperineal approach later in infancy or childhood.

Imperforate anal membrane and anal stenosis require simple incision and dilatation.

High lesions

A colostomy is usually performed at birth. At the age of 3 to 4 months the definitive surgery is undertaken. This is done using a midline perineal approach as described by Pena and DeVries. A muscle stimulator is used to identify the anal sphincter complex and the pelvic floor muscles with the levator ani sling. The muscles are divided in the midline. The terminal bowel is identified and any fistula is repaired. The bowel is brought down through the sphincters to the normal site of the anus. This 'pull through' operation provides the best anatomical reconstruction of the anorectal anomaly, yet despite this accurate reconstruction the results for normal faecal continence are still not good. Although the anorectal sphincter complexes are present in high anomalies, the muscles are often poorly developed or the nerve supply is deficient. Recurrent faecal impaction, major soiling or less severe but distressing minor soiling are still common problems. A carefully controlled diet to avoid diarrhoea along with a program of enemas or home bowel wash outs can give quite good 'assisted continence' in well-organised families. An occasional child needs antegrade enemas via an appendicostomy (Malone operation).

Imperforate anus is a difficult condition to diagnose and treat. Associated anomalies such as the VATER association can cause as much morbidity as the anorectal anomaly. Low lesions do reasonably well with minimal surgery, but high lesions require extensive reconstructive surgery and the results for continence in these high lesions depend as much on the long-term support and care of the family with bowel management as on the skill of the surgeon.

FURTHER READING

Davies M.R.Q. (1997) Anatomy of the nerve supply of the rectum, bladder, and internal genitalia in anorectal dysgenesis in the male. *J. Pediatr. Surg.* **32**: 536–41.

De Vries P.A. & Pena A. (1982) Posterior sagittal anorectoplasty. *J. Ped. Surg.* **17**: 638–43.

Goon H.K. (1990) Repair of anorectal anomalies in the neonatal period. *Pediatr. Surg. Int.* **5**: 246–9.

Kiely E.M. & Pena A. (1998) Anorectal Malformations. In: O'Neill J.A., Rowe M.I., Grosfeld J.L., Fonkalsrud E.W. & Coran A.G. (eds) *Pediatric Surgery*, 5th edn, Mosby, St. Louis, pp. 1425–48.

Matley P.J., Cywes S., Berg A. & Ferreira M. (1990) A 20-year follow-up of children born with vestibular anus. *Pediatr. Surg. Int.* **5**: 37–40.

Ong N.-T. & Beasley S.W. (1990) Comparison of clinical methods for the assessment of continence after repair of high anorectal anomalies. *Pediatr. Surg. Int.* **5**: 233–7.

Ong N.-T. & Beasley S.W. (1990) Long-term functional results after perineal surgery for low anorectal anomalies. *Pediatr. Surg. Int.* **5**: 238–40.

Ong-N.-T., de Campo M. & Fowler R. Jr (1990) Computerised tomography in the management of imperforate anus patients following rectoplasty. *Pediatr. Surg. Int.* **5**: 241–5.

Pena A. (1988) Surgical management of anorectal malformations: a unified concept. *Pediatr. Surg. Int.* **3**: 82–93.

Rich M.A., Brock W.A. & Pena A. (1988) Spectrum of genitourinary malformations in patients with imperforate anus. *Pediatr. Surg. Int.* **3**: 110–13.

Rintala R., Lindahl H. & Louhimo I. (1991) Anorectal malformations—results of treatment and long-term follow-up in 208 patients. *Pediatr. Surg. Int.* **6**: 36–41.

Rintala R.J., Pena A. & Ludman L. (1998) Anorectal malformations. In: Stringer M.D., Mouriquand P.D.E., Oldham K.T. & Howard E.R. (eds) *Pediatric Surgery and Urology: Long-term Outcomes*, W.B. Saunders, London, pp. 357–93.

Stephens F.D. & Smith E.D. (1986) Classification, identification and assessment of surgical treatment of anorectal anomalies. *Pediatr. Surg. Int.* **1**: 200–5.

— 12 —

The Scalp, Skull and Brain

CASE 1

A 3-month-old, ex-prem infant presents with a big head.

> *Q. 1.1*   *When should you be concerned about the enlargement of an infant's head?*

CASE 2

A 4-year-old boy presents with early morning headaches, vomiting and ataxia.

> *Q. 2.1*   *When does a child with headaches need a CT scan?*
>
> *Q. 2.2*   *Can we be optimistic about the outcome of children with brain tumours?*

CASE 3

A 7-year-old girl with a V-P shunt is complaining of vomiting and drowsiness.

> *Q. 3.1*   *Does the palpation of a shunt valve indicate whether a shunt is blocked?*

CASE 4

You are called to the postnatal ward to see a baby, just born, with a lump on the glabella.

> *Q. 4.1*   *What do you say to the parents of a newborn child with an encephalocele?*

CASE 5

A 4-month-old infant has a flattened occiput on one side.

> *Q. 5.1*   *What could the diagnosis be and what treatment is required?*

THE INFANT WITH A LARGE HEAD

Measurement of head circumference is an essential component of the routine examination of the young child. The growth curve of the head's circumference must be interpreted along with the weight and length curves. This is done using standard percentile charts. When suspicion arises that an infant's head is enlarging too rapidly,

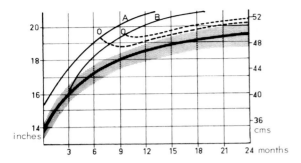

Fig. 12.1 Variations in the growth curve of the infant head, showing the mean, 90th and 10th percentiles. The additional curves represent: (a) hydrocephalus present from birth; (b) acquired hydrocephalus after meningitis at 3 months. In each case, operation (O) is followed by a return towards normal.

measurements must be repeated over a period of weeks or months, and compared with the normal curve for this dimension. Deviations from normal (Fig. 12.1) are grouped as follows:

(1) A steadily increasing divergence above the normal curve, commencing at birth.

(2) A normal curve interrupted by some event, for example, a subdural haemorrhage or an infection, with a subsequent increase greater than normal.

(3) An accelerated rate of growth initially, followed by less rapid growth that continues at a high level but parallel to the normal curve.

(4) The head circumference commences at a high level and remains high but grows at the appropriate rate.

The first two groups need treatment, but in the third, unless the accelerated growth in the initial period is very great, the operation may be deferred, and surgery is not usually required for the fourth.

An enlarging head may be the result of factors other than the accumulation of CSF, although these are uncommon. The infant's head may enlarge because of a thickening of the skull bones, as in diffuse fibrous dysplasia, and be readily recognizable in X-rays. The brain itself may be large, without any increase in the size of the ventricles. This type of macrocephaly is diagnosed by finding ventricles of normal size. The intelligence is often subnormal. One cerebral hemisphere may be larger (hemimegalencephaly) and is associated with cortical dysplasia, developmental delay, epilepsy and hemihypertrophy of the body. Localized expanding lesions, for example, subdural haematoma, simple intracerebral or arachnoid cysts or, very occasionally, a cystic neoplasm, may also cause enlargement of the head.

Benign enlargement of the subarachnoid space

This is a cause of macrocephaly and is due to a widening of the subarachnoid space and must be distinguished from chronic subdural haematoma. The head will usually grow at the normal rate and no treatment is required.

Hydrocephalus

Most infants with a large head suffer from excess CSF caused by: (i) excessive production, (ii) obstruction along the CSF pathway or (iii) impaired absorption into the veins.

Increased production of CSF causing hydrocephalus is rare and is caused by a papilloma of the choroid plexus.

Obstruction to the flow of CSF is the commonest cause of hydrocephalus, and is further subdivided as follows:

(1) *Non-communicating or obstructive hydrocephalus* in which there is no communication between the ventricles and the subarachnoid space. The ventricles are greatly enlarged without distension of the basal cisterns or cerebral sulci (Fig. 12.2).

The most frequent causes of obstruction are: (i) primary developmental anomalies such as aqueduct stenosis or a congenital cyst; for example, suprasellar arachnoid cyst, or posterior fossa cyst with hypoplasia of the vermis (Dandy–Walker syndrome); (ii) haemorrhage or infection — intracerebral and intraventricular haemorrhage in premature babies, which is now common;

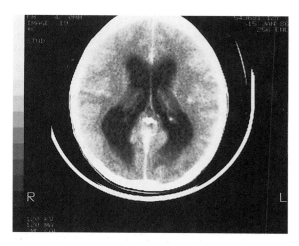

Fig. 12.2 Non-communicating hydrocephalus. CT scan showing massive dilatation of the ventricles.

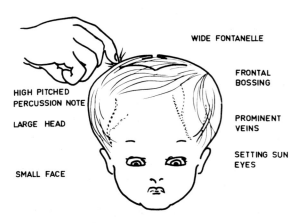

Box 12.1 Causes of childhood hydrocephalus

(1) Communicating hydrocephalus
    haemorrhage
    infection

(2) Stricture of cerebral aqueduct

(3) Tumours/cysts

(iii) tumours obstructing the ventricular system in the older child, but only 5 per cent of cases of hydrocephalus in infancy are caused by a neoplasm.

(2) *Communicating hydrocephalus* in which the ventricles communicate with the basal cisterns, but there is an obstruction in the subarachnoid spaces or in the arachnoid villi/ sagittal sinus.

Failure of absorption of the CSF may occur temporarily, as a result of inflammatory exudate around the basal cisterns and arachnoidal villi following meningitis, or as a result of haemorrhage in the subarachnoid space. Permanent and severe derangement follows thrombosis of the sagittal or lateral sinuses in the newborn as a result of dehydration; the result is a sudden enlargement of the head. Inadequate absorption of CSF also may occur rarely when the intracranial venous pressure is raised; for example, an arteriovenous malformation involving the venous sinuses.

The history, physical signs, a chart of the rate of head growth (Fig. 12.1) and special investigations such as ultrasonography, CT or MR imaging are all considered to determine a cause (Box 12.1), plan of treatment and estimate of the prognosis of the child with a large head.

Clinical signs

A head circumference that is increasing faster than the normal increments for the age of the infant is the main clinical feature and the indication for investigation and treatment. The deviation is depicted by plotting the measurements of the circumference obtained at regular intervals on a graph of the normal curve (Fig. 12.1). Auscultation for a bruit is a useful clinical sign for an underlying vascular malformation.

The shape of the head becomes abnormal (Fig. 12.3). The frontal region is prominent in

Fig. 12.3 Hydrocephalus. Seven clinical signs in a severe case.

all types, but in the stricture of the aqueduct, expansion of the lateral ventricles produces an 'occipital overhang' above the small posterior fossa as well. The opposite occurs when the fourth ventricle is expanded as a result of occlusion of its foramina; the external occipital protuberance is pushed upwards. Raised intracranial pressure produces a wide anterior fontanelle, palpable separation of the cranial sutures and a raised or drum-like note on percussion of the skull.

Abnormal neurological signs from hydro-cephalus alone are unusual. The sixth cranial nerve is vulnerable because of its long course and a lateral rectus palsy causing internal strabismus may occur. Persistent downward deviation of the eyes ('setting sun' sign) is present with advanced hydrocephalus causing pressure on the quadrigeminal plate. There may be brain-stem signs when the obstruction is acute and hydrocephalus develops rapidly, with increased extensor tone, rigidly extended lower limbs and clenched hands with the fingers over the infolded thumb. Retraction of the head and opisthotonus may be also present.

Transillumination of an infant's head by a beam of bright light in a darkened room often will show characteristic patterns. General transillumination indicates a gross and uniform dilatation of the ventricles. Unilateral translucency may indicate a subdural collection of fluid, and other localized bright areas may indicate large cysts or a large dilated fourth ventricle.

Investigations

Ultrasonography imaging is a non-invasive means of diagnosing hydrocephalus in infancy and is done by placing the ultrasonography probe on the anterior fontanelle. Little or no special preparation is required; the procedure is risk free and can be repeated as often as necessary. Once closure of the fontanelle occurs, the technique is no longer applicable.

Computed tomography (CT) or magnetic resonance (MR) are used in the older child and infants if more detail is required. These provide a clear image of the intracranial anatomy and a precise means of detecting the presence of hydrocephalus, determining its extent and frequently demonstrating the site and cause of obstruction.

The CSF dynamic scan involves the injection of a radionuclide tracer into the CSF pathway. Its passage through the ventricles and subarachnoid space is followed. Obstructions and abnormalities in the passage of CSF, from production to final absorption, can be recorded.

In more complex cases, intracranial pressure monitoring may help to determine the need, or otherwise, for treatment.

Plain X-rays are generally of no great value but may be used to confirm a diagnosis of raised intracranial pressure.

Treatment

Not all infants with enlargement of the head require operation, but if there is evidence of a continued deviation from the normal curve and/or signs of raised intracranial pressure the child should be investigated. Operation is indicated when there is sustained deviation from the normal curve in infants without obvious evidence of severe brain damage.

There are various methods of controlling an expanding head that depend on three principles:
(1) Reduction of CSF production. Production of CSF can be reduced by a drug that acts directly on the choroid plexus (carbonic anhydrase inhibitor) or by an osmotic agent. Control is frequently incomplete and of short-term benefit only.
(2) Reconstitution of CSF pathways within the cranium. Removal of a mass may allow CSF to return to a normal flow pattern. Tumours in the posterior fossa frequently cause hydrocephalus and excision of the tumour leads to a rapid resolution in most cases. The placement of an endoscope into the ventricles via a burr hole (neuro-endoscopy) is an important technique for inspection, biopsy and therapeutic manoeuvres such as

fenestration of a cyst into the ventricle, or the creation of an opening in the floor of the third ventricle (*third ventriculostomy*) that may correct an obstructive hydrocephalus.

(3) Diversion of CSF to a site outside the cranium. External removal of CSF is the usual method of treating this disorder. In communicating hydrocephalus, particularly in premature infants, removal may be undertaken intermittently, via lumbar puncture, or via a ventricular reservoir; this controls the hydrocephalus until normal pathways are re-established.

A *ventriculo-peritoneal shunt* is usually the definitive operation of choice in children of all ages. This shunt comprises a ventricular catheter, a valve or flushing device beneath the scalp, and a long kink-resistant tube passing along the chest wall to enter the peritoneal cavity. A long length of tube is placed within the peritoneal cavity to allow for subsequent growth of the patient. Less frequently, a ventriculo-atrial shunt to divert the CSF into the right atrium is performed.

Complications of shunts

Most children with shunts are 'shunt dependent' and they will not tolerate malfunction of these devices.

(1) Obstruction. Most frequently the ventricular catheter becomes occluded with choroid plexus or cerebral tissue. The lower end may be obstructed by the growth of the child that displaces the lower end into an unsuitable position, by adherence to the greater omentum or by fracture of the tube. Rarely will the valve malfunction. Revision of the shunt is required.

(2) Infection. The shunt system becomes colonized by pathogenic organisms that require removal of the shunt and temporary external drainage of the CSF until it is sterilized with antibiotics, and then replacement of the shunt.

(3) Disconnection. The peritoneal catheter may become disconnected from the valve under the scalp due to vigorous neck movements.

The tube may slide down the subcutaneous tunnel into the abdomen, and no longer will be palpable on the side of the head. Reconnection is necessary.

(4) Overdrainage. The ventricles become small and the child may develop chronic headache due to low intracranial pressure. The opening pressure of the valve may need to be raised.

A child with a shunt must be reviewed at regular intervals during the growing years. In general, if the diagnosis is established before hydrocephalus is advanced, if there are no other significant brain anomalies, and if the treatment is appropriate and maintained, then the patient has every chance of developing normally. A child with a shunt is not restricted in activities, except for vigorous twisting movements.

CONGENITAL ABNORMALITIES OF THE CRANIUM

Errors in the development of the scalp, skull and brain are not as common as those of the spinal cord, but they present the same variety of abnormalities. Only the more common or important ones are described here.

Dermoid sinus

This is found most frequently in the mid-occipital region and may communicate with a more deeply situated dermoid cyst containing sebaceous material and hairs. The sinus may have some fine hairs (often a different colour) protruding from it and usually discharges sebaceous material. The deeper component can cause all the signs of an intracranial tumour with cerebellar signs predominating; it may also become infected.

An intracranial dermoid can occur without an external sinus. Infection is uncommon and the cyst presents by causing local pressure or obstruction of the CSF. Rarely does the cyst rupture and cause aseptic meningitis.

Epidermoid cysts of the scalp are common near the orbital margin and are described in Chapter 16.

Craniosynostosis

Premature closure of the cranial sutures, which act as lines of growth, restricts development of the region; compensatory growth occurs at other suture lines. The subsequent distortion in the shape of the skull results in severe cosmetic deformities, but only occasionally does it cause sufficient diminution of the intracranial capacity to limit the growth of the brain. A description of the different deformities is given in Chapter 15 (craniofacial anomalies).

Treatment

The abnormal appearance and the risk of mental handicap are the two indications for surgery. Mental handicap probably occurs in only 10 per cent of these children, and its likelihood is to be suspected when radiographs show signs of increased intracranial pressure; that is, increased cerebral convolutional markings (*copper beating*) and separation of the unfused sutures. Headache, vomiting and papilloedema are rare, but exophthalmos and ophthalmoplegia are not infrequent.

Early operation, before 3 months of age, results in a head of almost normal size and shape. The operation consists of either simple linear craniectomy (excision of a strip of bone along the fused suture) or radical removal and repositioning of the vault bones (Chapter 15).

Plagiocephaly

This is a common deformity that skews the entire skull. One frontal region and the opposite occipital region are flat and the contralateral areas are full and rounded. The effect is that the longest diameter is displaced from the sagittal axis towards the side with the prominent frontal contour.

Congenital plagiocephaly may be caused by contact of the fetal head with the maternal pelvis or with irregularity of the uterine wall; for example, fibroids. Acquired plagiocephaly in the first 3 to 4 months after birth has become common, probably because mothers are advised to ensure their babies are put to sleep in a supine position. There may also be torticollis causing one occipital area to bear the weight of the cranium and the brain, which determines the shape of the thin and largely membranous calvarium (Chapter 16). X-rays may show some sclerosis along the lambdoid suture line without fusion. This is the *'sticky' lambdoid suture*. The deformity can be minimized by placing babies with postural or sternomastoid torticollis in such a way that they sleep on each side alternately and never directly supine.

The deformity tends to improve after the age of 6 months. A minor degree probably persists indefinitely, though this is not readily detected when hair obscures the contours of the skull. Surgery generally is not indicated except in infants with a significant cosmetic deformity.

Premature fusion of the lambdoid suture is an uncommon cause of plagiocephaly. Operative repair is required

Cranium bifidum (including encephalocele)

Defects at the cephalic end of the neural tube of the embryo are much less common than in the thoraco-lumbar region. The same basic deformities occur, mostly in the occipital region, but in some countries, for example, Thailand, they are more common in the frontal (sincipital) area.

The herniations are in the midline (Fig. 12.4), well covered with skin and lined by meninges, and may contain CSF alone (meningocele) or, more frequently, brain (encephalocele). Occasionally, the herniation occurs in the nasal cavity and the sac is then covered by mucosa, not skin.

Other intracranial abnormalities also may be present, and imaging is necessary to detect these before surgical repair.

Simple excision of the sac, replacement of viable herniated cerebral contents, and sound closure of the dura and the bony defect usually can be effected. Occipital encephaloceles may cause severe brain dysfunction (mental retardation,

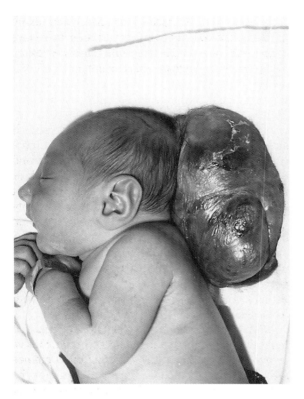

Fig. 12.4 Encephalocele. An example of a severe midline herniation with cranium bifidum, which is a neural tube defect.

visual defects, hydrocephalus) that may preclude treatment. The sincipital encephaloceles are repaired using a craniofacial technique with good cosmetic results and usually a good neurological outcome (Chapter 15).

INTRACRANIAL TUMOURS

Tumours of the central nervous system are the largest group of malignancies, excluding leukaemia, in childhood. Radical surgery and adjuvant chemotherapy or radiotherapy in selected cases may produce long-term survival. There are also many benign and slowly growing intracranial tumours that may be cured following surgery.

Table 12.1 Cerebral tumours: percentage distribution of 300 consecutive tumours, Royal Children's Hospital, Melbourne

Group 1	Cerebral hemispheres	18%
Group 2	Third ventricle	17%
	optic chiasm	5%
	craniopharyngioma	5%
	pineal tumour	5%
	glial tumours	2%
Group 3	Posterior fossa	53%
	medulloblastoma	
	solid/cystic astrocytoma	
	brain stem glioma	
	Spinal tumours	12%

Mode of presentation

The mode of presentation in children differs in many ways from that seen in adults:

(1) The common types of tumour and their sites of origin are different; for example, the preponderance of tumours in the posterior fossa in childhood (Table 12.1).

(2) Young children adapt better to an expanding intracranial lesion because of the expansion of the skull; accommodation for weeks or even months is possible, but once this fails the final decline is often rapid and catastrophic.

(3) Many tumours arise close to the CSF pathways in relatively 'silent' areas, so neurological signs are few or absent until the flow of CSF is obstructed, when signs of raised intracranial pressure, for example, headache, vomiting and papilloedema, develop with alarming suddenness.

(4) Early signs often affect the vision, but loss of acuity or diplopia are not appreciated in early childhood and never arise as symptoms in infants.

(5) Neurological signs may present early, while evidence of raised intracranial pressure appears much later. In infants and younger children the dramatic development of raised

intracranial pressure may initiate a search for localizing signs that only then are recognized.

Intracranial tumours can be divided into three main groups, each of which produces a more or less typical clinical pattern.

Group 1 Glial tumours of the cerebral hemispheres

These are less common than those in the posterior fossa and cover the full spectrum of gliomas varying from benign to highly malignant, although histology is a much less reliable guide to prognosis than in adult gliomas.

The clinical picture is similar to that of adults and diagnosis and management follow the same lines. The tumour is surgically debulked as far as possible without causing deficit.

Group 2 Tumours in the region of the third ventricle

These form a very important group in childhood. Their progress is often insidious until there are signs of ventricular obstruction but localizing neurological signs may be detected early. Those situated anteriorly produce defects in vision and endocrine disturbance; and those posteriorly cause hydrocephalus, disturbances in ocular movements and in rare cases a precocious puberty.

Gliomas of the optic chiasm

Gliomas of the optic chiasm and optic nerves are associated with neurofibromatosis in 30 to 50 per cent of cases. They cause bizarre field defects, loss of visual acuity, optic atrophy, squint and sometimes proptosis before obstructing the third ventricle. Infants may present with hydrocephalus or with involvement of the hypothalamus causing wasting and anorexia known as the 'diencephalic syndrome', and a similar lesion in older children may cause precocious puberty.

They usually behave in a very indolent manner, but a large or progressively enlarging tumour may be surgically debulked and many are sensitive to chemotherapy. Shunts to relieve ventricular obstruction are sometimes necessary. Long-term survivals are not uncommon.

Craniopharyngioma

The craniopharyngioma grows insidiously. It arises in, above or behind the sella turcica from a remnant of the primitive Rathke's pouch and compresses the pituitary gland, pituitary stalk or hypothalamus, slowing growth and development and gradually depressing vision. It is variably comprised of solid epithelial components and cysts filled with brown turbid fluid described as 'machine oil'. The tumour is usually not suspected until the child has had defective sight for years, growth and development have lagged behind or the child tires easily and is unable to keep up with his or her peers.

Small craniopharyngiomas can be removed totally without damage to the adjacent optic nerve or the pituitary gland. Large craniopharyngiomas are one of the most challenging problems for the paediatric neurosurgeon. There is controversy over whether to attempt a complete excision, with the chance of a cure but in risking serious morbidity, that includes visual pathway injury and persistent pituitary deficiency. Hormone replacement therapy and DDAVP (arginine vasopressin) have improved the outlook for these patients. Radiotherapy is used for recurrent tumours.

Pineal region tumours

The main types of pineal tumours are:
(1) Germ cell origin — germinoma, embryonal carcinoma, yolk sac tumour, choriocarcinoma and teratoma.
(2) Pineal cell tumours — pineocytoma and pineoblastoma.
(3) Glial tumours.

Pineal tumours often obstruct the aqueduct before local signs develop so that headache, vomiting, papilloedema and impaired consciousness are the presenting features. Later, pressure on the upper brainstem causes a loss of upward gaze, a distinctive localizing sign. Precocious puberty is an uncommon feature. These tumours range from highly malignant to benign. Treatment is controversial but pineal tumours may be biopsied or excised. The hydrocephalus may also require treatment. Chemotherapy and radiotherapy are often employed postoperatively. The prognosis depends on the histology and tumour burden following the primary treatment. Even though germinomas are malignant, they may be cured with chemotherapy or radiotherapy.

Group 3 Tumours of the posterior fossa

These form about 50 per cent of all intracranial tumours in childhood, but only 25 per cent in adulthood, and those in the cerebellum cause ventricular obstruction early, so that headache and vomiting — characteristically in the early morning — appear before neurological signs such as inco-ordination, ataxia, hypotonia and tremor. In brain-stem gliomas, gross inco-ordination, ataxia and cranial neve palsies precede signs of increased intracranial pressure. There are four common tumours in this region.

Medulloblastoma

This is a malignant tumour of the vermis forming a large mass that blocks the fourth ventricle (Fig. 12.5). It may spread out into the basal cisterns and characteristically disseminates widely throughout the CSF pathways, particularly in the spinal canal.

The tumour occurs more often in males at about 2 years of age, with a typical history of morning headaches and vomiting, change in

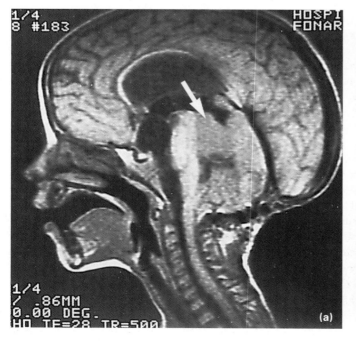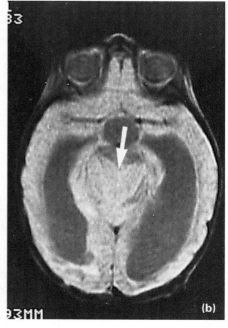

Fig. 12.5 Medulloblastoma. An MRI scan showing a massive posterior fossa tumour blocking the fourth ventricle in (a) sagittal section and (b) transverse section. The tumour is arrowed.

personality and clumsiness of gait. Papilloedema and truncal ataxia are the common neurological signs and there may be a tilting of the head when the child sits up. The tumour may recur locally and disseminate unless it responds to adjuvant chemotherapy and craniospinal radiotherapy in children over the age of 3 years. There is a 50 to 75 per cent 5-year survival rate where the tumour is completely excised at the first operation and adjuvant therapy is administered.

Astrocytoma of the cerebellum

An astrocytoma may be a solid tumour, a nodule of tumour in the wall of a cyst or even form the lining of a simple cyst. These develop in children who are older (about 5 years) than those with a medulloblastoma; the length of the history is 3 to 6 months rather than weeks, beginning with morning headaches and vomiting. Much later, usually in the 2 to 3 weeks before diagnosis, squint, inco-ordination and ataxia appear. The clinical signs are fairly constant: papilloedema, squint, mild ataxia and inco-ordination of hand movements.

There is usually a localized tumour, in one lateral lobe, which is often completely excised. Radiotherapy is reserved for tumours with more aggressive histological grades that have recurred. There is a high rate of cure of the benign (pilocytic) astrocytomas following surgery alone.

Brainstem glioma

This usually causes diffuse brain-stem enlargement without much evidence of a localized tumour. The age incidence is wide and the signs are caused by cranial nerve palsies and involvement of the long tracts passing through the brain-stem: gross strabismus, facial weakness, difficulty in swallowing, hemiparesis and ataxia occur. The child is miserable and pathetic, quite different from those with other types of posterior fossa tumours. Hydrocephalus is uncommon.

The diagnosis is confirmed by MR scan and surgery is usually not indicated. Radiotherapy and chemotherapy are used. In most patients the signs are resolved rapidly during treatment but recur within 3 to 6 months. The prognosis of the diffuse malignant brainstem glioma is very poor despite this therapy. A few patients with less aggressive tumours achieve a longer period of survival. There are some focal and benign tumours of the brainstem that can be largely excised with a good prognosis.

Ependymoma

The mode of presentation is similar to medulloblastoma. At the point of operation the tumour is frequently attached to the floor of the fourth ventricle and, like the medulloblastoma, it has the same tendency to metastasize in the CSF pathways. The overall prognosis is worse than medulloblastoma with a 40 to 50 per cent 5-year survival in the complete excision, radiotherapy group.

TUMOURS IN THE SPINAL CANAL

In infancy neuroblastoma is the commonest. Primary vertebral and intrathecal tumours are uncommon. In the first 2 to 3 years of life the commonest lesion is a metastasis from a medulloblastoma. These lesions may present following a short history of poor limb movement and general malaise.

In later childhood other intrathecal tumours appear; for example, neurofibromas of the nerve roots and astrocytomas and ependymomas of the spinal cord. The child presents variably with chronic spine pain that may be severe and unremitting, scoliosis, slowly progressive weakness of the limbs with abnormal reflexes, and sphincter disturbance. The diagnosis is established by MR. Surgical decompression, biopsy and excision of the tumour are performed. The child with a spinal tumour may also present acutely with spine pain and signs of spinal cord compression: paralysis, sensory loss and sphincter disturbance. This is a surgical emergency.

INTRACRANIAL VASCULAR DISORDERS

Arteriovenous malformations

Arteriovenous malformations (AVMs) are congenital
developmental vascular lesions of the brain,
which comprise abnormal arteriovenous fistulas,
that subsequently lead to dilated arteriolised
veins, multiple tortuous feeding arteries and a
central nidus of capillary-like fistulous vessels.

Aneurysms may develop on the feeding vessels
due to the high flow rates, and the lesions may
vary in size considerably. The presentation is
often with rupture and an intracerebral and
sometimes subarachnoid haemorrhage (Box 12.2)
(Fig. 12.6). This is the commonest cause of
spontaneous intracranial haemorrhage in children.
The children present with sudden severe headaches,
focal neurological signs, epileptic seizure and rapid
obtundation, if the clot enlarges sufficiently. The
treatment involves the evacuation of the clot
and excision of the AVM. Elective excision of
an unruptured AVM is complex. It may involve
surgical excision, preceded by embolisation. Some
small deep-seated AVMs may be treated with
focused radiotherapy (stereotactic radio surgery).

Intracranial aneurysms

Intracranial aneurysms occur at all ages but
are generally rare in children. The causes are:
(i) congenital 'Berry' aneurysms — these occur at
branch points of the major basal cerebral artery
at the Circle of Willis; in children these often reach
giant proportions; (ii) related to connective tissue

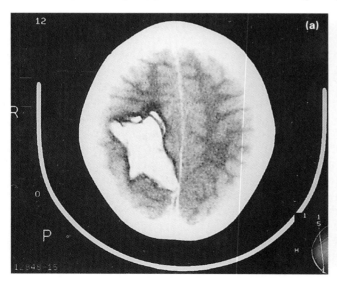
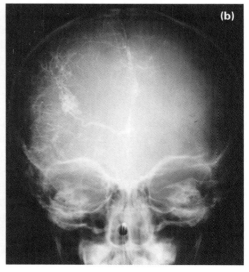

Fig. 12.6 Arteriovenous malformation (AVM). (a) CT scan with large acute intracerebral haemorrhage in the right
parietal region; (b) AP angiogram showing AVM fed by the middle cerebral artery and the single anterior cerebral artery
branch.

disorders; for example, Ehler's–Danlos syndrome; (iii) post-traumatic, 'false' aneurysms either from blunt or penetrating trauma; (iv) mycotic aneurysms, which result from infected emboli; for example, following endocarditis. Subarachnoid haemorrhage results from aneurysm rupture and craniotomy and clipping of the aneurysm is the definitive treatment.

Vein of Galen malformations

Vein of Galen malformations are rare. Congenital arteriovenous fistulas arising in the region of the Vein of Galen may result in a large dilatation of this vein, the straight sinus and the posterior venous sinuses. These high-flow fistulae may cause congestive heart failure in newborn infants, or may present later with an enlarging head, hydrocephalus, failure to thrive and epilepsy. Their management is complex but there is an increased trend to neuro-radiological embolisation of the feeding vessels, or of the vein of Galen aneurysm itself. Surgical division of major feeders may also be required. The outlook for the child depends on the completeness of fistula obliteration and how much ischaemic damage is present in the surrounding brain.

FURTHER READING

Berger M.S. (1992) Paediatric neuro-oncology. *Neurosurg. Clin. N. Amer.* **3**: 4.

Cheek W.R. (ed.) (1994) *Pediatric Neurosurgery. Surgery of the Developing Nervous System,* 3rd edn, W.B. Saunders, Philadelphia.

Cheek W.R. (1996) *Atlas of Pediatric Neurosurgery,* W.B. Saunders, Philadelphia.

Cohen M.E. & Duffner P.K. (1994) (eds) *Brain Tumours In Children. Principles of Diagnosis and Treatment,* 2nd edn, Raven Press, New York.

David D.J., Poswillo D. & Simpson D. (1982) *The Craniosynostoses: Causes, Natural History, and Management,* Springer Verlag, Berlin.

Drake J.M. & Sainte-Rose C. (1995) *The Shunt Book,* Blackwell, London.

Edwards M.S.B. & Hoffman H.J. (eds) (1989) *Cerebral Vascular Disease In Children And Adolescents. Current Neurosurgical Practice Series,* Williams and Wilkins, Baltimore.

Persing J.A., Edgerton M.T. & Jane J.A. (eds) (1989) *Scientific Foundations And Surgical Treatment Of Craniosynostosis,* Williams and Wilkins, Baltimore.

Roach E.S. & Riela A.R. (1988) *Pediatric Cerebrovascular Disorders,* Futura, Mount Kisco, New York.

— 13 —

The Eye

CASE 1

A 3-year-old girl is brought to you because her parents are concerned that her eyes are misaligned.

Q. 1.1   *Why should this be taken seriously?*

Q. 1.2   *How can you determine if the parents' observations are correct?*

CASE 2

The parents of a 3-month-old boy are worried that he cannot see properly and that at times his eyes seem to wobble uncontrollably.

Q. 2.1   *Do the parents have anything to be really worried about?*

Q. 2.2   *What are you going to do with this child?*

CASE 3

A 6-month-old baby has had a sticky eye since the age of about 1 week. Her mother has to clean the affected eye several times a day.

Q. 3.1   *How are you going to advise this child's parents and what treatments are available?*

Q. 3.2   *Should this child be prescribed topical antibiotic eye drops?*

CASE 4

A six-year-old boy is brought to see you with a three-hour history of a painful red eye.

Q. 4.1   *How are you going to assess this child?*

Vision loss may have profound effects on a child's development. A systematic clinical approach allows rapid diagnosis of most conditions affecting a child's eye and vision (Box 13.1). Timely and appropriate management will then reduce the chance of permanent visual loss.

Accurate diagnosis is dependent on obtaining a good history and appropriate clinical examination (see below) supplemented where necessary by further investigations.

EXAMINATION OF THE CHILD'S VISION AND EYE

Measurement of vision in preverbal children is by

Box 13.1 Common ocular symptoms and signs in children

(1) Suspected poor vision

(2) Misaligned eyes

(3) Wobbly eyes

(4) Inflamed eyes

(5) Droopy eyelids

(6) Watery or sticky eyes

(7) White reflex (leukocorea)

(8) Big or small eye

(9) Injured eye

(10) Headache

Box 13.2 Measuring vision

Parents' assessment

Fix on face/light through 90°	6 weeks
Fix on moving objects	6 months
Pick up coloured sprinkles	12 months
Name simple pictures	2 years
Letter/shape matching	3–4 years
Snellen eye chart	5–6 years

observation rather than formal testing. Asking the parent 'How well does your child see?' or 'What do you think your child sees?' will provide useful clues to the level of vision.

At birth, an alert infant can fix on a face briefly. By 6 weeks of age most infants smile in response to a face, and also will be able to follow a face or light through an arc of 90°. By 6 months of age an infant can reach for a small object and actively follow moving objects in the environment. By 12 months a child can pick up tiny objects such as hundreds-and-thousands ('sprinkles') (Box 13.2).

At 2 years of age most children can name simple pictures to more accurately document visual acuity. Letter- or shape-matching tests of vision are possible at about 3 to 4 years of age. Formal Snellen measurement of acuity is managed by most children once they reach school age (5 to 6 years).

Always document the estimate of vision for each eye. For a preverbal child this may consist of statements like: 'Fixes on a face with left eye but not with right.' If more formal measurement is possible, document the Snellen fraction. For example, 'right eye — 6/9'. This means that at a distance of 6 metres the child can read the '9' line of letters or symbols. Most tests are performed at 3 or 6 metres, but if the child's vision is reduced the chart can be brought closer to the child.

Reduced visual acuity in a child is often the result of amblyopia. Amblyopia occurs when one eye (or rarely both) is ignored by the visual cortex, for example, the squint, when the two eyes point in different directions, and to avoid diplopia one is ignored. If the two eyes have an unequal refractive error, one will generally have a more blurry retinal image and thus a poor signal will be sent to the visual cortex, causing amblyopia. Amblyopia only arises during development of the visual cortex and when 'defective' information is being sent from the eye to the brain. Similarly, amblyopia is only treatable when the visual cortex is still immature and adaptable: visual cortical maturation occurs at about 7 years of age.

Inspection will provide much useful information. Significantly misaligned eyes, abnormal eye movements (such as nystagmus), inflamed eyes, droopy eyelids, red, watery or discharging eyes will all be obvious on a simple inspection.

Examining the red reflex with a direct ophthalmoscope will reveal much about the internal structure of the eye. The red reflex is examined with a direct ophthalmoscope set to the zero power lens and by observing the child's

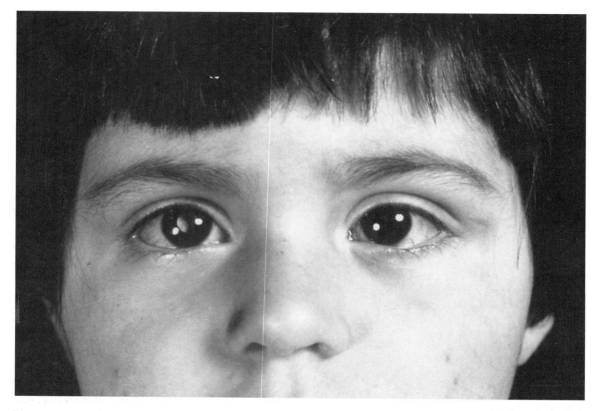

Fig. 13.1 The 'white' reflex. The normal red reflex is replaced by a white reflection in the right eye in this child with retinoblastoma.

eyes from a distance of about 1 metre. A normal red reflex is red to orange and uniform over the pupil, and should be the same in each eye. Children with darker iris pigmentation will tend to have duller red reflexes than those with lightly pigmented eyes.

A white reflex (Fig. 13.1) generally indicates significant pathology within an eye and the need for urgent dilated fundus examination by an ophthalmologist. In children over 1 year of age, the pupils can be safely dilated with cyclopentolate 1 per cent or tropicamide 1 per cent. In children less than 1 year of age, 0.25 per cent or 0.5 per cent preparations should be used.

Observing the corneal light reflections will indicate strabismus in a child who is not co-operative with cover testing. When a light is

positioned directly in front of a child's face the corneal light reflections should be symmetric. Asymmetry of the corneal light reflections suggests that the eyes are misaligned.

Cover testing is the method of choice to determine if a child has strabismus (misaligned eyes or squint). The cover test is done by first getting the child to fix on an object while the observer determines which eye appears to be misaligned. The eye that appears to be fixing on the object (and not misaligned) is then covered while the apparently misaligned eye is observed. If strabismus is present a corrective movement of the misaligned eye will be seen as this eye takes up fixation on the object of regard (Fig. 13.2). If no movement is seen the eye is uncovered. The cover test is then repeated but the other eye is

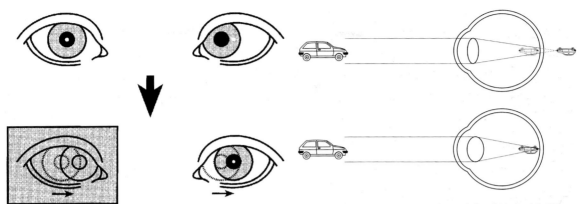

Fig. 13.2 Cover test. The child's attention is attracted with a toy or light (top). Once the eye that appears to be looking directly at the toy is covered, the other eye is observed for a refixation movement (bottom). In convergent squint there is outward movement of the uncovered eye (pictured). In divergent squint the eye moves inward. If no movement is seen, cover the other eye first.

Fig. 13.3 Hypermetropia (long-sightedness). (a) When the eye is relaxed the image of a distant object is 'focused behind' the retina, producing a blurred retinal image. (b) By accommodation (changing focal length) the image is focused on the retina.

covered this time. The eye that is not covered is again observed for a corrective movement and to confirm present strabismus. The test can be repeated as many times as necessary. If no movement follows repeated covering of either eye, then no strabismus is present. Care must be taken to let the child fix with both eyes open before covering either eye, otherwise normal binocular control may be prevented and a small latent squint (phoria) may be detected. Latent squints are normal variants and of no significance.

Eversion of the upper eyelid is helpful if a foreign body is suspected to be the cause of a red irritable eye. The upper eyelid is everted by first asking the child to look down. A cotton-bud is then applied about 1 centimetre from the lid margin to act as a fulcrum about which the eyelid will be everted. Finally, to evert the eyelid the eyelashes are gently pulled initially downward and then rotated upward. The subtarsal conjunctiva can then be inspected and any foreign body removed with a second moistened cotton-bud.

REFRACTIVE ERRORS (FOCUSING PROBLEMS)

A basic understanding of refractive errors helps a great deal in making sense of ophthalmology. There are three principal refractive errors, these are hypermetropia (long-sightedness), myopia (short-sightedness) and astigmatism. The easiest way to understand refractive errors is to consider the eye in a relaxed state.

When relaxed, a hypermetropic eye focuses light from a distant object behind the retina. To bring such an image into clear focus on the retina, accommodative effort has to be used or a converging (plus) lens placed in front of the eye (that is, the focal length of the eye has to be changed) (Fig. 13.3). Conversely, a myopic eye, when relaxed, focuses light from a distant object in front of the retina. No amount of further relaxing will enable the eye to lessen its focal length to bring such an image into clear focus. A diverging (or minus) lens will do this, thus a myopic eye can only 'see' a distant object clearly with the aid of some type of lens (Fig. 13.4). Astigmatism is more complex but it can be thought of as a regular distortion of the image on the retina by an eye that has different focal lengths in different axes.

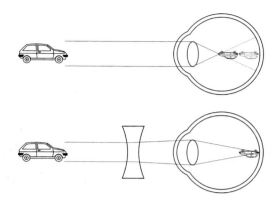

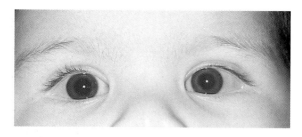

Fig. 13.5 Pseudostrabismus. This infant has prominent epicanthic folds giving the appearance of misaligned eyes. Note that the corneal light reflections are symmetrical. Cover-testing failed to reveal misalignment of either eye.

Fig. 13.4 Myopia (short-sightedness). (a) When the eye is relaxed the image of a distant object is focused in front of the retina, producing a blurred image. (b) Only by placing a diverging lens in front of the eye can a distant object be focused clearly on the retina.

Refractive errors can be compensated for by the use of glasses. In young children refractive error can be measured accurately with the aid of cycloplegic eye drops and retinoscopy. This method of measuring refractive error is objective, and requires minimal co-operation from the child. It can be done very easily on preverbal children to determine the need for glasses. Focusing problems of all types are relatively common in childhood. During primary school years approximately 5 per cent of children wear glasses.

Most children are born a little hypermetropic, and because of a child's prodigious accommodative capability he or she can easily overcome this to see clearly and hence glasses are not necessary. If a child is excessively hypermetropic, large amounts of accommodative effort will be required to focus clearly. Such large amounts of accommodation may result in excessive convergence and the child will develop a convergent squint (see 'Turned eyes' below).

TURNED EYES (STRABISMUS OR SQUINT)

Strabismus is one of the commonest eye problems in childhood. An understanding of strabismus is important because a turned eye may, in the rare case, indicate a major problem with one eye (for example, cataract or retinoblastoma); more commonly, it is associated with reduced vision (amblyopia) in one eye. Thus a turned eye may be secondary to poor vision or may be the cause of reduced vision (amblyopia). Early diagnosis of squint and appropriate intervention increases the chance of restoring or preserving vision.

The initial assessment of a child suspected of having strabismus involves confirmation of the misalignment (observation, corneal light reflection and cover testing), measurement of vision in each eye and examination of red reflex to detect major structural defects in either eye. All children with confirmed or suspected strabismus should be referred to an ophthalmologist. If a major structural defect is suspected on the basis of an abnormal red reflex, specialist opinion should be obtained urgently.

Infants have relatively broad and flat nasal bridges, and if this is associated with prominent epicanthic folds a very strong impression of convergent strabismus can arise. This is known as pseudostrabismus (Fig. 13.5) and is quite common. Careful assessment, as outlined above, will enable pseudo and true strabismus to be distinguished.

Most children with strabismus have a full range of eye movement and thus the misaligned eyes are not the result of a muscular abnormality or nerve damage. Childhood strabismus is usually

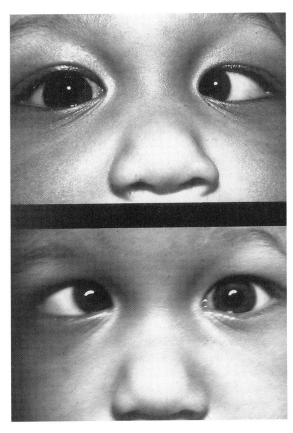

Fig. 13.6 Infantile esotropia. This infant has a large angle alternating esotropia. Note the marked asymmetry of the corneal light reflections.

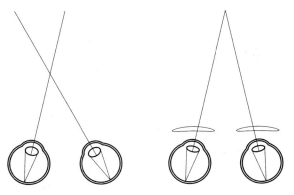

Fig. 13.7 Accommodative esotropia. (a) Excessive accommodation of the hypermetropic eye may result in excessive convergence and esotropia. (b) By placing corrective (plus) lenses in front of the eyes, the amount of accommodation needed to see the object is reduced and so is the convergence. As a result, the eyes are now correctly aligned.

the result of failure of the development of normal binocular co-ordination of the eyes. There may be a primary failure of such co-ordination. This is seen with early onset convergent strabismus (known as infantile esotropia).

Strabismus associated with a full range of eye movement is called concomitant strabismus. If the eyes converge excessively it is known as esotropia, and if the eyes diverge it is called exotropia. Vertical misalignment is called hypertropia, if the eye goes up, and hypotropia if the eye goes down.

Infantile esotropia is seen before 6 months of age and is generally a large angle convergent strabismus (Fig. 13.6). These infants seldom have

any significant refractive error and surgery is usually required to realign the eyes successfully. Patching may be necessary for the treatment of amblyopia.

Accommodative esotropia usually has its onset between 18 months and 4 years of age, and is often intermittent at the initial stage. It occurs in children who are excessively hypermetropic (long-sighted). To overcome hypermetropia and to focus a clear image on the retina, accommodative effort is used. Accommodation consists of the combination of changing focal length of the lens and converging the eyes (so that both are directed at the nearer object of regard). Thus in children with excessive hypermetropia there is increased focusing and at times excessive convergence (causing accommodative esotropia) (Fig. 13.7): this can be corrected by prescribing glasses that compensate for the appropriate amount of hypermetropia. Amblyopia is often seen with accommodative esotropia and requires treatment. If glasses only partly correct the esotropia, surgery may be indicated to obtain optimal alignment.

Intermittent divergent strabismus is unusual before 18 months of age. It is often more noticeable on distance fixation and may be associated with closure of the deviating eye, especially in bright light. Amblyopia is uncommon as the deviation is intermittent, and presumably when the eyes are straight normal visual development proceeds. In some cases the divergence becomes more constant, and in such situations surgery may be undertaken to improve alignment.

All children with strabismus have to be reviewed periodically until about age 10 to 12 years, to detect any amblyopia and to monitor ocular alignment. Even after successful realignment with surgery or glasses, amblyopia may occur and the eyes may also deviate again.

Children require a general anaesthetic (day surgery) for strabismus surgery to be undertaken. The principle of such an operation is to align the eyes correctly by weakening and/or strengthening extra ocular muscles so as to rotate one eye relative to the other. Simple analgesia, such as paracetamol, is sufficient for postoperative pain management. Postoperative nausea and vomiting is not unusual in older children (over 5 years of age). This is generally self-limited and not a major problem; it settles with restriction of oral intake and a little patience.

WOBBLY EYES

Nystagmus is to-and-fro movement of the eyes; it is almost always involuntary. In childhood most nystagmus is a primary defect in the child's ability to keep the eyes still, or the result of early failure of normal development of vision. Nystagmus in childhood is seldom the result of medication, cerebral degeneration, cerebrovascular disease or cerebral tumour as is the case in adults.

Congenital nystagmus is a primary defect in the mechanism that stabilises the eyes and results in mild to moderately reduced vision (6/9 to 6/24). It is seldom evident before 6 to 8 weeks of age, and will often reduce or dampen in a particular direction of gaze (called the null point). Thus to maximise vision a child may adopt a compensatory head posture to take advantage of the null point. If the compensatory head posture is extreme, surgery may be necessary to manipulate the null point so that it is closer to the primary position of the gaze.

Sensory nystagmus is caused by poor vision and is usually obvious by 3 months of age. Causes include bilateral congenital cataracts, albinism and congenital retinal dystrophy (Leber's congenital amaurosis). These conditions are rare, but immediate recognition will result in a better final visual outcome, and early intervention will minimise developmental problems associated with lifelong reduced vision (for example, in albinism and congenital retinal dystrophy).

WATERY (EPIPHORA) AND STICKY EYES

An eye will become watery and sticky because of the failure of tear drainage or because of an inflammatory response (increased production of tears, mucus and cellular response). Congenital nasolacrimal duct obstruction and bacterial conjunctivitis are typical examples of each cause. It is possible that the two problems may coexist in the one child. An irritated eye may be painful and erythematous, depending on the cause (Table 13.1).

Congenital nasolacrimal duct obstruction affects about 10 per cent of newborn infants and resolves itself in about 95 per cent of cases by the first year. It presents as a watery and sticky eye in the first two weeks of life. Despite the persistent discharge the eye is generally neither red nor inflamed. The differential diagnosis includes trauma, conjunctivitis and infantile glaucoma (see 'Big and small eyes' below). An inflamed eye suggests infective conjunctivitis.

If the obstruction persists the lower lid will often redden and sometimes become slightly scaly as a result of the skin being constantly moist. If obstruction persists beyond 12 months of age, probing under a general anaesthetic is indicated and generally curative.

Ophthalmia neonatorum presents with copious discharge from the eyes in the first few days of

Table 13.1 Watery and sticky eyes: common symptoms, signs and causes

Problem	Symptoms	Signs
Neonatal conjunctivitis (*ophthalmia neonatorum*)	Severe pain	Moderate epiphora Copious discharge Mod. to severe erythema
Congenital nasolacrimal duct obstruction	Painless	Mild to mod. epiphora Mild to copious discharge Minimal erythema
Infantile glaucoma	Photophobia	Mod. epiphora No discharge Minimal erythema Enlarged and cloudy cornea
Viral conjunctivitis	Moderate discomfort	Mod. epiphora Mild discharge Mild to mod. erythema
Bacterial conjunctivitis	Mod. to severe discomfort	Moderate epiphora Copious discharge Mod. to severe erythema
Allergic conjunctivitis	Itch is often prominent	Mild to mod. epiphora Stringy discharge Mild erythema
Chemical conjunctivitis	Intense pain	Severe epiphora Mild discharge Mod. to severe erythema
Corneal abrasion	Intense pain	Mod. epiphora No discharge Variable erythema Fluorescein staining
Foreign body	Intense pain	Mod. epiphora No discharge Variable erythema Variable fluorescein staining
Preseptal cellulitis	Mod. pain	Minimal epiphora Variable discharge Marked erythema and swelling of eyelids — the eye is white
Orbital cellulitis	Severe pain Reduced eye movements	Minimal epiphora Variable discharge Marked erythema and swelling of eyelids — the eye is often inflamed and proptosed.

life, and is the result of infection acquired during birth (for example, Neisseria gonorrhoea and Chlamydia trachomatis). Gonococcal conjunctivitis is serious because of the risk of spontaneous perforation of the cornea, loss of vision and generalised sepsis. Chlamydial conjunctivitis is important because of the risk of more generalised chlamydial sepsis. For accurate and prompt diagnosis, conjunctival swabs should be directly inoculated on to culture medium plates and conjunctival scrapings taken for Gram staining and immunofluorescent staining. Systemic, as well as topical, antibiotic therapy is indicated.

Bacterial conjunctivitis occurring beyond the first few days of life is generally the result of relatively innocuous organisms (for example, *Staphylococcal spp.* and *Haemophilus spp.*). Microbiological investigation is not indicated initially and a broad spectrum topical antibiotic should be prescribed (such as neomycin/polymixin or chloramphenicol). Topical chloramphenicol preparations have an extremely low risk of secondary agranulocytosis.

Viral conjunctivitis is relatively common at all ages, and may be very difficult to differentiate from bacterial conjunctivitis. There may be somewhat less discharge with viral conjunctivitis. When there is uncertainty as to aetiology, topical antibiotics as for bacterial conjunctivitis should be used.

Preseptal cellulitis is a bacterial infection of the skin and soft tissue of the eyelids; it will present with redness and swelling. Often there is discharge and watering as well. This infection may respond to oral antibiotics but frequently parenteral antibiotics are needed. Less commonly, an infection spreads to the orbital tissues from the surrounding nasal sinuses. This is orbital cellulitis, which is a more serious infection than preseptal cellulitis, and which presents with proptosis (forward protrusion of the eye), redness of eye and eyelids, and painful limitation of eye movements. If untreated, orbital cellulitis will frequently result in loss of vision because the raised pressure in the orbit will interfere with the blood supply to the globe, which in turn may lead to infarction of the optic nerve or retina. Treatment involves parenteral antibiotics, an urgent CT scan to define the extent of any orbital abscess and the drainage of any significant collection of pus.

BIG AND SMALL EYES

A young child's eye will become bigger if the pressure within it is raised, as in infantile glaucoma. Less commonly, the eye is enlarged as in megalocornea (literally 'big cornea'). Small eyes in children result mainly from defects in growth of the eye, and there may be other major anomalies of the eye.

Infantile glaucoma (buphthalmos, or 'ox eye') is a rare condition with deficient drainage of aqueous fluid from the anterior chamber. The intraocular pressure rises and the infant's sclera and cornea stretch and the eye enlarges. The stretching of the cornea damages the inner corneal layers (Descemet's membrane and associated endothelium), allowing the cornea to become oedematous and opaque. This damaged cornea causes irritation and light sensitivity. Thus the features of infantile glaucoma are an enlarged, cloudy cornea with watering and photophobia. There is no significant discharge, which differentiates infantile glaucoma from nasolacrimal obstruction and conjunctivitis.

Treatment for infantile glaucoma requires surgery to restore aqueous fluid drainage from the anterior chamber. Such surgery is usually successful, though the stretched cornea will remain and the eyes will be often myopic (short-sighted).

An eye that is small but otherwise normal is termed a nanophthalmic eye. If the eye is associated with an ocular anomaly, the eye is microphthalmic. Microphthalmos is frequently associated with a failure of development of part of the uveal coat of the eye (iris and choroid). Such a defect in the iris or choroid is called a coloboma. Microphthalmic eyes often have poor vision that cannot be improved.

INJURED EYES

Trauma to the eye can be physical (blunt or sharp), radiation (thermal or electromagnetic) or chemical.

Direct blunt trauma to the eye may disrupt iris blood vessels, cause bleeding in the anterior chamber of the eye (hyphema), tear the iris, dislocate the lens, rupture the choroid and (rarely) rupture the eye wall (sclera) if the force is sufficient. Simple inspection of the eye will reveal most of these injuries, and choroid and globe rupture may be suspected on the basis of the nature of the injury and associated poor vision. Referral to an ophthalmologist is necessary in these cases for confirmation of the injury and further management. The prognosis for vision is poor with severe injuries.

Blunt trauma to the eye may result in a blow out fracture of the bones of the orbital wall rather than a rupture of the globe: the orbital floor and medial wall are most often fractured, as they are thin bones. The extraocular muscles and/or their fascial connections may become entrapped in a blow out fracture, leading to restrictive strabismus. Surgery may be needed to free the entrapped tissue and repair the fracture.

Sharp trauma may result from tiny objects, such as a subtarsal foreign body that causes a corneal abrasion, or fingernail scratches, through to the penetration of the eye by sharp objects such as scissors or knives. Surface trauma can be easily diagnosed with the help of fluorescein stain and a cobalt blue light. Areas of epithelial abrasion will fluoresce green. If a round ulcer and/ or vertical linear abrasions are seen, a subtarsal foreign body should be suspected and the upper lid should be everted and the foreign body removed with a moistened cotton bud. Superficial trauma is treated with antibiotic ointment and a patch, and reviewed daily until the ulcer or abrasion is healed.

In penetrating injuries of the eye (cornea or sclera) the intraocular contents may prolapse out through the wound, the iris and pupil may appear distorted or the anterior chamber may be shallowed. Any suspected penetration of the eye must be referred to an ophthalmologist for further investigation and management. The eye should be protected with a cone that does not exert any pressure on the eye. If vomiting is likely or occurs, an antiemetic should be given to reduce the chance of further prolapse of intraocular tissue.

Thermal injuries to the eye itself are rare as the eyelids protect the eye. Facial burns may cause scarring that interferes with the lid function, leading to the exposure and drying of the eye's surface. If a primary thermal injury to the eye is suspected, fluorescein dye should be used to detect any ulceration. If ulceration is found the treatment is with antibiotic ointment and a patch.

Radiation injuries to the eye are rare in childhood, and most are the result of intentional irradiation as part of medical therapy for facial and ocular neoplasm. Typical injuries are cataract, dry eye syndrome, radiation retinopathy and optic neuropathy. These changes become obvious a considerable time after the irradiation.

Chemical burns to the eye are unusual in childhood, but potentially very serious, especially if the chemical is alkaline. Many domestic cleaning agents are alkaline. Strong alkali will denature and dissolve protein, and penetrate deeply into the surface of the eye. Acids tend to coagulate surface structures and this often prevents deeper penetration of the acidic chemical into the eye. Immediate first aid consists of copious irrigation with water for at least 10 minutes. Local anaesthetic eye drops relieve pain while the eye is irrigated. All chemical burns of the eye should be referred to an ophthalmologist.

WHITE PUPIL

The pupil is normally black because very little light is reflected back out of the eye. Any abnormal reflecting surface in the eye increases reflected light and causes the pupil to appear coloured rather than black. Cataracts, retinal tumours and colobomas are the most common causes of a white pupil. These conditions are all rare, but important because of their affect on vision and, in some instances, the importance of early recognition and treatment.

A cataract is any opacity within the lens. Cataracts will frequently present because a white pupil has been noted. Bilateral congenital cataracts cause poor vision in infancy, while unilateral congenital cataracts may go unrecognised as one eye has normal vision. Both bilateral and unilateral congenital cataracts are treatable if diagnosed early. Cataracts are readily detected by inspection of the red reflex with the direct ophthalmoscope.

Most cataracts in childhood are congenital and causes include: hereditary (dominant, recessive and X-linked), metabolic (for example, galactosaemia), association with systemic syndrome (for example, Down syndrome) and congenital infection (for example, rubella embryopathy). Many, especially unilateral cataracts, are idiopathic.

Management of cataracts in children involves surgical removal of the cataract and visual rehabilitation with glasses or contact lenses. In older children an intraocular lens can be implanted in the eye but in children under 2 years this is not possible. These children often develop amblyopia and require long-term follow-up.

Retinoblastoma most often presents with a white pupil (the white tumour is seen immediately behind the lens) (Fig. 13.1). Other presentations are with strabismus, poor vision or a known family history of retinoblastoma. Prompt recognition and treatment is vital to preserve vision and life.

Sporadic and hereditary forms of retinoblastoma are recognised. The sporadic form is the result of two separate mutations that negate the action of the retinoblastoma gene ('Rb gene') within a single retinoblast cell and thus is always unilateral. The hereditary form arises when the first of these two mutations occurs within a germ cell (most often a sperm). The second mutation occurs within the retinoblast. As all retinoblasts descended from an affected germ cell have the first mutation, more than one retinoblastoma will usually develop and hence the hereditary form is often bilateral.

Treatment of retinoblastoma may involve removal of the eye (enucleation), chemotherapy, freezing of the tumour (cryotherapy), laser heating of the tumour in association with chemotherapy (thermochemotherapy) or irradiation (both external beam or a local implanted source of irradiation — plaque brachytherapy). Current 5-year survival is about 98 per cent.

LUMPY EYELIDS

Swellings in the eyelids are common in childhood. Most are the result of minor infections, obstructed oil glands or bruising. Benign tumours occur occasionally and malignant tumours very rarely.

Lid infections are common in children and most arise in the lash follicles (stye or hordeolum externum) and meibomian glands (hordeolum internum). Unless there is significant secondary erythema of the surrounding lid, topical and systemic antibiotics are not indicated. Occasionally, severe preseptal cellulitis will follow a focal lid infection and systemic (often intravenous) antibiotics will be needed.

Chronic inflammation of a meibomian gland (chalazion) is generally chemical inflammation rather than infection, and occurs when the gland contents escape into the lid following blockage of the duct. A chalazion will appear as a lump in the substance of the lid and is often not particularly inflamed in appearance. Topical antibiotics seldom hasten resolution. Warm compresses may give symptomatic relief and help drainage. Chalazia may persist for many months; some will discharge through the conjunctiva or the skin. On occasions surgical drainage is indicated for a persistently inflamed and large chalazion.

Angular dermoids occur at inner or outer aspects of the upper lid (Fig. 16.7, Chapter 16). These are benign hamartomas that grow in proportion with the rest of the child. Rarely will direct trauma cause a rupture of a dermoid and significant inflammation ensue. A deep extension necessitating extensive surgery more often occurs with medial angular dermoids. A CT scan should

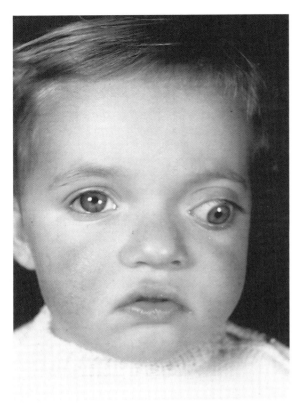

Fig. 13.8 Neuroblastoma is the commonest cause of metastatic tumour of the orbit with proptosis.

be undertaken before planned excision if a deep extension is suspected.

Malignant tumours of the eyelid and orbit are rare. Rhabdomyosarcoma is the most frequent, and presents with rapidly progressive (days to weeks) eyelid swelling and/or proptosis. The overlying skin may appear reddened but other signs of acute inflammation (pain and fever) are absent. Management includes imaging to delineate site and extent of the lesion, incisional biopsy, chemotherapy and often external beam irradiation. This management is multidisciplinary. The overall survival rate for this form of rhabdomyosarcoma is excellent. Metastatic orbital tumours occur, with neuroblastoma being the most common (Fig. 13.8).

DROOPY LIDS

Ptosis (or blepharoptosis) is a droopy upper eyelid and results from innervational or muscular defects of the *levator superioris* or Muller's muscles. Innervational defects include third cranial nerve palsy, Horner's syndrome (sympathetic nervous system) and myaesthenia gravis. Most ptosis in childhood is congenital and has no other systemic associations. Acquired ptosis in childhood requires a thorough investigation to find a cause.

Most congenital ptosis is an isolated abnormality in the function of one or both levator muscles. The affected muscle is often described as being 'dystrophic' but there is in general no association with more widespread muscular dystrophies. Congenital ptosis will appear worse when the child is tired or unwell; this is not evidence of ocular myaesthenia gravis. A child with ptotic eyelids will often adopt a compensatory chin-up head posture to look straight ahead or to look up.

Ptosis will cause visual defects if the lid occludes the visual axis or if it induces astigmatism by altering the corneal curvature. Ptosis is also a cosmetic concern, in that it may make an affected child look sleepy or dull. Surgical correction is possible in most cases. Early surgery is indicated when the ptotic eyelid is interfering with the development of vision. If intervention is primarily for reasons of appearance, surgery is usually undertaken just prior to school commencement.

HEADACHE

Headache in children occasionally is caused by an ocular abnormality. Astigmatism and high hypermetropia (long-sightedness) are rare causes of childhood headache. Sustained attention to a near object will often cause some visual discomfort and headache. This is really a fatigue or tension headache and in general does not indicate any significant eye problem. These headaches are often described as a tightening around the head and are not associated with other symptoms.

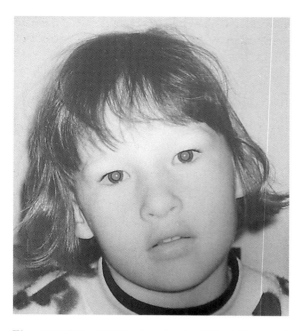

Fig. 13.9 This child developed a head-tilt at 5 years of age. Investigation revealed a pineocytoma compressing the quadrigeminal plate

(pseudotumour cerebri) and tumours causing obstructive hydrocephalus.

ABNORMAL HEAD POSTURE

Children will adopt abnormal head postures for many reasons. Structural abnormalities, hearing loss, visual defects, habit and (rarely) central nervous system tumours can all cause abnormal head posture. Sternocleidomastoid muscle 'tumour' or hemivertebra are examples of structural abnormalities causing abnormal head posture.

If vision is improved with the head held in a particular position, a child will characteristically adopt this position (Fig. 13.9). Visual stimuli for abnormal head posture include strabismus, where binocular depth perception is improved or diplopia is avoided, loss of vision in one eye, dampening of nystagmus, ptosis and severe photophobia.

POSTOPERATIVE CARE OF THE CHILD AFTER EYE SURGERY

The principles of postoperative eye care for children are: (i) maintaining general comfort; (ii) protecting the eye when necessary; (iii) minimising specific complications; and (iv) returning the child to normal activities as soon as is reasonable.

Pain is usually minimal after paediatric eye surgery. Paracetamol is sufficient for most postoperative pain relief. Immediately after strabismus procedures, children are often distressed and disoriented. This phase may last minutes to an hour or so, and in most instances will settle with comforting alone. Older children are more likely to require postoperative analgesia than infants.

Nausea and vomiting may occur after strabismus procedures. Avoidance of pre- and intra-operative narcotic analgesia and intra-operative anti-emetic will minimise these problems. Limited oral intake in the early postoperative

Migraine headaches are common in childhood and may be associated with visual symptoms. The typical visual aura is the blurring of central vision with zig-zag bright lines (fortification spectra). These headaches are recurrent; they are often associated with nausea and/or vomiting and settle with simple analgesia (paracetamol) and rest. A family history of migraine is common.

Eye examination may help determine the cause of some headaches. Raised intracranial pressure will usually cause headache that is often worse in the morning and after lying down. The pain is often described as dull, pounding and persistent. It may be associated with nausea and vomiting and sometimes transient blurring of vision (visual obscurations). If the intracranial pressure is raised, fundus examination will reveal papilloedema in most cases. The commonest causes of raised intracranial pressure that present with headache are 'benign' intracranial pressure period will lessen the occurrence and severity of nausea and vomiting. Severe vomiting that requires re-admission and rehydration will occur rarely.

Patches to protect the eye are generally only needed after intraocular surgery (cataract and glaucoma) and eyelid surgery (ptosis repair and drainage of chalazion). Patches will often annoy a child and should be avoided following strabismus surgery.

Postoperative eye drops (antibiotic and steroid preparations) minimise the risk of infection and inflammation, especially following intraocular surgery. The benefit that follows strabismus procedures is less evident. Lubricating ointment is used for days or weeks after ptosis repair, to protect the ocular surface during healing.

Swimming should probably be avoided for one to three weeks after most eye operations because of the eye irritation from chlorinated or salt water. Care must be taken with face- and hair-washing; soap or shampoo will be more irritating after an eye operation.

FURTHER READING

Beasley S.W., Hutson J.M. & Myers N.A. (1993) *Paediatric Diagnosis*, Chapman & Hall, London, pp. 118–27.

Isenberg S.J. (1994) *The Eye in Infancy,* 2nd edn, Mosby, St. Louis.

Robinson M. & Roberton D.M. (1998) *Practical Paediatrics,* 4th edn, Churchill Livingstone, Edinburgh.

Taylor D. (1997) *Pediatric Ophthalmology,* 2nd edn, Blackwell, Boston.

Wright K.W. (1995) *Pediatric Ophthalmology and Strabismus*, Mosby, St. Louis.

— 14 —

The Ear, Nose and Throat

CASE 1

An 18-month-old girl who has had an upper respiratory tract infection for a week has been irritable for the past 2 days, particularly at night. She has had 3 ear infections over the past 3 months and has not yet developed any speech. She presented to the emergency department with a temperature of 37.8°C and was mildly unwell. Otoscopy revealed pale, opaque tympanic membranes but the view was difficult. Her mother thinks she has another ear infection.

> Q. 1.1   *Why is the tympanic membrane pale and opaque?*
>
> Q. 1.2   *What is the treatment for otitis media?*
>
> Q. 1.3   *Is hearing impaired in this child?*

CASE 2

A 6-year-old boy presents to his local doctor with yet another episode of acute tonsillitis and has also been snoring heavily at night. His mother wonders whether or not it is time for him to have his tonsils and adenoids removed.

> Q. 2.1   *What advice would you give?*

CASE 3

A 4-week-old infant presents with a history of stridor since birth. The child is noisy but appears well and is thriving.

> Q. 3.1   *How is stridor assessed?*
>
> Q. 3.2   *What causes congenital stridor?*

OTITIS MEDIA

Introduction

The term otitis media implies the presence of a middle ear effusion. Fluid develops because of dysfunction of the eustachian tube that normally provides ventilation and drainage of the middle ear, together with protection of the middle ear from nasopharyngeal contamination. For both infective and structural reasons, otitis media is very common in young children, particularly over the winter months.

The tympanic membrane is a window to the middle ear and is usually translucent. Ascertaining its translucency is the most important step in diagnosing otitis media by otoscopy. An opaque tympanic membrane may be due to fluid in the middle ear or simply thickening of the membrane itself (Fig. 14.1). The diagnosis of otitis media can

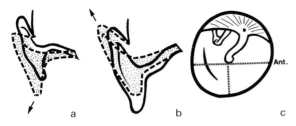

Fig. 14.1 The tympanic membrane. (a) The direction of the canal in infants and young children: to visualise the membrane, pull the pinna downwards and outwards; (b) in older children and adults the pinna is drawn upwards and backwards; (c) the normal eardrum is transparent, with the Incus and Stapes visible in the background. The site for the myringotomy or tympanostomy tube is shown.

be confirmed by demonstrating impaired mobility of the tympanic membrane by either pneumatic otoscopy or tympanometry.

Otitis media presents clinically as a spectrum of diseases that are all characterised by the presence of a middle ear effusion. At either end of the spectrum the child may be labelled as having:
(1) acute suppurative otitis media
(2) otitis media with effusion.

Acute suppurative otitis media (ASOM)

ASOM is diagnosed on the basis of the presence of a middle ear effusion associated with features of inflammation that are either local (pain) or systemic (fever, irritability), provided there is no other explanation for the systemic symptoms. Using this diagnostic criterion, bacteria are cultured in approximately 80 per cent of cases and are usually *Streptococcus pneumoniae*, non-typable *Haemophilus influenzae* and *Branhamella catarrhalis*. Antibiotics should be administered if there are significant symptoms. Amoxycillin (40 mg per kg per day in 3 divided doses for 5 days) is recommended. Broader spectrum antibiotics may provide greater *in vitro* cover; however, there is no proven benefit, and side effects may be greater with broader spectrum antibiotics. Spontaneous perforation is usually associated with relief of pain

and treatment is the same as when perforation does not occur. Most cases of ASOM will settle spontaneously even if antibiotics are withheld, and therefore treatment may not be required when symptoms are only mild.

The follow-up of ASOM involves a review within 48 hours in case the child fails to respond to medical treatment (Box 14.1), and longer term review to document resolution of the middle ear effusion.

Acute drainage of the ear should be considered if local or systemic symptoms persist despite adequate antibiotic treatment. This not only relieves pain immediately but also should prevent the development of suppurative complications (Box 14.2). The middle ear effusion associated with ASOM persists for a variable period of time beyond resolution of the infective features (Table 14.1).

Otitis media with effusion (OME)

Middle ear effusion is typically associated with mild hearing loss. When bilateral, this may lead to delayed speech development, behavioural problems and educational difficulties. Bacteria can be cultured in 25 per cent of cases and as a consequence, antibiotic treatment may be of some benefit.

Surgical intervention by way of insertion of tympanostomy tubes is indicated when OME is associated with symptomatic hearing loss or

Table 14.1 Duration of effusion after ASOM

Period after ASOM	Percentage middle ear effusion
2 weeks	70%
1 month	40%
2 months	20%
3 months	10%

recurrent ear infections, and the clinical situation is thought unlikely to improve spontaneously in the near future. Factors contributing to persistence of OME include the length of time the effusions have been present, seasonal factors (OME is associated with upper respiratory tract infections over the winter months) and anatomical factors such as the presence of a cleft palate or other craniofacial anomalies.

Tympanostomy tubes are usually designed to last between 6 to 18 months and reinsertion of tubes is necessary in 25 per cent of cases (Fig. 14.2). The longer the tubes remain *in situ*, the higher the rate of tympanic membrane perforation, which is approximately 1 per cent per year. Tubes may discharge intermittently, particularly with upper respiratory tract infections, and this is best treated by topical antibiotics.

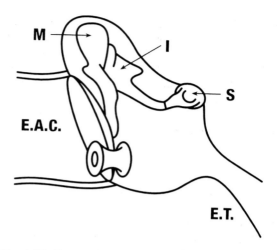

Fig. 14.2 Tympanostomy tube. The tube is sitting in the tympanic membrane and has a central lumen that ventilates the middle ear, equalizing pressure between the middle ear and external auditory canal (EAC). The malleolus (M), incus (I) and stapes (S) convey vibrations to the inner ear. The eustachian tube (ET) ventilates the middle ear to the nasopharynx.

CHOLESTEATOMA

The presence of squamous epithelium (skin) in the middle ear constitutes cholesteatoma. This squamous epithelium may cause bone destruction due to a combination of enzymatic action and infection, and may result in conductive hearing loss, sensori-neural hearing loss, facial paralysis and intracranial infection.

Cholesteatoma may be congenital or acquired. Congenital cholesteatoma may be recognised in the early phase by the presence of a white mass deep to the tympanic membrane usually in the antero-superior quadrant.

Acquired cholesteatoma usually occurs due to the tympanic membrane retraction associated with eustachian tube dysfunction. This may involve the tympanic membrane inferior to the lateral process of the malleus (pars tensa) or superior to it (pars flaccida). The development of a retraction pocket can be observed clinically and cholesteatoma formation prevented by the insertion of a tympanostomy tube. Acquired cholesteatoma may also occur due to traumatic or iatrogenic implantation of squamous epithelium, medial migration of squamous epithelium from the external auditory canal and squamous metaplasia of the middle ear mucosa. When extensive, removal of cholesteatoma usually requires a combined surgical approach to both the mastoid and middle ear.

ACUTE TONSILLITIS

Bacterial tonsillitis is caused by the Group A haemolytic streptococcus. The clinical features include fever and systemic upset, sore throat, inflamed tonsils and cervical lymphadenitis. Streptococci can be cultured from the surface of the tonsil in 10 to 40 per cent of healthy carriers and routine pre- and post-treatment throat swabs are therefore not routinely obtained.

Acute tonsillitis is usually seen in the 4- to 14-year-old age group and is uncommon in young children. The diagnosis of acute tonsillitis needs to be differentiated from a viral upper respiratory tract infection or pharyngitis, and specific viral causes of acute tonsillitis, particularly infectious mononucleosis.

Rheumatic carditis and post-streptococcal glomerulonephritis are now very uncommon complications of acute tonsillitis. Treatment of acute tonsillitis generally aims to minimise morbidity and decrease suppurative complications, and is dealt by a 10-day course of penicillin.

Infection may extend beyond the tonsil into a peritonsillar cellulitis or abscess (quinsy) (Box 14.3). A peritonsillar abscess must be drained (local anaesthetic may suffice in older children).

Tonsillectomy may be considered for recurrent attacks of acute tonsillitis in children over 4 years of age (younger children usually have a viral upper respiratory infection) (Box 14.4). There is a 2-week recovery period following surgery when spontaneous bleeding may occur (2 per cent). Secondary haemorrhage settles spontaneously in the majority of cases, while immediate postoperative

> ### Box 14.3 Signs of quinsy
>
> (1) Increased systemic symptoms.
>
> (2) Drooling of saliva.
>
> (3) 'Hot potato speech'.
>
> (4) Trismus.
>
> (5) Bulging tonsil and soft palate.
>
> (6) Fluctuance on palpation.

> ### Box 14.4 Indications for tonsillectomy ± adenoidectomy
>
> (1) Recurrent, severe acute tonsillitis in a child > 4 years old, if predicted to have ongoing severe morbidity before natural resolution in adolescence:
> (e.g. > 7 infections in 1 year, or
>   > 5 per year in 2 years, or
>   > 3 per year in 3 years).
>
> (2) Peritonsillar abscess (quinsy) needing drainage under GA.
>
> (3) Obstructive sleep apnoea syndrome (> 10 seconds/episode) (± failure to thrive, daytime drowsiness, cor pulmonale).
>
> (4) Suspected tonsillar malignancy (lymphoma).

haemorrhage is best treated by haemostasis in the operating theatre.

ADENOTONSILLAR HYPERTROPHY

Symptomatic enlargement of the adenoids and/or tonsils is commonly seen in children; however,

Box 14.5 Increasing symptoms of adenotonsillar hypertrophy

(1) Snoring alone.

(2) Symptomatic nasal obstruction.

(3) Sleep disturbance (laboured breathing, restlessness).

(4) Sleep apnoea.

(5) Failure to thrive.

(6) Cor pulmonale.

the tonsils and adenoids tend to involute towards the end of the first decade of life. The severity of associated obstructive symptoms depends not only on the size of the adenoids and tonsils, but also on the degree of neuromuscular control of the airway during sleep (Box 14.5).

The decision to go ahead with surgery depends on the severity of the symptoms, and the likelihood that this will continue in the immediate future. The presence of apnoea suggests that both removal of tonsils and adenoids is necessary; however, when the tonsils are small and the adenoids only are enlarged, adenoidectomy alone is a lesser procedure and should be adequate to relieve symptomatic nasal obstruction. Adenoidectomy should not be performed in the presence of a structural or functional abnormality of the palate (for example, cleft palate) because of the likelihood of causing velopharyngeal incompetence with hypernasal speech.

SINUSITIS

Sinusitis is often difficult to diagnose in children because of frequent upper respiratory tract infections characterised by symptoms suggestive of sinusitis that include rhinorrhoea, nasal congestion, cough and craniofacial pain. This difficulty is exacerbated by the fact that CT scans may reveal sinus abnormalities in up to half of otherwise healthy children.

The organisms causing acute sinusitis are the same as those causing ASOM and a similar antibiotic regime is usually recommended, together with nasal decongestants.

Sinusitis may present with a suppurative complication and be responsible for complications in the orbit and brain. Central nervous system complications include extradural, subdural and frontal lobe abscess.

Periorbital and orbital inflammation is usually a complication of acute sinusitis. Periorbital cellulitis (see Fig. 16.3, Chapter 16) is characterised by inflammation of the eyelids and usually settles with IV antibiotics. Orbital cellulitis needs to be differentiated from periorbital cellulitis and this can be recognised by the presence of increased systemic symptoms, chemosis, proptosis, ophthalmoplegia and decreased visual acuity. The spread of infection into the orbit may be associated with a presence of a subperiostial abscess usually along the medial wall of the orbit adjacent to the ethmoid sinus, and therefore a CT scan must be performed in all cases. If there is no abscess, medical treatment should be continued; however, if an abscess is present, surgical drainage via an external approach is necessary.

CONGENITAL STRIDOR

In assessing stridor, its timing is most important. Inspiratory stridor suggests an abnormality at or above the level of the cervical trachea while expiratory stridor suggests an abnormality in the thoracic trachea. Severity of the stridor can be judged by the presence of associated laboured breathing and retractions. Longstanding airway obstruction in young children leads to the failure to thrive.

An assessment of the airway can be performed in the awake patient by flexible laryngoscopy; this provides a view of the upper airway down

Box 14.6 Causes of congenital stridor

Nose/Nasopharynx	Choanal atresia Nasal stenosis Mucosal congestion
Oropharynx	Glossoptosis (Pierre Robin sequence)
Supraglottis	Laryngomalacia (neuromuscular disorder)
Glottis	Bilateral vocal cord paralysis
Subglottis	Subglottic stenosis (post-intubation)
Trachea	Tracheomalacia (dysplastic rings)

to and including the larynx. Radiologic imaging by airway fluoroscopy and barium swallow may reveal tracheal collapse or compression. When no diagnosis has been made and the child has significant symptoms, assessment under general anaesthesia by bronchoscopy is required.

Depending on the severity of the obstruction, treatment may be required which includes temporary airway support by nasopharyngeal or endotracheal intubation, surgical correction, or bypassing the obstruction by tracheostomy.

The causes of stridor can be classified according to whether they are structural or functional. Obstruction is usually functional in neonates, the commonest cause of inspiratory stridor being laryngomalacia. Neonates are obligate nose breathers for the first 3 months of life and nasal obstruction will cause significant upper airway obstruction. The causes of congenital stridor can also be classified according to the site of obstruction (Box 14.6).

TRAUMA

Fractured base of skull with temporal bone fracture

A fractured base of the skull may present with bleeding from the ear following a head injury. This may also be associated with the leakage of cerebrospinal fluid. Alternatively, blood or cerebrospinal fluid may collect behind an intact tympanic membrane. Temporal bone fractures may cause conductive hearing loss, sensori-neural hearing loss and facial paralysis.

Nasal trauma

Nasal trauma, even without a nasal fracture, may be associated with the development of a septal haematoma. This should be recognised and drained before a septal abscess can develop, which can cause the destruction of the nasal septum and a collapse of the nose.

The nose should be assessed for a cosmetic deformity due to bone displacement once the initial oedema has settled (around 5 days). Radiology is of no benefit as the decision to reduce the fracture is based on the presence of a cosmetic deformity. Fracture reduction should be performed within 10 days of the nasal injury.

Oropharyngeal injury

Oropharyngeal injury typically occurs as a consequence of a child falling with a stick in their mouth, causing injury to the palate or posterior pharyngeal wall. Initial assessment involves nasal endoscopy to assess the integrity of the posterior pharyngeal wall, and a lateral neck X-ray to detect any air in the retropharyngeal tissues, the presence of foreign material and any associated cervical spine injury.

Hospital admission is required when there is:
(1) Significant palatal laceration that requires repair.
(2) Significant bleeding.

(3) A child unable to feed.

(4) Upper airway obstruction.

(5) Significant retropharyngeal injury with the risk of a retropharyngeal abscess developing.

(6) The possibility of internal carotid artery damage from an injury immediately posterior to the tonsil. Blunt trauma, which may cause intimal disruption and carotid thrombosis, is as potentially dangerous as penetrating trauma.

COMMON CONDITIONS OF THE MOUTH

Mucus retention cysts

Goblet cells in the buccal mucosa may become blocked and form a pale pedunculated retention cyst up to 1 cm in diameter on the inner aspect of the lip, the gingivo-labial sulcus or the lining of the cheek. They sometimes evacuate spontaneously, but usually they annoy the patient, worry the parents and occasionally interfere with feeding. They are best removed if troublesome.

Ranula

A ranula, a larger sessile cyst 2 to 3 cm in diameter in the floor of the mouth under the tongue, arises as an extravasation cyst of the sublingual gland. It is lax, bluish-grey or translucent, and may grow large enough to interfere with speech and swallowing. It should be deroofed (marsupialised) or excised together with the sublingual gland.

Tongue-tie

In tongue-tie the lingual frenulum is short and may be attached to the very tip of the tongue. It never interferes with the infant's sucking or swallowing, and only rarely interferes with speech. When tongue protrusion is not possible in a child over 2 years of age, the tight frenulum can be divided under general anaesthesia.

FURTHER READING

Glasziou P.P., Hayem M. & Del Mar C.B. (1997) Antibiotic versus placebo for acute otitis media in children. In: Douglas R., Bridges-Webb C., Glasziou P., Lozano J., Steinhoff M. & Wang E. (eds), *Acute Respiratory Infections Module of the Cochrane Database of Systemic Reviews*. Available in the Cochrane Library (database on disk and CD-ROM). The Cochrane Collaboration; Issue 1, Oxford, Update Software. Updated quarterly.

NSW Health Department Working Party (1993) Guidelines on the management of paediatric middle ear disease. *Med. J. Aust.* **159**; Suppl. 4, 1–8.

Pichichero M.E. (1995) Group A *Streptococcal Tonsillopharyngitis*: cost-effective diagnosis and treatment. *Ann. Emerg. Med.* **25**: 390–403.

— 15 —

Cleft Lip, Palate and Craniofacial Anomalies

CASE 1

A term neonate has a small jaw, wide cleft palate and airway obstruction when supine.

    Q. 1.1   *What is the diagnosis?*

    Q. 1.2   *How should this be managed in the next few hours, days and in the long term?*

CASE 2

A child is born with a unilateral cleft lip and palate.

    Q. 2.1   *What is the risk of a sibling being born with a similar problem?*

    Q. 2.2   *What is the risk if a parent is also affected?*

CASE 3

An ultrasonography at 16 weeks of gestation shows syndactyly of all digits of all limbs and significantly decreased anterior–posterior cranial dimensions.

    Q. 3.1   *What is the most likely cause?*

    Q. 3.2   *What are the principles of management?*

    Q. 3.3   *Will the IQ be normal?*

CLEFT LIP AND PALATE

A cleft lip is a cleft of the 'primary' palate and involves the lip, the alveolus between the lateral incisor and the canine, and the anterior portion of the hard palate as far back as the incisive foramen. The cleft is caused by the failure of the mesoderm to merge between the frontonasal process and the maxillary process of the first branchial arch, between 4 and 7 weeks of gestation.

The 'secondary' palate forms the hard and soft palate behind the incisive foramen. Palatal clefts are caused by the failure of fusion of the two hemipalatal shelves between 7 and 10 weeks of gestation.

Incidence, aetiology and risk

Congenital clefts of the lip and palate are common malformations. They occur in approximately 1 in

600 live births. A cleft lip, with or without a cleft palate (CL ± P) makes up about 70 per cent of patients, and is seen more commonly in boys. CL ± P is more commonly found in Asians and least frequently in black people. Cleft palate alone (CP) accounts for 30 per cent of cases, is more common in girls, and has no racial differences. CL ± P is a different clinical group from CP. Clefts are inherited in a multifactorial, polygenic way. There is a positive family history in 25 per cent of cases, particularly CL ± P. The risk of having a second child with a cleft is 2 per cent for CP and 4 per cent for CL ± P, with one child affected and 16 per cent if the parent is affected as well. The risk of a cleft patient having a child with a cleft is also 4 per cent.

Other congenital anomalies should be looked for; they may occur in up to 30 per cent of patients and some may be life-threatening. The initiating cause of the Pierre Robin sequence is under-development of the mandible, causing elevation of the tongue that prevents fusion of the palatal shelves at 10 weeks of gestation. The resulting wide U-shaped cleft is associated with a small jaw and upper airway obstruction by the tongue base. These patients have feeding difficulties, failure to thrive and apnoeic episodes.

A submucous cleft palate is often overlooked. In these patients the uvula is bifid and the soft palate is grooved in the midline where there is a cleft in the muscle. There is also a palpable notch in the posterior margin of the hard palate. These patients require careful assessment and may need surgical repair or a pharyngoplasty in the same manner as an overt cleft palate. Isolated cleft of the uvula is present in 1 in 80 white people and 1 in 10 Asians and is asymptomatic.

Classification

Clefts of the lip may be incomplete, complete, unilateral or bilateral (Fig. 15.1). Bilateral clefts need not be symmetrical. Two-thirds also have a cleft of the secondary palate involving both the hard and soft palate posterior to the incisor foramen.

Management

Clefts of the lip and palate are managed by neonatal referral to the surgical team. The deformity affects not only the patient's appearance but also feeding, hearing, speech, dental and maxillofacial development. The cleft lip and palate team includes specialists from many disciplines, so that problems in all of these areas can be diagnosed, assessed and treated. Careful nursing of children with the Pierre Robin sequence in a neonatal unit should allow these children to outgrow their anatomical problems. Occasionally, an oropharyngeal airway or an operation to produce a tongue-lip adhesion may be required to prevent the tongue from falling back before the palate is repaired.

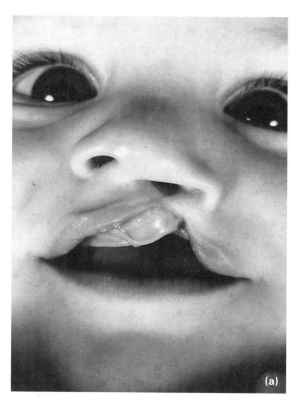

Fig. 15.1 Classification of cleft lip and palate: (a) left unilateral complete cleft lip involving the nose, lip, alveolus and primary palate;

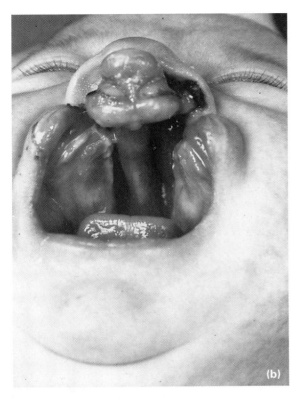 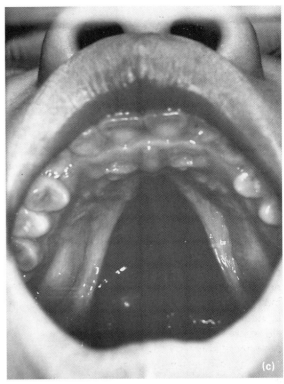

Fig. 15.1 (cont.) (b) bilateral complete cleft lip and palate; (c) isolated complete cleft of secondary palate.

The proposed management is discussed with parents as early as possible. The presence of a cleft can be a severe shock for parents, and considerable support and explanation of the likely outcome are necessary. This can be facilitated by a prompt referral to a plastic surgeon. Obstetric ultrasonography often makes the diagnosis of facial clefting in the early second trimester, prompting a prenatal consultation.

Feeding

Sucking presents no difficulty for the baby with a cleft of the lip alone. Breast-feeding is normal. However, babies with clefts involving the secondary palate are unable to generate enough negative intra-oral pressure to make suction through the mouth possible. These babies swallow normally. A bolus of feed is delivered to the back of the tongue, usually by means of a squeeze bottle (Fig. 15.2) with a spoon-shaped mouth-piece. There are also a number of specially designed teats that deliver milk as they are compressed in the mouth. Nasogastric feeding is unnecessary in an otherwise normal infant with a cleft palate.

Cleft lip repair

Repair of the lip is carried out at about 3 months of age in otherwise fit babies. In patients with bilateral clefts or wide unilateral clefts, presurgical orthodontics can be used to guide the palatal segments into a better position prior to surgery. The aim of lip repair is to obtain definitive closure of the skin, vermilion and *orbicularis* oris muscle, as well as creating a normal buccal

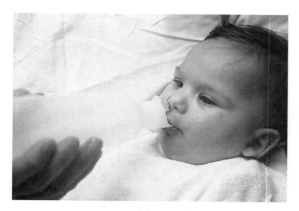

Fig. 15.2 Infant feeding bottle for patients with cleft palate (the infant has had lip repair also).

sulcus. Nasal deformity can be corrected. If the cleft includes the primary palate, this and the nasal floor are also closed (Fig. 15.3). A bilateral cleft is usually repaired at one operation, although there are two-stage procedures.

Cleft palate repair

Clefts of the secondary palate are repaired between 6 and 9 months of age, prior to the acquisition of speech. Unnecessary delay in palate repair may affect the prognosis for normal speech, as the child develops compensatory speech patterns that are difficult to correct later with speech therapy. The aims of the procedure are to lengthen the palate and repair the soft palate musculature (*levator palatini*). The oral and nasal cavities can then be separated during speech and swallowing by normal elevation of the soft palate against the posterior pharyngeal wall.

Speech

Approximately 80 per cent of patients with cleft palate will achieve normal or acceptable, intelligible speech. Speech should be assessed periodically following surgery. Speech therapy will benefit patients with articulation problems, or those who use compensatory mechanisms to produce certain sounds. Palatopharyngeal incompetence allows

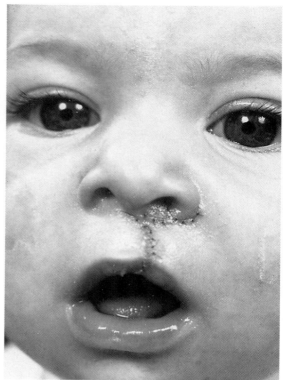

Fig. 15.3 A repair of cleft lip.

nasal escape of air during speech, and is due to a soft palate that is too short and/or moves poorly. Significant palatopharyngeal incompetence is managed with a pharyngoplasty where local pharyngeal tissue is mobilised and repositioned either into the upper surface of the soft palate or into the posterior pharyngeal wall. This helps the soft palate to close off the narrow nasopharyngeal space during speech. Pharyngoplasty is indicated also for patients with palatopharyngeal incompetence due to unoperated clefts in later childhood, in some submucous cleft palates, as well as other conditions such as idiopathic palatopharyngeal incompetence.

Problems in the ear, nose and throat

Children with a cleft palate have abnormal eustachian tube function, leading to a very high incidence of otitis media and most will require tympanostomy tubes for middle ear ventilation. Tubes often are inserted at the time of palate repair. Hearing may be impaired, and these patients require frequent otoscopic and audiological evaluation. Tonsils and adenoids occupy a significant space in the pharynx. Their removal is discouraged in cleft palate patients except when severe recurrent infections cannot be controlled.

Dental and orthodontic treatment

Virtually all children with cleft lip and/or palate will require orthodontic treatment necessitating good dental hygiene. The cleft alveolus usually is bone-grafted at about 9 years of age to allow for proper eruption of the adult canine tooth. Supernumerary or abnormal teeth in the cleft may require removal.

When growth is complete, some patients require orthognathic surgery to re-position the hypoplastic maxilla to obtain functional occlusion and improve appearance. Rarely will surgery be required on both jaws.

Secondary surgery

Secondary surgery may be required to correct residual cosmetic functional problems, particularly of the nose. Initial procedures are performed prior to school entry to minimise obvious deformity, particularly in a bilateral cleft lip where the columella is distinctively short. A deficient philtrum can be reconstructed by transposing a central V-shaped wedge of the lower lip to the upper lip in a two-stage procedure (Abbé flap). Nasal and septal correction is usually reserved until the completion of nasal growth in the late teens.

Minor procedures on the lip and vermilion, and closure of palatal fistulae, can be performed at any time.

CRANIOFACIAL ANOMALIES

Facial appearance is to a large extent determined by the underlying bony skeleton. Soft tissues of the face and orbits can be elevated beneath the periosteum, providing safe access to osteotomise, reshape and reconstruct the cranial and/or facial skeletons. Similar techniques can be utilised to resect tumours and reconstruct the ensuring deficit without deforming the patient. Craniofacial trauma can be managed by using the same principles, with immediate or delayed surgery.

Congenital craniofacial deformities

Principles of dysmorphology

Congenital anomalies may result from malformations, deformations or disruptions. Craniofacial *malformations* are the result of intrinsically abnormal development; for example, cranial suture synostosis and clefts of the lip and face. *Deformations* are the result of extrinsic compression *in utero*; for example, deformational plagiocephaly. *Disruptions* are the result of an extrinsic disruptive intrauterine mechanical force; for example, amniotic bands producing bizarre facial clefts (fitting no particular pattern) and constriction ring syndrome.

Cranial growth

The cranial sutures are not centres of growth, but rather 'gaps' that allow the cranial bones to be pushed out by the growing brain. Bony growth occurs secondarily by desposition of bone at the sutures (sutural growth) and at the pericranial surface (appositional growth), as well as by absorption of bone from the dural surface. Pathological fusion of a suture restricts growth perpendicular to the suture, with compensatory growth occurring in other non-restricted areas of open sutures.

The growth of the brain and its surrounding cranium is rapid in the first two years of life, reaching half adult size by 9 months and three-quarters by the age of 2 years. In cranial suture synotosis the ensuing deformity will worsen with ongoing cranial growth in the first two years of

Table 15.1 Craniofacial deformities: nomenclature and aetiology

Plagiocephaly	Flattened forehead and/or occiput	Coronal/lambdoid synostosis
		Intra-uterine compression
		Torticollis
		Sleeping position
Scaphocephaly	Long, narrow head (boat-shaped)	Sagittal synostosis
Trigonocephaly	Triangular forehead	Metopic synostosis
Brachycephaly	Short head	Bicoronal synostosis
		Crouzon, Apert and other syndromes
Turricephaly	Towering forehead	Apert syndrome
Kleeblatschadel	Cloverleaf skull	Crouzon syndrome with multiple synostoses
Hypertelorism	Orbits too far apart	Encephalocele, tumours, clefts and other syndromes

life. If more than one suture is involved, the volume of the cranial or orbital cavities may be restricted, causing secondary effects on the brain or eyes. In contrast, in deformational plagiocephaly of an otherwise normal skull with normal sutures, once the deforming force is removed, growth of the brain may be expected to decrease the deformity without surgical correction. Disruptions, such as bizarre facial clefts, are not likely to be modified by further growth.

Craniosynostosis

The commonest form of craniosynostosis (Table 15.1) is isolated non-syndromal sutural synostosis. This may be unicoronal, metopic, sagittal, lambdoid or bicoronal, and is not usually associated with other malformations, although some 15 per cent may have raised intracranial pressure. Secondary growth effects may be seen in the face. The aetiology is unknown and the condition is not inherited, although occasionally there is a positive family history. It may occasionally be seen after rapid decompression of hydrocephalus, maternal ingestion of Epilim and thyrotoxicosis. The differential diagnosis of unilateral coronal or lambdoid synostosis includes deformational plagiocephaly, which tends to improve with ongoing cranial growth once the deforming forces are removed (Figs 15.4 and 15.5).

Syndromal craniosynostosis is rare, more severe and inherited (frequently autosomal dominant). Bicoronal synostosis with mid-face hypoplasia occurs in Crouzon syndrome, and a similar picture, associated with symmetrical polysyndactyly of the hands and feet, is seen in Apert syndrome. These are the commonest of several hundred syndromes. In syndromal cranial synostosis there is an associated risk of raised intracranial pressure, hydrocephalus, primary brain anomalies and cervical spine anomalies.

Craniofacial microsomia

Craniofacial microsomia is the most common term for hemifacial microsomia, first and second branchial arch syndrome, Goldenhaar syndrome, oral-mandibular-auricular syndrome, oculoauriculovertebral syndrome and dysostosis otomandibularis.

It consists of a variable hypoplasia of all craniofacial elements, in particular auricular, mandibular and maxillary hypoplasia, as well as other structures embryologically derived from the first and second branchial arches, such as the facial nerve. These are associated with deficiencies of the skin, muscles and nerves. Thus cleft lip and palate, preauricular skin-tags and sinuses, macrostomia, epibulbar dermoids, cranial nerve palsies (especially facial nerve) and plagiocephaly may all be associated. It is usually unilateral, but 15 per cent of cases are bilateral.

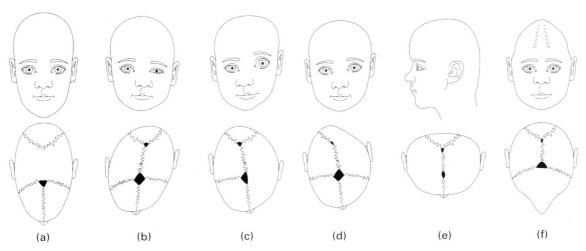

(a)   (b)   (c)   (d)   (e)   (f)

Fig. 15.4 Descriptive names are applied to various head shapes that do not necessarily reflect the aetiology: (a) scaphocephaly ('boat-shaped') with fusion of the sagittal suture; (b–d) plagiocephaly ('flattened forehead') may be due to deformation (b), unilateral coronal synostosis (c), or unilateral lambdoid synostosis (d); (e) brachycephaly ('short head') is usually due to bicoronal synostosis, commonly Apert's or Crouzon's; (f) trigonocephaly (triangular forehead) is seen with isolated metopic suture synostosis.

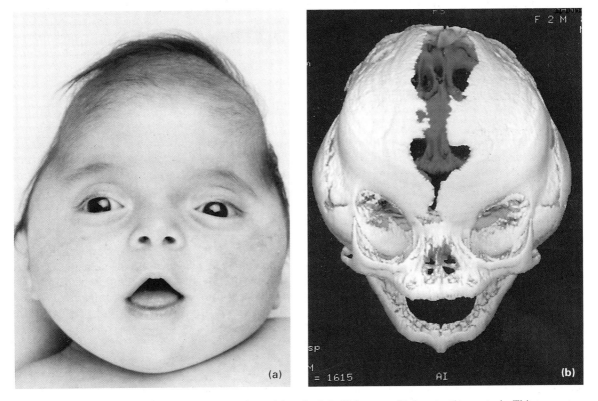

Fig. 15.5 An infant with Kleeblatschadel deformity, or 'cloverleaf skull' due to multiple sutural synostosis. This may occur in several craniofacial syndromes, the commonest being Crouzon's: (a) pre-operative at age three months; (b) 3-D CT scan.

Encephaloceles

Encephaloceles are congenital lesions consisting of a herniation of intracranial contents from the cranial cavity (see Chapter 12). Sincipital (anterior) encephaloceles pass into the face, through the region of the foramen caecum, and may give rise to secondary craniofacial deformities, such as hypertelorism, trigonocephaly, orbital dystopia, elongation of the face and dental malocclusion. Anterior encephaloceles are usually associated with normal intelligence and development.

Facial clefts

Facial clefting is classified into three categories: cleft lip and palate, the Tessier clefts (see Further Reading for details) and bizarre facial clefting.

Clefts may be complete soft tissue and bony clefts, or incomplete. For example, a 0–14 Tessier midline cleft may be incomplete, presenting as a pseudo-encephalocele, as hypertelorism with a bifid nose, or as a complete facial cleft (Fig. 15.6). Defects in the eyebrows may indicate a *forme fruste* facial cleft and a widow's peak in the hairline often points to the cleft.

Bizarre facial clefts fit into no particular pattern and are frequently severe. They are thought to be a disruption produced by amniotic bands.

Craniofacial neoplasia

Neoplasia is rare in the craniofacial region in infants. Benign lesions include fibro-osseous lesions and dermoids. Neoplasms are best treated with a wide resection and reconstruction to prevent local recurrence and secondary growth deforming effects; with utilisation of craniofacial principles this can be achieved without deforming the patient. Ewing's Sarcoma, for example, is treated with induction chemotherapy until the maximum reduction in tumour size is achieved. This is followed by a craniofacial resection of the remaining tumour mass and reconstruction, prior to maintenance chemotherapy, with excellent results. Radiotherapy is avoided, where possible,

as it is frequently associated with deforming growth restriction, as well as the late induction of new tumours.

Trauma

Extensive craniofacial trauma is seen with horse-kick injuries, falls from balconies, bungy-jumping injuries and motor vehicle accidents. Complex fractures are best treated primarily by utilising craniofacial techniques, with an accurate reduction of fractures, rigid fixation with mini-plates, primary bone grafts as required, and reconstruction of all soft tissue layers. Secondary deformities, such as enophthalmos, orbital dystopia and secondary deformities relating to growth (for example, failure to develop a frontal sinus unilaterally due to a fracture of the fronto-orbital region in childhood), are also best addressed with craniofacial techniques.

Management of craniofacial anomalies

Conservative management

Although deformational craniofacial malformations (for example, plagiocephaly) tend to improve spontaneously, many do not completely correct, and severe deformations may have significant residual deformities. All should have plain skull X-rays by experienced radiologists to exclude synostosis. Mild to moderate cases may be reassured and managed with an altered sleeping position; however, severe cases are likely to benefit from helmet moulding. Helmet moulding directs growth, and is thus most effective between 3 and 6 months of age, and of little benefit after 9 months, so early referral for assessment is encouraged. Very severe cases of deformational plagiocephaly may require surgery.

Operative management

Cranial synostosis requires surgery, with suturectomy combined with cranial vault remodelling. The best age for surgery is about 6 months

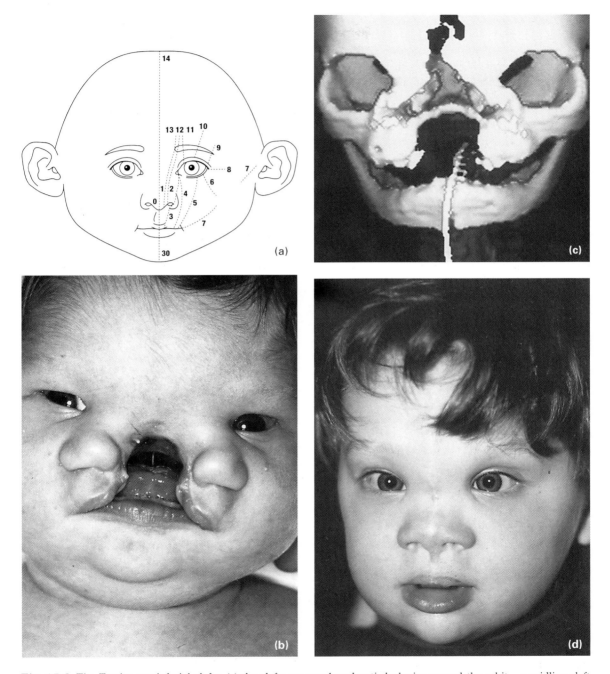

Fig. 15.6 The Tessier craniofacial clefts: (a) the clefts are numbered anti-clockwise around the orbit — a midline cleft below the level of the orbits is a Tessier 0 cleft, and above the level of the orbit a 14 cleft; (b) an example of an 0–14 Tessier cleft; (c) 3-D CT scan with endotracheal tube *in situ*. The bony cleft continues in the 14 position, despite intact skin in this region. Hypertelorism secondary to the cleft is demonstrated; (d) postoperative appearance.

when the secondary growth effects are not too pronounced, and the continuing growth of the brain can be utilised to maintain the normal shape. However, with multiple sutural synostosis and subsequent craniostenosis, such as is seen in Kleeblatschadel deformity, it may be necessary to operate as early as 1 month of age to allow room for the growing brain to develop.

FURTHER READING

Aston S.J., Beasley R.W. & Thorne C.H.M. (eds) (1997) *Grabb and Smith's Plastic Surgery*, 5th edn, Lippincott-Raven, Philadelphia, chaps 19–32.

Dufresne C.R. & Manson P.N. (1990) Pediatric facial trauma In: McCarthy J.G. (ed.) *Plastic Surgery*, Vol. 2, chap. 28, W.B. Saunders, Philadelphia, pp. 1142–87.

Dufresne C.R., Carson B.S. & Ziinereich S.J. (eds) (1992) *Complex Craniofacial Problems*, Churchill Livingstone, New York.

Holmes A.D., Klug G.L. & Breidahl A.F. (1997). The surgical management of osseous cranial base tumours in children. *Aust. NZ J. Surg.* **67**: 722–30.

McCarthy J.G. (ed.) (1990) Cleft lip and craniofacial anomalies. In: *Plastic Surgery,* Vol. 4, W.B. Saunders, Philadelphia, chaps 5–6.

— 16 —

Abnormalities of the Neck and Face

CASE 1

Thomas is 2 years old; he was well until two days ago when he developed fever and a tender lump under the right side of his jaw.

> Q. 1.1   *What is the differential diagnosis?*
>
> Q. 1.2   *Is surgery required, and if so, when?*

CASE 2

Anita was first noticed to have a small, hard lump on her eyebrow at six months. Since then it has grown gradually larger.

> Q. 2.1   *What is the lesion and how is it treated?*

CASE 3

Ahmed (18/12) has a lump under his chin in the midline. It varies in size a little and recently became red and sore.

> Q. 3.1   *What is the differential diagnosis of midline neck lumps?*
>
> Q. 3.2   *What treatment does Ahmed need?*

The neck is one of the commonest sites for cystic and solid swellings during childhood. Lesions are either 'developmental anomalies' arising from remnants of the branchial arches, the thyroglossal tract, the jugular lymphatics or the skin; or 'acquired', as in diseases in the lymph nodes, salivary glands or the thyroid gland (Box 16.1).

BRANCHIAL CYSTS, SINUSES, FISTULAE AND OTHER REMNANTS

These arise from the branchial arch system. Persisting branchial clefts give rise to an epithelial-lined branchial cyst, branchial sinus (blind-ending tract) or branchial fistula (communication between two epithelial-lined surfaces). The branchial arch itself may give rise to mesodermal remnants, usually cartilaginous, lying along the line of development of the arch.

Sinuses and fistulae most commonly arise from the second branchial cleft, occasionally from the first and rarely from the third branchial cleft. In second branchial cleft defects, the tract commences in the tonsillar fossa and passes with the glossopharyngeal nerve between the internal and external carotid arteries to end in the skin at the anterior border of the lower third of the sternomastoid muscle. First, cleft fistulae run from the external auditory canal to the skin below the lower border of the mandible. The rare third

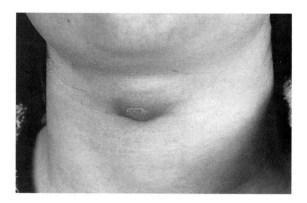

Fig. 16.1 Thyroglossal cyst that has become infected.

> ## Box 16.1 Swellings in the neck
>
> **Developmental anomalies**
>   Branchial cleft: cyst, sinus or fistula
>   Branchial arch: cartilage
>   Thyroglossal cyst
>   Ectopic thyroid
>   Cystic hygroma
>   Epidermal cyst
>
> **Acquired lesions**
>   Inflammation of cervical lymphatics:
>   • acute lymphadenitis

branchial cleft fistula opens internally into the piriform sinus and externally on the skin overlying the lower end of the sternomastoid muscle.

Branchial fistulae usually present in early childhood when a drop of mucus is observed leaking from the external orifice or when a persisting damp patch is noticed on the clothing. Sinuses may present at any time during childhood and sometimes may be complicated by infection. The treatment for both is surgical excision.

Branchial cysts are uncommon in childhood. They usually arise from the second cleft and emerge from beneath the anterior border of the sternomastoid in the upper third of the neck. They may extend upwards behind the angle of the jaw to the base of the skull or antero-inferiorly towards the midline, lying on the carotid sheath. The fluid contents are milky and contain cholesterol crystals. They may become infected and these cysts should be excised.

Branchial arch remnants usually arise from the second branchial arch and present as a skin tag at the anterior border of the lower third of the sternomastoid. These lesions are excised for cosmetic reasons.

THYROGLOSSAL CYST

The descent of the thyroid anlage from the floor of the fetal mouth leaves a track from the foramen caecum of the tongue to the thyroid isthmus. A cyst lined by respiratory epithelium may arise anywhere along the track, but it is usually close to and adherent to the hyoid bone (75 per cent). Typically, there is a tense rounded cyst in the mid-line or just to one side, which moves on swallowing and on protrusion of the tongue. The cysts also may be submental (15 per cent), lingual (2 per cent) and suprasternal (8 per cent) in position. Infection may supervene (Fig. 16.1) and an infected thyroglossal cyst may be mistaken for acute bacterial lymphadenitis in the submental lymph nodes. The thyroglossal cyst and the entire thyroglossal track should be excised, preferably before infection occurs; this excision should include the middle third of the hyoid bone to minimise the risk of recurrence (Sistrunk operation).

ECTOPIC THYROID

Ectopic thyroid is a rare cause of midline neck swelling, as it presents as 'low thyroid function' on neonatal screening. The swelling tends to be softer than that of a thyroglossal cyst, but the diagnosis may not be apparent until at operation, when the lesion is found to be solid and vascular. If this lesion is suspected pre-operatively, a thyroid isotope scan should be performed to determine the distribution of all functioning thyroid because the ectopic thyroid may be the only thyroid tissue present. In this situation it is not excised: the mass is divided in the midline and rotated on its pedicle laterally to lie behind the strap muscles. Other thyroid swellings in children are rare. Neonatal goitre may result from excessive maternal iodine ingestion. Thyrotoxicosis is rare in young children. Adenoma and papillary carcinoma are seen occasionally in older children.

CYSTIC HYGROMA

A cystic hygroma is a hamartoma of the jugular lymph sacs. It presents in infancy and is more common in boys than girls (Fig. 16.2). Cystic hygromas are of two types: either a simple or multicystic lesion merely compressing adjacent structures; or a complex lesion that infiltrates other structures including the mouth, pharynx, larynx or mediastinum, and which may contain cavernous haemangiomatous elements. This type resembles lymphangiomas found elsewhere in the body.

Simple cystic hygromas are commoner, and are usually found as unilateral fluctuant, transilluminable swellings centred on the anterior triangle. The cysts are of varying sizes and contain clear fluid (lymph). They may enlarge suddenly and rapidly, due to viral or bacterial infection or haemorrhage. The effect of this will depend on the site and size of the cysts. A clinical emergency may arise if the increased swelling compromises the airways. In the absence of these complications, surgical excision is undertaken for cosmetic reasons.

Complex cystic hygromas are less common, and complications arise because of extensive soft-tissue involvement. These malformations may involve the oropharynx, leading to difficulty with speech and swallowing, or the larynx and trachea, leading to a life-threatening respiratory obstruction. Involvement of the mediastinum and pleural cavity likewise may lead to respiratory embarrassment. They present on the first day of life and emergency care may necessitate the insertion of an endotracheal tube, and sometimes a tracheostomy. Surgical excision is undertaken early, and involves debulking the lesion.

EPIDERMOID CYSTS

Inclusion dermoids arise from ectodermal cells detached during fetal growth. They are often in the midline or along lines of fusion; for example, the midline cervical dermoid, which may be mistaken for a thyroglossal cyst. They contain sebaceous 'cheesy' material surrounded by squamous epithelium. They enlarge slowly and should be removed. The commonest inclusion dermoid is at the orbital margin (see pp. 121–2).

Less common varieties include the sublingual dermoid that lies between the *mylohyoid* and *genioglossus* muscles in the floor of the mouth. It may interfere with speech and swallowing and can be excised through a submental incision. It may be confused with a ranula or mucocele of the floor of the mouth, which contains mucus.

A rare developmental anomaly of this region is the midline cervical cleft, a vertical open groove that results from failure of fusion of the branchial arches. Surgical repair is undertaken.

PERIORBITAL CELLULITIS

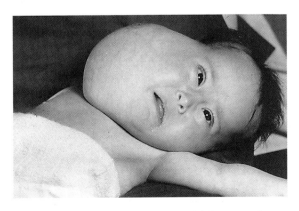

Fig. 16.2 Cystic hygroma in a baby with Down syndrome.

Infection in the soft tissues and sinuses around

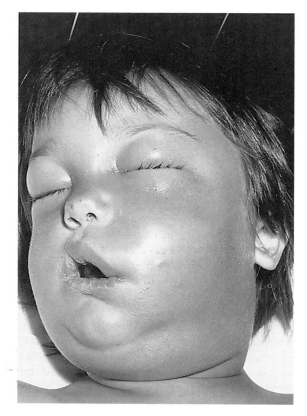

Fig. 16.3 Periorbital cellulitis: sinusitis is the common source of infection.

the eye can cause periorbital cellulitis with rapid extension across the face (Fig. 16.3). The danger with this infection is that it may spread to the cavernous sinus, which is potentially lethal. Children with periorbital cellulitis should be admitted to hospital for ophthalmological assessment and treatment with intravenous antibiotics (Chapter 13), and may need ENT opinion regarding drainage of pus from the orbital cavity (Chapter 14).

DISEASES OF THE LYMPH NODES

Infection is the commonest cause of lymph node enlargement in childhood. It may be caused by bacteria, viruses or non-tuberculous mycobacteria. In many cases the lymph nodes are reacting to an upper respiratory tract or ear infection; this is known as non-specific reactive hyperplasia. Lymph nodes also may become enlarged due to primary or secondary malignancy. A surgical biopsy is indicated when the diagnosis is in doubt, or if lymph nodes are persistently enlarged (> 3 cm) or present for longer than 4 to 6 weeks.

Reactive hyperplasia

Persistently enlarged lymph nodes are seen in many children with frequent upper respiratory tract infections. These nodes are not painful and are a normal response to infection. Occasionally, a markedly enlarged hyperplastic node (> 3 cm) may come to excision biopsy to exclude tumour or other diagnoses.

Acute lymphadenitis

Acutely tender enlarged lymph glands are commonly seen during upper respiratory tract infections. Lymphadenitis usually settles with rest, analgesia and, if bacterial infection is suspected, antibiotics.

Acute lymph node abscess

Lymphadenitis may progress to an abscess, particularly in children aged 6 months to 3 years. The swelling enlarges over 3 or 4 days and may become fluctuant. An abscess in deeper nodes may not exhibit fluctuation. The overlying skin is red and, if untreated, the abscess will eventually point and discharge. The management of an abscess in a child is incision and drainage under general anaesthesia. Damage to the mandibular branch of the facial nerve must be avoided when submandibular abscesses are incised.

'MAIS' lymphadenitis

Mycobacterium avium, *intracellulare* and *scrofulaceum* (MAIS) cause chronic cervical lymphadenitis and 'collar stud' abscesses in children. In most Western countries, human TB and bovine TB strains have been nearly eradicated. However, MAIS lymphadenitis is still a problem in the preschool child. The MAIS mycobacteria are found in the soil and infection is from the child's dirty hand to the mouth and then to the tonsillar or parotid lymph node. Initially the node is enlarged and firm, but non-tender. Over a period of 4 to 6 weeks the node produces a collar stud abscess in the subcutaneous tissue causing the overlying skin to become a characteristic blue-purple colour. Untreated, the collarstud 'cold' abscess will ulcerate through the skin and lead to multiple discharging sinuses. MAIS mycobacteria do not respond to antibiotics and require surgical excision to remove the infected lymph nodes. The mandibular branch of the facial nerve may be at risk during excision of an affected jugulodigastric lymph node. The diagnosis of MAIS lymphadenitis is confirmed by histological examination of the lymph node and culture of the pus and lymph node tissue.

Lymph node tumours

Primary neoplasia

Hodgkin's and non-Hodgkin's lymphomas may occur in cervical lymph nodes in older children.

Secondary neoplasia

Nasopharyngeal and thyroid tumours and neuroblastoma may present with cervical node enlargement. In most cases the marked enlargement and rocky hardness of the lymph nodes makes the diagnosis of neoplasia obvious. In other circumstances the differential diagnosis between a large hyperplastic lymph node and a neoplastic node is difficult and necessitates excision biopsy.

THE SUBMANDIBULAR GLAND

The commonest cause of enlargement is a small calculus in the submandibular duct. It produces rapid and painful enlargement of the gland during eating. The gland becomes hard and tender and fluctuates in size. The submucous part of the duct in the floor of the mouth should be inspected for a tiny calculus impacted near the orifice under the tongue. An X-ray of the floor of the mouth may show an opaque calculus that is too small or too proximal to be seen with the naked eye. The submandibular calculus can be removed by a simple incision of the duct.

THE PAROTID GLAND

Recurrent enlargement is common in the parotid gland and is due to recurrent parotitis associated with sialectasis, a condition analogous to bronchiectasis, which affects the lesser ducts and their tributaries. Parotid calculi are extremely rare.

Symptoms of sialectasis usually commence at 2 to 4 years of age, and the first attack may be misdiagnosed as mumps, although both sides are seldom swollen at the same time. One or both parotids are affected and the attacks are unilateral or alternate from side to side. The gland becomes generally enlarged and mildly tender: fever and malaise are mild or absent.

Purulent fluid issues from the orifice when the duct is compressed, and *Streptococcus viridans* or other weakly pathogenic organisms may be found on culture. The attacks are self-limiting and last 3 to 4 days, but the symptoms may persist intermittently for several years.

The diagnosis is clinical. However, if a sialogram is performed, it will show a snowstorm of sacculations 2 to 4 mm in diameter along the radicles of the gland (Fig. 16.4) but no duct obstruction. The changes are often present in both glands, even when the symptoms have been confined to one side.

The condition is self-limiting and treated by massage of the parotid, tart drinks to promote the flow of saliva and chewing-gum. Most children improve by about 10 years of age, and sialograms during adolescence often show that the sialectasis has disappeared. Parotidectomy is not necessary.

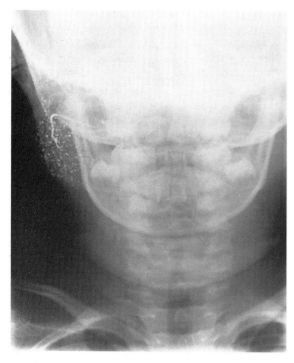

Fig. 16.4 Sialogram showing sialectasis. A contrast X-ray of the parotid duct showing a 'snowstorm' of saccular dilatations of the lesser ducts in the enlarged parotid.

TORTICOLLIS

The common causes of torticollis in infants and children are, in order of frequency:
(1) fibrosis in the sternomastoid muscle
(2) postural torticollis (a legacy of the position *in utero*)
(3) cervical hemivertebrae; and
(4) imbalance of the ocular muscles.
Postural torticollis is present from birth and disappears in a few months. Likewise, the associated plagiocephaly (Chapters 12 and 15) and scoliosis do not require treatment — they are caused by intrauterine moulding.

Cervical hemivertebrae produce a mild angulation of the head and neck. The cause is readily seen in X-rays, which should be taken in all cases of torticollis where the sternomastoid muscle is not tight. No treatment is necessary, for the degree of torticollis is mild and the course is not progressive.

Ocular torticollis is not detectable until the age of 6 months and is usually not noticed until the child is at least 1 or 2 years old. Strabismus suggests that this is the cause, but it is not always obvious and may be latent or intermittent. An ocular imbalance is the most likely cause of torticollis in a child without hemivertebrae, with normal sternomastoid muscles and a full normal range of passive rotation (that is, the chin can be made to touch each acromion). Treatment is the correction of the imbalance by adjusting the attachment of the eye muscles to the globe.

STERNOMASTOID FIBROSIS

This is found in two groups of patients:
(1) Infants 2 to 3 weeks old present with a localized swelling in one sternomastoid muscle; that is, a sternomastoid 'tumour' (Fig. 16.5).
(2) Older children present with torticollis and a tight, short fibrous sternomastoid muscle. Rotation of the head towards the affected side

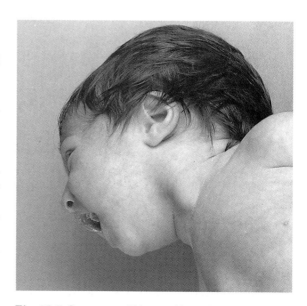

Fig. 16.5 Sternomastoid 'tumour' in an infant.

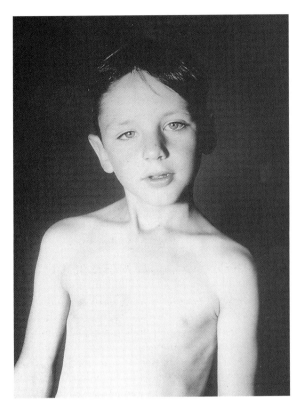

Fig. 16.6 Sternomastoid torticollis. A tight (scarred) right sternomastoid muscle is apparent with secondary hypoplasia of the right side of the face.

is limited, growth of the face on the side of the affected muscle is reduced (hemihypoplasia of the face, Fig. 16.6) and the ipsilateral trapezius muscle is wasted.

The aetiology is unknown, but prenatal or perinatal trauma is suspected in some cases. On histology, there is endomysial fibrosis around individual muscle fibres, which undergo atrophy.

Clinical features

The 'tumour' is so characteristic that it is diagnostic; that is, a hard, painless spindle-shaped swelling 2 to 3 cm long in the substance of the sternomastoid muscle. Sometimes the fibrosis may affect the whole length of the muscle.

Angulation of the head is not always present, and the infant can turn the head towards the opposite side without angulation. Plagiocephaly (Chapters 12 and 15) is evident in the first 3 months of life as a result of this preferred position, and can be limited by putting the infant down to sleep on each side in turn.

Hemihypoplasia of the face (Fig. 16.6) describes the decreased growth of one side that may occur as a non-specific result of any type of immobilisation and is not directly attributable to fibrosis in the sternomastoid.

Treatment

Babies with a sternomastoid 'tumour' should be managed non-operatively because in 90 per cent of cases it will subside completely in 9 to 12 months.

In the remaining few cases the fibrosis causes permanent muscle shortening and persistent torticollis. Division of the sternomastoid muscle is indicated if there is persistent torticollis after the age of 12 months or hemihypoplasia of the face. The symmetry of the face improves after operating but this may take several years; however, it probably never recovers completely.

DEVELOPMENTAL ANOMALIES OF THE FACE

External angular dermoid

This is a common anomaly of fusion between the frontonasal and maxillary processes during formation of the head and face (Chapter 12). The cyst is noticed in infancy as it enlarges gradually and progressively (Fig. 16.7). Often it is beneath the pericranium, which gives it a firmer consistency than may be expected. Occasionally it is misdiagnosed as a bony lump. Excision through a small eyebrow incision is curative.

Many varieties of facial clefts have been described and classified, but most of them are rare. Cleft lip and palate, by contrast, are very common. Clefts are described in Chapter 15.

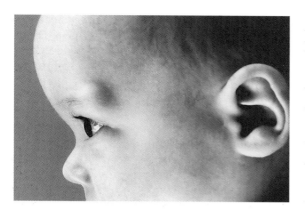

Fig. 16.7 External angular demoid.

Microsomia

Malformations of the structures derived from the first pharyngeal arch may cause microstomia, a misshapen ear, absence of the external auditory canal, a rudimentary middle ear, hypoplasia of the mandible and its teeth, hypoplasia of the malar-maxillary complex and, sometimes, facial paralysis. The condition may be bilateral.

Children with Treacher Collins syndrome have bilateral absence of the malar bone, microtia, colobomata of the eyelids and hypoplasia of the masseter and temporalis muscles. Complex defects of the facial skeleton, such as this, are managed by craniofacial surgery (Chapter 15).

DEFORMITIES OF THE EAR

Accessory auricles

Small tags of skin and cartilage may be present, usually close to the tragus, but sometimes along a line extending to the angle of the mouth. They are removed for cosmetic reasons.

Pre-auricular sinus

This is a common condition (1/50 in children of Asian origin), often bilateral and asymptomatic. There is a tiny hole just in front of the upper crus of the helix, from which an epithelial track extends deeply forwards. The track is often short, but sometimes extends more deeply.

Where there are no symptoms, or only an occasional bead of watery discharge, it is best left alone. If it becomes infected with purulent discharge and the opening becomes sealed, a large abscess may develop. In such cases the abscess should be deroofed and the sinus excised, which is curative.

Microtia

A rudimentary ear of irregular skin and cartilage is associated with absence of the external auditory canal, a rudimentary middle ear and a small mandible on the same side (Fig. 16.8). When the site of the ear is acceptable, it can be used as the basis for reconstruction, which is preferable to an artificial prosthetic ear.

Only when the condition is bilateral is it necessary to create an external auditory canal and it is important to provide a hearing aid within the first few months of life to enable the infant to hear and develop speech. Further operations are required in later years.

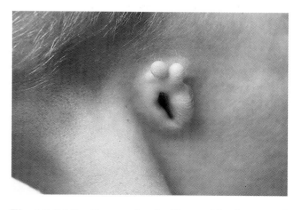

Fig. 16.8 Microtia, associated with a maldevelopment of the dorsal ends of the first and second branchial arches. The external auditory canal is a shallow pit.

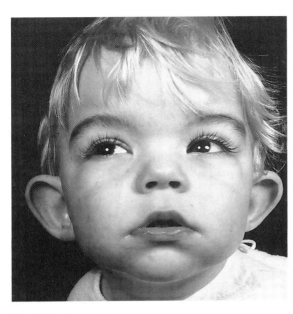

Fig. 16.9 Bat ears.

Bat ears

Bat ears, both unilateral and bilateral, are common and often familial (Fig. 16.9). The concavity of the concha extends to the rim, which stands out farther than normal. The ear is often bigger than normal, as well as more protruberant.

Corrective surgery is advisable when there is gross protrusion, particularly when there are adverse comments from other children. Strapping in the neonatal period achieves nothing, and removal of skin from the post-auricular groove is inadequate. The fold of the antihelix must be fashioned, shaping and fixing the cartilages in a new relationship, and held in position for an approximate period of 3 weeks for the cartilages to unite. Surgery can be performed any time after infancy.

'Shell' ears

Shell ears, like bat ears, protrude from the scalp, but they are small and the rim of the helix is so short that the ear cannot be readily folded back into the normal position. Surgical repair usually has to be done in stages and is much more difficult than in bat ears.

FURTHER READING

Doi O., Hutson J.M., Myers N.A. & McKelvie P.A. (1988) Branchial remnants: a review of 58 cases. *J. Pediatr. Surg.* **23**: 789–92.

Joshi W., Davidson P.M., Jones P.G., Campbell P.E. & Roberston D.M. (1989) Non-tuberculous mycobacterial lymphadenitis in children. *Eur. J. Pediatr.* **148**: 751–4.

Merriman T., Davidson P.M. & Myers N.A. (1992) The spectrum of cervical cystic hygroma. *Pediatr. Surg. Int.* **7**: 253–5.

Muir I.F.K. (ed.) (1987) Other conditions of the face. In: *Plastic Surgery in Paediatrics*, pp. 93–104, Lloyd-Luke (Medical Books) London.

Muir I.F.K. & McKay K.A. (1987) The ear. In: Muir I.F.K. (ed.) *Plastic Surgery in Paeditarics*, pp. 82–92, Lloyd-Luke (Medical Books), London.

Nathanson L.K. & Gough I.R. (1989) Surgery for thyroglossal cysts: Sistrunk's operation remains the standard. *Aust. NZ J. Surg.* **59**: 873–5.

— 17 —

The Umbilicus

CASE 1

The baby appeared normal at birth. The umbilical cord desiccated and detached at 1 week, but a few weeks later the mother noticed an intermittent swelling at the umbilicus, which was covered with skin. It became quite large and the baby would cry often; the parents grew concerned over a possible rupture. The lump often gurgled when compressed, but did not seem to upset the infant.

    Q. 1.1   *Is this lesion dangerous and what is its natural history?*

    Q. 1.2   *Is surgery needed?*

    Q. 1.3   *Why is there a hole in the abdominal wall?*

CASE 2

A week or two after separation of the cord stump, the umbilicus is still slightly red and damp. Despite careful drying the dampness persists and, at 6 weeks, a cherry red mass is seen protruding from the umbilical scar.

    Q. 2.1   *Why is this occurring and how is it treated?*

CASE 3

On the day of birth a small defect is noted near the base of the umbilical cord that drains some fluid. Close inspection reveals a mucosal surface at the site of the defect.

    Q. 3.1   *What are the possible causes of this problem?*

    Q. 3.2   *How are they distinguished and treated?*

CASE 4

A six-year-old boy presents with a small, tender lump 5 cm above the umbilicus. He has a history of recurrent epigastric pains over several years. The mother first noticed the lump in infancy, but did not seek attention as it appeared to be harmless.

    Q. 4.1   *What are the contents of the lump?*

    Q. 4.2   *Is it dangerous?*

    Q. 4.3   *Does it need treatment?*

EMBRYOLOGY

Prior to birth, two umbilical arteries (via internal iliac arteries) and one umbilical vein (via falciform ligament and ductus venosus) form the umbilical cord. Vestigial connections between the midgut and yolk sac (vitello-intestinal duct), and between the bladder and allantois (urachus) may persist. After birth, the cord desiccates and separates and the umbilical ring closes. Delayed contraction of the fibromuscular ring allows the peritoneum and abdominal contents to bulge through the defect. Residual necrotic tissue from the cord stump may be colonised by bacteria to produce a low-grade, subacute infection with a secondary response of granulation tissue formation. Gaps in the criss-crossing fibres of the linea alba superior to the umbilicus may allow extra-peritoneal fat to protrude. When the gap is immediately adjacent to the umbilical scar it may contain a peritoneal sac.

Failure of the normal folding of the embryo to produce the umbilical ring, or rupture of the physiological hernia, may produce the more serious but rare conditions of exomphalos and gastroschisis respectively (Chapter 8).

UMBILICAL HERNIA

Some degree of umbilical herniation is present in almost 20 per cent of newborn babies: this is even more frequent in premature infants, or when there is any increase in intra-abdominal pressure; for example, in ascites, Down Syndrome or cretinism. Because the anomaly occurs after involution of the umbilical cord, associated anomalies are rare, and the hernia is covered by skin and the umbilical cicatrix.

While the infant lies quietly the umbilical skin merely looks redundant. When the infant cries or strains, the bowel fills the hernia and the lesion enlarges to become tense and bluish beneath the thin shiny skin (Fig. 17.1). The bowel can be reduced easily, often with an audible gurgle.

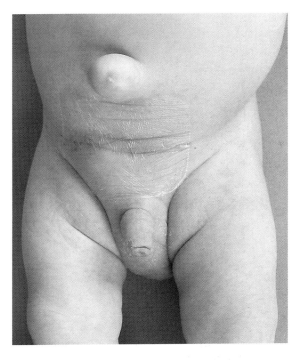

Fig. 17.1 Umbilical hernia in a baby with repaired inguinal hernias.

Most umbilical hernias close spontaneously. However, there are several practical points that must be explained to the parents:
(1) The time of natural closure. In the first 3 to 4 months of life the bulge may actually increase a little before getting smaller. Resolution usually occurs in the first 12 months but it may take up to 3 years.
(2) The skin never ruptures, and the thin skin of the first 4 weeks gradually becomes thicker.
(3) Strangulation is virtually unknown and it is safe to wait. The tenseness of the hernia when the infant cries is often interpreted incorrectly as causing pain: umbilical hernias probably are symptomless.

Treatment

The use of strapping does not induce closure when this would not otherwise have occurred spontaneously, and because strapping may cause complications it is contraindicated.

Surgery should be considered if the hernia is still present after the age of 2 to 3 years.

If the neck of the sac is less than 1 cm in diameter at 12 months of age, eventual spontaneous closure is still likely, and surgery should be deferred until at least 2 to 3 years of age. Even if the neck is 2 cm or more in diameter at 12 months, and spontaneous closure is less likely, surgery is deferred until the third year.

PARA-UMBILICAL HERNIA

This is a defect in the linea alba separate from but adjacent to the umbilical cicatrix. Most are just above the umbilicus, rarely to one side or below it. The defect is a transverse elliptical slit with sharp edges, in contrast to the rounded shape and blunt edges of a central umbilical hernia. Spontaneous closure is unlikely and surgery is required in nearly all cases, as an elective procedure after the first year of life.

EPIGASTRIC HERNIA

Extraperitoneal fat from within the falciform ligament may protrude through a tiny defect in the decussating fibres of the linea alba. The small lump is tender from oedema/ischaemia and it may be missed in obese children. Recurrent, vague epigastric tenderness is the usual presentation. A tender nodule is found in the midline of the epigastrium on careful examination. This is treated by excising the protruding fat and closing the defect in the linea alba.

THE INFANT WITH A DISCHARGE FROM THE UMBILICUS

A discharge from the umbilicus may be pus, urine or faeces.

Purulent discharge

The commonest cause of purulent discharge is a localised infection, and the rarest an abscess in a urachal or vitello-intestinal remnant.

Umbilical sepsis

Umbilical sepsis (omphalitis) is a dangerous infection that occurs in the neonatal period in the exposed stump of the cord. Consequently, an important aspect of preventive medicine is to keep the stump dry and dressed with antiseptics. The commonest causative organisms are *Staphylococci*, *Escherichia coli* and *Streptococci*. In minor infections, the navel is red and swollen with a seropurulent discharge, but responds well to local and systemic antibiotics.

There may be little superficial evidence of inflammation when infection has spread further, via lymphatics or the umbilical vessels. Drainage of any abscess and local and general antibiotics are required. Septicaemia and/or peritonitis result when organisms enter the bloodstream through the superficial vessels, or through the recently patent vessels in the umbilicus: the two umbilical arteries retain a lumen for some time after birth and provide a route of infection to the internal iliac arteries. An abscess along this pathway is more common than entry of micro-organisms into the circulation or into the peritoneal cavity.

Infection can also travel along the lumen of the umbilical vein to the portal vein and via the ductus venosus to the vena cava. Clinically overt infections in these structures are rare but serious, and latent infection can lead to thrombophlebitis and thrombosis of a segment of portal vein. Portal hypertension ensues with recanalization and opening collaterals, leading to a cavernomatous malformation of the portal vein.

Umbilical granuloma

An umbilical granuloma is an extremely common lesion that presents as a small mass of heaped cherry-red granulations, accompanied by a seropurulent discharge. It is granulation tissue produced in response to subacute bacterial colonization of the cord stump. If there is a definite stalk, it can be ligated without anaesthesia, but if it is soft, deep or too broad, topical application of silver nitrate will enable epithelium to cover the surface and it is curative. Sometimes, a small area of ectopic bowel mucosa at the base of the umbilicus has a similar clinical appearance and is treated in the same way (see below).

URINARY DISCHARGE

Urinary discharge from the umbilicus results from a rare persistent communication through the urachus to the bladder (Fig. 17.2). Persistent urachus may occur in association with obstruction in the lower urinary tract, for example, posterior urethral valves, and occasionally with imperforate anus.

The surgical treatment is excision of the urachal remnant after investigation and treatment of any underlying anomalies.

A mass or abscess in the midline, at or below the umbilicus, also may develop from a partly obliterated urachus; drainage and excision are required.

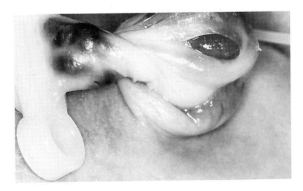

Fig. 17.2 A patent vitello-intestinal duct and patent urachus may look similar: the diagnosis depends on whether the discharge is urinary or faecal.

MUCOUS OR FAECAL DISCHARGE

Ectopic mucosa

Discharge of mucus from the umbilicus may be caused by a small sequestrated nodule of ectopic alimentary mucosa, which appears shiny, spherical, bright red and is situated in the depths of the umbilical cicatrix. Crusts form on the cicatrix and surrounding skin, and a persistent vitello-intestinal (omphalomesenteric) tract may be suspected.

Careful inspection will show the 'pseudopolyp', and the application of silver nitrate on one or two occasions is all that is needed to remove the alimentary epithelium, which is replaced rapidly by normal skin.

Persistent vitello-intestinal duct

Persistence of the vitello-intestinal (omphalo-mesenteric) duct, a rare condition, produces a communication between the intestinal tract and the umbilicus, reflecting the embryonic communication between the yolk sac and the mid-gut that normally disappears at about the sixth week of fetal life. Persistence of part or all of this tract gives rise to a group of lesions that usually present in early infancy, but on occasions not until some years later.

A vitello-intestinal duct represents patency of the whole tract, and the contents of the ileum may discharge intermittently. Very rarely, when the channel is short and broad, the ileum may intussuscept through it on to the surface of the umbilicus as a Y-shaped segment of bowel, inside out, with two orifices.

A sinus or cyst is the result of partial obliteration of the duct; these may become infected, form an abscess and discharge pus.

A vitello-intestinal band is the remnant of the duct and runs from the deep surface of the umbilicus to the ileum. It may cause no symptoms throughout life or it may, at any age, cause intestinal obstruction when a loop of bowel becomes entangled beneath it.

Meckel's diverticulum is the patent inner segment of the duct, and very rarely a band attaches it to the underside of the umbilicus. The presenting features and complications are described in Chapter 23.

All remnants of the vitello-intestinal duct are excised, which may necessitate a laparotomy to search for discontinuous segments of the tract.

FURTHER READING

Campbell J., Beasley S.W., McMullin N.D. & Hutson J.M. (1986) Umbilical swellings and discharges in children. *Med. J. Aust.* **145**: 450–3.

Cilley R.E. & Krummel T.M. (1998) Disorders of the umbilicus. In: O'Neill J.A., Rowe M.I., Grosfeld J.L., Fonkalsrud E.W. & Coran A.G. (eds) *Pediatric Surgery*, 5th edn, Mosby, St. Louis, pp. 1029–44.

— 18 —

Vomiting in the First Months of Life

CASE 1

Trevor, a 4-week-old breast-fed boy, was completely well until two days before presentation, when he began vomiting all feeds. He was otherwise well, and keen to feed despite the non-bile-stained vomiting. He had lost weight and had few wet nappies.

> *Q. 1.1*   *What physical signs would you wish to elucidate to confirm the diagnosis you suspect?*
>
> *Q. 1.2*   *If you were unable to demonstrate these signs, what would you do if you still suspected the diagnosis?*
>
> *Q. 1.3*   *What initial investigation would you perform to assist you in resuscitation?*

CASE 2

A 9-day-old girl, Iris, suddenly began severe bile-stained vomiting. There were no groin swellings. She would not feed. Previously, she had been completely well.

> *Q. 2.1*   *What diagnosis would you wish to exclude urgently?*
>
> *Q. 2.2*   *How would you do this?*
>
> *Q. 2.3*   *If this diagnosis was confirmed, what treatment is required and how urgent would it be?*

CASE 3

A 3-month-old boy, George, was always vomiting, irrespective of how frequently he fed. He had been breast-fed initially; now he was bottle-fed and his grandmother assisted with night-feeds. The vomitus was small volumes of milk. He was not distressed by the vomiting, weighed 8 kg and was growing well.

> *Q. 3.1*   *What is the most likely diagnosis?*
>
> *Q. 3.2*   *What measures could be suggested to reduce the vomiting?*

Box 18.1 Causes of vomiting at 1 month of age

Septic	Meningitis
	Urinary tract infection
	Septicaemia
Mechanical	Gastro-oesophageal reflux
	Pyloric stenosis
	Strangulated inguinal hernia
	Malrotation with volvulus
	(bile-stained vomitus)
Other	Overfeeding
	Congenital adrenal hyperplasia

Vomiting is common in the first months of life, when the evaluation of its significance is particularly important. The temptation to disregard it must be resisted: it is a symptom, not a diagnosis, and its cause must be established (Box 18.1).

Vomiting is significant when it is:

(1) bile-stained
(2) persistent
(3) projectile
(4) blood-stained; that is, 'coffee grounds', flecked with altered blood
(5) accompanied by loss of weight or failure to gain weight.

Vomiting most commonly is due to non-surgical conditions or feeding difficulties. Neonatal infections, for example, septicaemia, meningitis or urinary tract infection, may present with a wide variety of clinical features, including vomiting, convulsions, diarrhoea, pallor, cyanosis and hypothermia. Gastroenteritis may be seen in bottle-fed babies but is uncommon in fully breast-fed infants. In approximately 25 per cent of those with the rare syndrome of congenital adrenal hyperplasia there is a salt-losing metabolic disturbance with severe vomiting and genital abnormalities in females (Chapter 10).

Malrotation with volvulus is a rare but dangerous cause of vomiting. It usually presents in the first week or so of life with bile-stained vomiting, but may occur at any age. The possibility of malrotation with volvulus must be entertained in any child with a sudden onset of green vomiting. An urgent barium meal will diagnose malrotation. If volvulus goes unrecognised the entire mid-gut may be lost from ischaemia and the child will die (Chapter 7).

Strangulated inguinal hernias are common in infants and they are easily diagnosed on examination. A hard, tender irreducible swelling at the external inguinal ring will confirm the diagnosis.

PYLORIC STENOSIS

Pyloric stenosis is the most common cause of vomiting that requires surgery in infants, and it affects 1 : 450 children of whom 85 per cent are boys.

Congenital hypertrophic pyloric stenosis is an important surgical condition in infancy because it is common, there is a risk to life and permanent relief is obtained by a relatively simple operation. The aetiology remains obscure and is partly genetic. Almost 20 per cent of cases have a family history of pyloric stenosis.

Symptoms

The usual presentation is with severe vomiting, which commences between 3 and 6 weeks of age in an otherwise well baby. Pyloric stenosis is rare in infants younger than 10 days or older than 11 weeks.

The vomiting occurs after all feeds and is copious. The vomitus contains milk with some added gastric mucus, and is practically never bile-stained. It may contain some brown coffee-ground flecks of altered blood, reflecting the gastritis secondary to the gastric outlet obstruction. Often the vomiting is projectile, and may occur well after the last feed. Initially, the child is active and hungry, and a key feature is his readiness and ability to feed again immediately after vomiting. Later, with increasing dehydration and electrolye

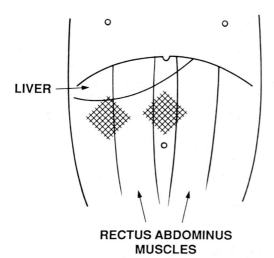

LIVER

RECTUS ABDOMINUS
MUSCLES

Fig. 18.1 Schema showing the two places to palpate a pyloric tumour.

imbalance, he becomes weak, lethargic and listless, not unlike the clinical picture seen in a child with sepsis. He loses weight and looks malnourished. If untreated, he may ultimately die of dehydration and metabolic alkalosis.

Signs

Peristaltic waves of gastric contraction indicate hypertrophy of the gastric muscle secondary to slowly progressive obstruction: their presence makes pyloric stenosis very likely. Palpation of the thickened pylorus in the epigastrium, however, confirms the diagnosis. The hypertrophic and thickened pylorus is traditionally called a 'pyloric tumour'. It feels like an olive or a small pebble and has been likened to the terminal segment of the little finger. It is relatively mobile. It is palpable most easily in the angle between the liver and the lateral margin of the right rectus abdominus muscle or in the gap between the two recti midway between the umbilicus and the xiphisternum (Fig. 18.1). It is felt most easily when the baby is relaxed and not crying, and when the stomach is empty. When difficulty is experienced in feeling the 'tumour', a nasogastric tube should be passed to empty the stomach.

Box 18.2 Tips in palpating pyloric tumours

1   Help the baby relax
    • be patient
    • repeat examination
    • flex hips
    • wait until crying stops or the infant is asleep
    • allow it to feed or suck a dummy
    • palpate at the start of a feed.

2   Empty stomach
    • pass NG tube to empty stomach.

3   Is the diagnosis wrong?
    • check for sepsis/hernias if peristaltic waves are absent.

4   Is pyloric stenosis suspected (because gastric peristalsis is present) but tumour not felt?
    • ultrasonography
    • barium meal.

Failure to palpate the pyloric tumour

If the initial palpation is not conclusive, further observation is necessary and a second examination is made a few hours later. Other manoeuvres that may assist in the palpation of an elusive pyloric tumour are summarised in Box 18.2. When no tumour can be palpated and septic causes of vomiting have been excluded, a paediatric surgeon should be consulted, or radiological investigation may be required. Real-time ultrasonography may identify the hypertrophied pylorus (Fig. 18.2). A barium contrast meal performed under fluoroscopic control may show gastric outlet obstruction (Fig. 18.3) and may show other pathology, including gastro-oesophageal reflux. These investigations are required in a small minority of cases only.

The diagnosis may be delayed because vomiting has been attributed to a pre-existing

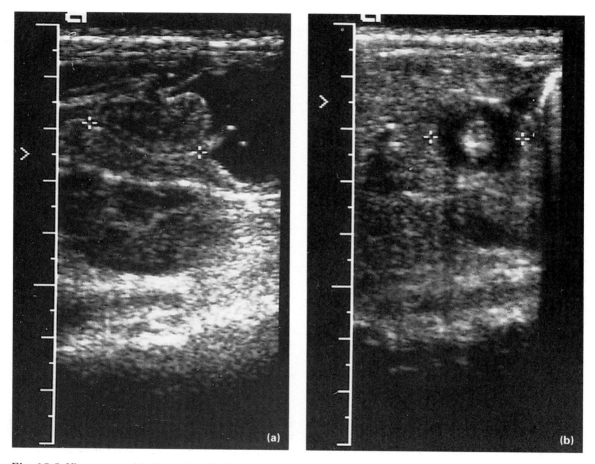

Fig. 18.2 Ultrasonographic diagnosis of pyloric stenosis shows the thickened circular pyloric muscle in (a) longitudinal and (b) the transverse plane.

gastro-oesophageal reflux (which is extremely common in infants) or to feeding problems. Often there is a history of several changes in feeding patterns before the diagnosis is made. However, the palpation of a tumour is the *sine qua non* of diagnosis and excludes all other causes. Features such as visible gastric peristalsis are supporting evidence sufficient to warrant referral to a paediatric surgeon.

Investigation

The history and clinical findings reveal the degree of dehydration. The extent of the electrolyte and acid-base imbalance must be determined to guide appropriate resuscitation before operation. Further estimations of the serum electrolytes and acid-base parameters after resuscitation should confirm complete correction of the electrolyte disturbance before surgery.

Treatment

Treatment involves the correction of the fluid and electrolyte abnormality followed by pyloromyotomy, the Ramstedt operation. These infants should be resuscitated with 0.45 per cent sodium chloride in 5 per cent dextrose with supplementary potassium

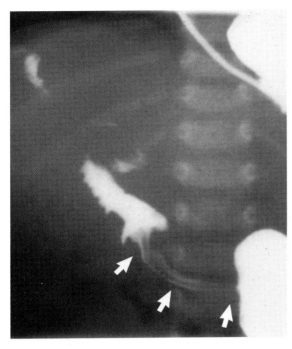

Fig. 18.3 Pyloric stenosis in a barium meal, showing the 'string sign'. The greatly narrowed pyloric canal (arrows) causes gastric outlet obstruction.

chloride. The rate of infusion is determined after estimation of the percentage dehydration, weight of the infant and maintenance requirements.

The Ramstedt operation involves splitting the hypertrophied pyloric muscle as far as the mucosa, enabling it to bulge through the gap, thus providing a wider channel into the duodenum. The best results are obtained when the muscle split includes the distal 1 cm of antrum. Normal oral feeds can be commenced 24 hours after the operation. The babies rapidly regain their lost weight.

GASTRO-OESOPHAGEAL REFLUX

Incompetence of the sphincteric mechanism at the oesophago-gastric junction causes vomiting in the neonatal period and tends to become less severe as the infant gets older. Vomiting occurs at any time during or between feeds and usually is neither projectile nor bile-stained. If oesophagitis is present, bleeding may occur as bright blood in the vomitus, or more commonly, as 'coffee ground' flecks of altered blood. In some infants severe gastro-oesophageal reflux is associated with repeated episodes of aspiration and pneumonia, or failure to thrive.

Gastro-oesophageal reflux affects many infants and the diagnosis is made on clinical grounds.

Management

There is a natural tendency towards spontaneous improvement with age. For this reason, the initial treatment should be conservative, including putting the infant prone with the head of the cot elevated on blocks. Thickening of feeds, Cisapride®, the use of mild antacids — Gaviscon® — and Maxolon® also may be helpful.

In severe cases, where there is evidence of oesophagitis, oesophageal stricture, anaemia, respiratory symptoms or failure to thrive, a barium swallow is advisable to confirm the presence of gastro-oesophageal reflux and to demonstrate any oesophageal stricture (Fig. 18.4).

Oesophagoscopy and oesophageal biopsy should be performed if haematemesis has occurred or when anaemia is present, to assess the extent and severity of the peptic oesophagitis, or when a barium swallow shows evidence of oesophageal obstruction. Further information may be gained from 24-hour pH monitoring and oesophageal manometry.

Surgery to control the reflux is indicated if the conservative regime fails, or there is an oesophageal stricture, or if a large 'sliding' hernia is present. This involves plication of the fundus of the stomach around the lower oesophagus (Nissen fundoplication), a procedure that can be performed laparoscopically. The oesophageal hiatus is repaired at the same time. Oesophageal strictures secondary to reflux normally resolve spontaneously once the reflux has been eliminated.

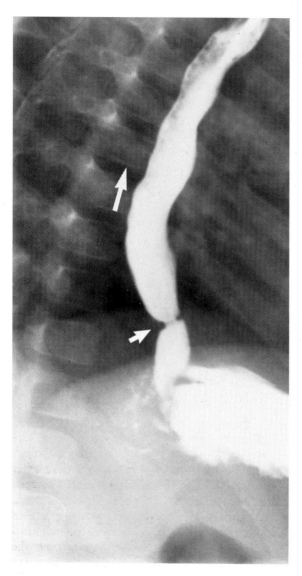

Fig. 18.4 Severe gastro-oesophageal reflux with an oesophageal stricture secondary to reflux oesophagitis (small arrow). The contrast can be seen to flow freely up the oesophagus (arrow).

FURTHER READING

Beasley S.W., Hudson I., Hok Psan Yuen & Jones P.G. (1986) Influence of age, sex, duration of symptoms and dehydration on serum electrolytes in hypertrophic pyloric stenosis. *Aust. Paediatr. J.* **22**: 193–7.

Hutson J.M. & Beasley S.W. (1988) Non-bile-stained vomiting in infancy. In: *The Surgical Examination of Children*, pp. 71–6, Heinemann Medical, Oxford.

Kobayashi H., Webster T. & Puri P. (1997) Age-related changes in innervation in hypertrophic pyloric stenosis. *J. Pediatr. Surg.* **32**: 1704–7

Ohshiro K. & Puri P. (1998) Pathogenesis of infantile hypertrophic pyloric stenosis: recent progress. *Pediatr. Surg. Int.* **13**: 243–52.

Rasmussen L., Anderson O.P. & Pedersen S.A. (1990) Intestinal malrotation and volvulus in infancy. *Pediatr. Surg. Int.* **5**: 27–9.

— 19 —

Intussusception

CASE 1

A 5-month-old boy is brought to you with a 48-hour history of being unwell and vomiting. At times he appears to have been in severe pain. He looks pale and lethargic. There is a vague impression of a mass on the right side of his abdomen.

Q. 1.1   *What is the likely diagnosis?*

Q. 1.2   *How can the diagnosis be confirmed?*

Q. 1.3   *Once treated, is it likely to happen again?*

CASE 2

Annabel, a 7-month-old infant, has been unwell for 5 days: she initially seemed irritable, vomited and refused further feeds, and became listless and dry. Her mother measured her temperature at 37.8°C. She has had few dirty nappies and has developed a distended and tender abdomen. There are no hernias.

Q. 2.1   *What surgical condition would be in your differential diagnosis?*

Q. 2.2   *What would be the initial management of this child?*

Q. 2.3   *What is the likely definitive treatment that will be required?*

In intussusception one segment of the bowel passes onwards inside the adjacent distal bowel. Once this telescoping phenomenon becomes established intestinal obstruction follows. Intussusception represents one of the more common surgical emergencies in the first 2 years of life.

AETIOLOGY

In 90 per cent of episodes there is no obvious cause (so-called 'idiopathic intussusception'), although in older children there is more likely to be a pathological lesion at the lead point of the intussusceptum; for example, a Meckel's diverticulum, a polyp or a duplication cyst.

In idiopathic intussusception, which usually affects infants, it is possible that enlarged submucosal lymphoid tissue in the distal ileum (Peyer's patch) becomes oedematous or undergoes reactive hyperplasia, possibly as the result of a viral infection, and becomes the apex of the intussusception. The apex moves through the ileocaecal valve into the colon and occasionally may reach the anus.

INCIDENCE

The peak incidence is in infants 4 to 7 months old, and 70 per cent of patients are between 3 and 12 months of age. Boys are affected more frequently than girls.

CLINICAL FEATURES (BOX 19.1)

Symptoms

Pain is the most important symptom (85 per cent) that typically commences as a colicky pain lasting 2 to 3 minutes during which the infant screams and draws up his or her knees. Spasms occur at intervals of 15 to 20 minutes. The infant becomes pale, clammy, exhausted and lethargic between

---

Box 19.1 Presenting features of intussusception

(1) Vomiting

(2) Abdominal colic

(3) Pallor

(4) Lethargy

(5) Abdominal mass

(6) Rectal bleeding

---

spasms. After 12 hours or so, the pain becomes more continuous.

Vomiting, the most frequent symptom, usually occurs once or twice in the first hours, and then reappears once the intestinal obstruction is fully established.

Signs

The children look pale and lethargic and are intermittently aroused by a spasm of severe pain. A mass (sometimes described as being 'sausage-shaped') is palpable in more than half the infants and is usually found in the right hypochondrium, although it may be anywhere between the line of the colon and the umbilicus (Fig. 19.1). The intussusception mass is felt most easily early in the course of the disease, before abdominal distension and increasing abdominal tenderness conceal it.

Normal or loose stools are often passed at or soon after the onset of symptoms, but any diarrhoea is of small volume and short duration. About half the patients pass a stool containing blood and mucus ('red currant jelly'), formed by the diapedesis of red cells through the congested

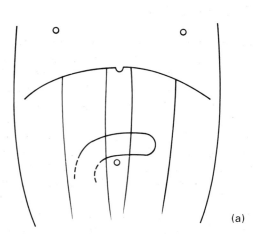

(a)

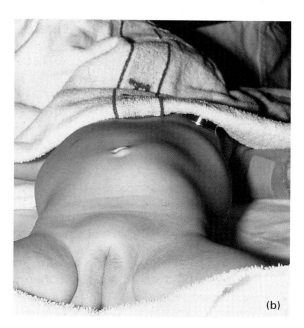

(b)

Fig. 19.1 The site of the sausage-shaped intussusception in the abdomen, shown schematically in (a) and in a patient (b).

mucosa of the intussusceptum. Blood may be identified on the glove following rectal examination in many patients. Rectal examination may disclose the apex of the intussusceptum within the rectum.

The infant is pale, limp and tired and has a tachycardia. If there is a delay in diagnosis the infant will become dehydrated, listless, febrile, have abdominal distension and look ill. These are late signs and the diagnosis should be made before they appear.

Differential diagnosis

Wind colic is common in the first 3 months of life but rarely lasts more than an hour and usually is not accompanied by vomiting. Persisting severe colic for more than 1 to 2 hours should arouse suspicion of an intussusception, particularly if accompanied by vomiting.

Gastroenteritis

Colic and the passage of blood and mucus in severe cases of gastroenteritis may mimic intussusception, except that the volume of diarrhoea is greater. In intussusception, the small loose stools passed early in the course of the disease simply represent evacuation of the colon distal to the obstruction. Persistent vomiting and pain without diarrhoea is unlikely to be gastroenteritis.

A strangulated inguinal hernia may present with abdominal pain, vomiting and distension, but is recognised easily on examination of the groins.

Investigations

A plain X-ray of the abdomen may be normal, show non-specific abnormality, or reveal a small bowel obstruction with air-fluid in the dilated small bowel. Occasionally, the apex of the intussusceptum can be seen (Fig. 19.2).

An air or barium contrast study will not only confirm the diagnosis, it also will be therapeutic. The diagnosis can be made on ultrasonography as well.

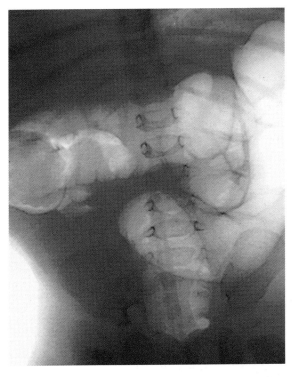

Fig. 19.2 Gas enema showing end of intussusception, which confirms the diagnosis of intussusception.

TREATMENT

Enema reduction of intussusception should be attempted in most cases, unless there is clinical evidence of dead bowel as demonstrated by peritonitis or septicaemia. Gas (air or oxygen) is more effective and probably safer than barium, and is the medium of choice if available (Fig. 19.2). Successful enema reduction is slightly less likely if there is a long duration of symptoms (> 24 hours), age extremes (< 3 months or > 24 months), or when there is an established small bowel obstruction with air-fluid levels on X-ray. If the child remains stable clinically after incomplete reduction on a first attempt, a delayed repeat enema 30 minutes to 2 hours later is performed.

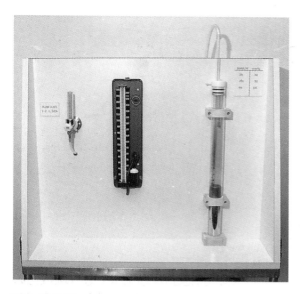

Fig. 19.3 The oxygen enema apparatus currently in use at the Royal Children's Hospital uses oxygen from the wall supply. There is an overflow valve so that the pressure cannot rise above a predetermined level (reproduced with permission from Phelan *et al.* 1988).

Technique of gas enema reduction

The infants should be resuscitated with intravenous fluids and kept warm. A Foley catheter is inserted into the rectum and the balloon inflated. The buttocks are strapped tightly together. Gas (usually oxygen from the wall supply) is introduced into the colon through the catheter, the pressure being controlled by a manometer (Fig. 19.3). Under continuous fluoroscopic control, progress of the reduction is monitored. Sudden filling of the small bowel with gas suggests reduction is complete. The infant can be fed within hours of the procedure.

Surgery

Surgery is indicated when the delayed repeat enema fails to reduce the intussusception, where there is peritonitis clinically or where there is strong evidence of a pathological lesion at the leadpoint; for example, circumoral pigmentation of Peutz–Jegher's syndrome. A laparotomy is performed through a transverse right supra-umbilical incision. The intussusception is reduced manually and resection may be required if there is gangrene, or for a pathological lesion at the leadpoint; for example, Meckel's diverticulum or polyp.

RECURRENT INTUSSUSCEPTION

Recurrence of intussusception occurs in about 7 per cent of patients. It is more likely after enema reduction than surgery. It usually occurs within 2 or 3 days of the first reduction. Recurrent intussusception usually presents early and is treated the same way as a first episode. The possibility of a lesion at the leadpoint should be considered.

FURTHER READING

Beasley S.W. (1996) Intussusception. In: Puri P. (ed.) *Newborn Surgery*, Butterworth-Heinemann, pp. 404–7.

Beasley S.W., Hutson J.M. & Auldist A.W. (1996) Intussusception. In: *Essential Pediatric Surgery*, Arnold, London, pp. 45–51.

Doody D.P. (1997) Intussusception. In: Oldham K.T. *et al.* (eds) *Surgery of Infants and Children: Scientific Principles and Practice*, Lippincott-Raven, Philadelphia, pp. 1241–8.

Hutson J.M. & Beasley S.W. (1988) Colic. In: *The Surgical Examination of Children*, pp. 77–84, Heinemann Medical, Oxford.

Ong N.-T. & Beasley S.W. (1990) The leadpont in intussusception. *J. Pediatr. Surg.* **25**: 640–3.

Phelan E., de Campo J.F. & Malecky G. (1988) Comparison of oxygen and barium reduction of ileocolic intussusception. *Amer. J. Radiol.* **150**: 1349–52.

Young D.G. (1998) Intussusception In: O'Neill J.A. & Rowe M.I. *et al.* (eds) *Pediatric Surgery*, 5th edn, Mosby, St. Louis, pp. 1185–97.

— 20 —

Abdominal Pain: Appendicitis?

CASE 1

Jeremy, a 6-year-old, developed central abdominal pain and high fever yesterday. Today he presents with pain in the right iliac fossa. He looks flushed and has tenderness in both iliac fossae (R > L), but no peritonism. There is a 'gurgle' on deep palpation.

> Q. 1.1   *What is the likely diagnosis?*
>
> Q. 1.2   *What tests are required?*

CASE 2

Alex, a 5-year-old, has been vaguely unwell with abdominal pain for two days. Today he has pain in the right iliac fossa. He limps into the consulting room but does not look flushed, and his temperature is normal (37.2°C). There is tenderness and guarding very lateral in the right flank.

> Q. 2.1   *What is the likely diagnosis?*
>
> Q. 2.2   *Is a rectal examination necessary?*

The knowledge that delay in diagnosis of appendicitis is potentially dangerous has probably been a major factor in reducing its morbidity in children. As a rule, abdominal pain in childhood lasting more than 3 to 4 hours should be regarded as evidence of a potential abdominal emergency until proven otherwise. Likewise, diarrhoea lasting more than 24 hours should suggest the possibility of a pelvic, retrocaecal or retroileal appendicitis, and even in gastroenteritis, diarrhoea does not preclude the possibility that appendicitis has supervened. Only a minority of children presenting with these features are found to have a genuine surgical cause. Where there is a high index of suspicion of appendicitis the child must be reassessed frequently with early referral to a paediatric surgeon.

THE INTERPRETATION OF ABDOMINAL PAIN IN CHILDREN

The presence of significant abdominal pain in small children tends to be recognised late by parents and professionals alike, largely because of young children's inability to voice their symptoms adequately, and partly because the pain of appendicitis may not be dramatic in this age-group.

If the infant shows unnatural immobility, refuses to be cuddled, wants to be left untouched and is reluctant to be examined, this suggests that movement exacerbates the pain, as in peritonitis.

If abdominal pain is persistent, observation must be continued and re-examination repeated until there are definite signs that indicate surgery, or until the pain has subsided. In most children whose pain is subsiding an operation should be deferred if the physical signs are not completely diagnostic.

ASSESSMENT OF PHYSICAL FINDINGS

Examination of the older co-operative child is straightforward, whereas in a young, sick and frightened child it requires great skill. The examination must be unhurried and gentle, and performed with warm hands, with the examiner seated beside the child. The child should be supine, straight and with arms at the side. Useful assessment can sometimes be made if the child is asleep when first seen or, in the toddler, if the abdomen is palpated from behind with both hands while the mother cuddles the child's front against her. However, with a continually crying child, adequate assessment is difficult and re-examination must be undertaken a short time later. Failure to acknowledge inadequate examination is likely to result in serious diagnostic delay.

Abdominal tenderness

Localised tenderness is found in conditions ranging from excess flatus, an overloaded colon or inflamed mesenteric lymph nodes, to acute appendicitis and strangulated gut; so that tenderness alone is an inadequate basis for operation.

In children, localised tenderness can be elicited by direct palpation over any distended or inflamed loop of the gut. This is a particular feature of the solitary distended loop in intestinal obstruction, but can also be observed in gastroenteritis. Irritated or inflamed visceral peritoneum will produce tenderness by direct, rather than by reflex, pathways.

Localised tenderness in the right iliac fossa, without guarding or a strongly suggestive clinical history, may be due to causes other than appendicitis. Although localised tenderness is often the earliest sign of appendicitis, children requiring operation soon develop guarding to support the diagnosis, whereas tenderness due to non-surgical conditions subsides in 1 to 2 days.

Guarding

Children with local or general peritonitis rarely display the board-like rigidity so often found in adults. More often there is a variable degree of involuntary increased muscle resistance, referred to as 'guarding'. Small differences in resistance in the lower and upper abdomen, or between right and left sides, may be significant when the findings are consistent.

Assessment of percussion tenderness is a sensitive test of peritoneal irritation in children. Likewise, pain in the abdomen during micturition is common in pelvic appendicitis, where the appendix lies close to the bladder.

There are no pathognomonic symptoms or signs of appendicitis itself, but when signs of peritonitis are localised to the right iliac fossa, appendicitis is likely.

Acute appendicitis may be missed when it presents with signs of local peritonitis other than in the right iliac fossa; the interposition of other tissues between the appendix and the anterior abdominal wall in pelvic, retrocaecal and retroileal appendicitis delays the appearance of abdominal signs until relatively late, and even then they may be atypical.

In retrocaecal appendicitis the signs are high and lateral on the right side, whereas in pelvic appendicitis, or in retroileal appendicitis, the signs are more central or may even be predominantly left-sided.

A palpable mass

Apart from faecal masses and symptomless masses in the loin (Chapter 25), the most common mass in the abdomen in childhood is an appendiceal abscess, particularly in children under 5 years of age, in the mentally handicapped child, or when the appendix is in an unusual position.

Rectal examination

When appendicitis has been diagnosed on the basis of the history and anterior abdominal signs, a rectal examination is not indicated. However, rectal examination is mandatory when: (i) the signs are equivocal; (ii) ovarian pathology is suspected; (iii) low and diffuse tenderness suggests pelvic appendicitis; or (iv) the duration of symptoms or the passage of blood, mucus or diarrhoea suggests a pelvic collection.

The lateral position is traditional in small children, but more information may be obtained when the digital examination is performed with the child in the dorsal position, combined wherever possible with bimanual palpation. It must be done gently: rectal palpation causes some stretching of the anal canal and sphincters, and pain from this source may be misinterpreted as pelvic or peritoneal tenderness. The little finger is used in small children. The parents should be informed about the rectal examination and should be present when it is performed.

The use of an enema

When the differential diagnosis includes constipation in a child with equivocal abdominal symptoms and signs, an enema may prove both diagnostic and therapeutic. There is no evidence that an enema is dangerous in early acute appendicitis.

Signs arising in other systems

Infections in the ear, the tonsils or the respiratory passages may be accompanied by abdominal pain and vomiting and may simulate an abdominal emergency. Measles or chicken-pox may produce abdominal signs, as can a wide range of viral infections, by causing mesenteric lymphadenitis. Acute appendicitis can coexist with other conditions, so that the finding of pneumonia, tonsillitis or generalised lymphadenopathy should not divert attention from any abdominal signs that also may be present. Similarly, gastroenteritis may progress to appendicitis, so that even a well-established and undoubted diagnosis of gastroenteritis should be subject to review. Special diagnostic difficulties can be presented by the abdominal crisis of diabetic acidosis, Henoch–Schönlein purpura and various haematological disorders, including haemophilia — in all of which surgical intervention generally is contra-indicated.

Repeated observation and re-examination for signs of peritoneal irritation is essential.

ACUTE APPENDICITIS

The mortality of acute appendicitis in children is less than 0.2 per cent, due to early diagnosis and the management of fluids and electrolytes before and after operation.

Clinical diagnosis

The abdominal findings are the crucial factors on which the diagnosis and the decision to operate is made. The value of history lies in arousing suspicion that an abdominal emergency is present, and in determining its most likely cause.

The clinical diagnosis is determined by the presence of objective signs of local or general peritonitis. However, acute appendicitis is not only a common abdominal emergency, but also a great imitator, and it may appear in a variety of guises (Box 20.1).

Differential diagnosis

A perforated appendix is the only common cause of general peritonitis in childhood. In most children with an appendiceal abscess there are signs of local or generalized peritonitis. Occasionally, however, an appendical mass may be present with little or no constitutional upset or localized signs of peritoneal irritation.

In acute appendicitis, mild pyuria (20 to 50 white blood cells/mm³) may be seen and this is due to an inflamed appendix adjacent to the ureter or the bladder. Conversely, acute pyelonephritis

Box 20.1 The variety of presentations of acute appendicitis: presentation and differential diagnosis

Local tenderness in the right iliac fossa
 Simple colic
 'Bilious attack'
 Gastroenteritis
 Acute constipation
 Mild mesenteric adenitis
 Urolithiasis
 Deep iliac lymphadenitis

Local peritonitis (most often in right iliac fossa)
 Severe mesenteric adenitis
 Primary peritonitis
 Meckel's diverticulitis
 Ruptured luteal cyst; that is, the 'apoplectic ovary'
 Torsion of an ovarian cyst or ovary
 Torsion of the omentum
 Suppurating deep iliac lymph nodes

Generalised peritonitis
 Primary peritonitis
 Perforated Meckel's diverticulum

An inflammatory mass
 Intussusception
 Duplication of the gut
 Ectopic kidney
 Retroperitoneal masses (Chapter 25)

Intestinal obstruction
 Adhesive bowel obstruction
 Internal hernia
 Meckel's band

'Gastroenteritis' (from retroileal or pelvic appendix)
 Gastroenteritis

'Urinary tract infection'
 Urinary tract infection
 Acute pyelonephritis

Acutely painful scrotum
 Torsion of testis
 Torsion of appendix testis

may be present without pus cells or bacteria in the bladder, and this must be distinguished from high retrocaecal appendicitis, in which tenderness and rigidity often extend into the loin.

Infections in the lower urinary tract, particularly those associated with vesicoureteric reflux, can mimic appendicitis in the right iliac fossa, but do not exhibit the guarding typical of peritoneal irritation. In pelvic appendicitis, the child may complain of low abdominal pain during micturition.

Peritonitis in the young child

Peritonitis is a frequent complication of appendicitis that may be difficult to recognize in infants and young children. Tenderness may be diffuse rather than localized and rigidity may be absent, even when there is advanced general peritonitis. More often, a lesser degree of involuntary muscular rigidity or 'guarding' is encountered. Differences between the right and left sides or between the lower and upper abdomen are highly significant.

As localised peritonitis progresses, the signs become more definite in the right iliac fossa. Paradoxically, as the peritonitis becomes more generalised and the abdomen more distended, the right iliac fossa signs may appear to diminish in some children. In this situation, abdominal distension and reluctance on the child's part to allow palpation of the abdomen are signs of great significance.

Even without distension, however, the persistence of pain, with or without accompanying diarrhoea, demands careful assessment, re-examination of the abdomen and, if required, rectal examination.

Treatment

The management involves:
(1) adequate pre-operative intravenous correction of fluid and electrolyte deficits
(2) surgical removal of the appendix
(3) irrigation of the peritoneal cavity to remove pus and contaminated free peritoneal fluid; and
(4) effective peri-operative antibiotic treatment.

Fluid and electrolyte deficits are replaced by intravenous infusions, and if there is marked abdominal distension and vomiting, the bowel is decompressed by nasogastric suction. A dehydrated, toxic child with severely depleted fluid and electrolytes is a poor candidate for anaesthesia and operation. Obstruction of the airways by inhaled vomitus, unexpected cardiac arrest and prolonged 'surgical shock' with peripheral circulatory collapse are less likely after fluid resuscitation.

The aim of surgery is to remove the appendix and perform intraperitoneal toilet.

Antibiotics are given to reduce the incidence of septic complications of appendicitis and peritonitis. Peritonitis is a polymicrobial infection caused by bowel organisms, so a wide spectrum of antibacterial activity is necessary. A combination of an anti-aerobic agent (cephaloridine derivative) and an anti-anaerobic agent (Metronidazole) is more effective than either alone. Wound infection results from intra-operative inoculation by peritoneal contaminants; they can be prevented by administering an effective concentration of an appropriate antibacterial agent at or just prior to operation.

ABDOMINAL PAIN OF UNCERTAIN ORIGIN

This represents a substantial group of children (Box 20.1) in which the final diagnosis remains in doubt. 'Indigestion', wind pains, acute constipation and other minor disturbances of bowel function are impossible to establish as objective diagnoses but are labels that tend to be attached to a number of children.

Perhaps the most troublesome condition is mesenteric adenitis ('non-specific viral infection') because of the difficulty in distinguishing some cases from acute appendicitis. The combination of high fever, minimal abdominal tenderness in two or more areas (which may vary), the absence of guarding and failure of the signs to progress all suggest mesenteric adenitis. A succussion splash in the right iliac fossa (consistent with an ileus), but no peritonism, is typical.

ABDOMINAL EMERGENCIES IN MENTALLY HANDICAPPED CHILDREN

Acute appendicitis is the commonest condition. Impaction, ulceration or perforation of the alimentary canal by an ingested foreign body is more frequent than in children of normal intelligence.

The degree of difficulty in diagnosis is dependent on the severity of the mental handicap. In the most severely affected children — those with hyperkinesia, hypertonia, inability to speak and a high threshold of pain — there may be few symptoms, and abdominal signs — for example, tenderness or rigidity — may be difficult to detect or evaluate. Distension and the absence of bowel sounds, although late developments, are usually present when attention is first drawn to the abdomen. Vomiting, fever and tachycardia may also be present.

As in normal children less than 5 years of age, appendicitis in mentally retarded children has usually progressed to a local abscess or to spreading peritonitis by the time the diagnosis is made. A palpable mass on rectal examination, traces of intestinal obstruction from involvement of a loop of small bowel in the wall of an appendiceal abscess or signs of paralytic ileus are common.

The delay in diagnosis leads to an increase in

the incidence of complications and consequently an increase in mortality.

INTESTINAL OBSTRUCTION

A common cause of obstruction is strangulation of an inguinal hernia that, if looked for, presents few problems in diagnosis or management.

In children who have not had a previous abdominal operation the cause of the obstruction may be a volvulus (Chapter 7), Meckel's band or diverticulum (Chapter 23), a duplication (Chapter 7), or very rarely, an internal hernia.

Most cases of obstruction in older children are due to bands or adhesions following a previous abdominal operation. Recurrent pain, accompanied by vomiting, generally causes these patients to present early. Clinical evidence of distended loops of gut, either visible and palpable, or as air-fluid levels in an X-ray of the abdomen, will confirm the diagnosis.

Bowel obstruction is less obvious and more likely to be overlooked: (i) in the early postoperative period when pain is difficult to interpret and delay in recovery from paralytic ileus may mask the presence of an early fibrinous obstruction from adhesions; and (ii) in children in whom vomiting alone is the presenting feature of a high small bowel obstruction in which pain and abdominal distension may be absent.

Treatment

Oral fluids are withheld, the stomach is aspirated by a nasogastric tube, and intravenous fluid and electrolytes are commenced. Some children respond promptly to this regimen and the symptoms and signs subside within a few hours.

Continuing or increasing volumes of aspirate or persistent localised abdominal tenderness are sufficient grounds for laparotomy, preferably before a rising pulse rate, severe pain and increasing abdominal tenderness that suggest impending strangulation of a loop of bowel.

MECKEL'S DIVERTICULUM

The commonest cause of major gastrointestinal bleeding in childhood (Chapter 23), Meckel's diverticulum may also be suspected before an operation on intestinal obstruction in a child who has not undergone a previous abdominal operation. The clinical manifestations of Meckel's diverticulitis are indistinguishable clinically from appendicitis and the true diagnosis only becomes apparent at operation.

PAEDIATRIC GYNAECOLOGIC EMERGENCIES

In menarchal or pubertal girls a gynaecologic disorder may be unsuspected or it may present signs that are not recognized. This group of conditions includes the exaggerated intraperitoneal bleeding at the normal time of ovulation (mittelschmerz bleeding) or the rupture of a small luteal cyst. Tubal menstruation, torsion of the ovary, acute salpingitis and primary peritonitis are all uncommon and rarely diagnosed unless they come to operation.

If carefully sought for by bimanual palpation in the dorsal position, differences in the size and degree of tenderness of the tube and ovary on each side can be detected, for pelvic peritoneal tenderness in the pouch of Douglas often is more marked than the abdominal signs in the hypogastrium. Typically, extreme tenderness in the pelvis contrasts with the relative absence of abdominal signs.

Distinction between rupture of a follicular or luteal cyst and acute pelvic appendicitis can be difficult. Pelvic ultrasonography can detect ovarian cysts 1 cm in diameter or less with accuracy, and save many of these children from unnecessary exploration. However, in all cases with abdominal peritonism or a palpable mass, including a painful pelvic swelling, surgical exploration is necessary. Increasingly, this involves laparoscopy in the first instance.

FURTHER READING

Anderson K.D. & Parry R.L. (1998) Appendicitis. In: O'Neill J.A., Rowe M.I., Grosfeld J.L., Fonkalsrud E.W. & Coran A.G. (eds) *Pediatric Surgery*, 5th edn, Vol. 2, Mosby, St. Louis, pp. 1369–80.

Auldist A.W. (1967) Acute appendicitis in children less than 5 years of age. *Aust. Paediatr. J.* **3**: 144–50.

Beasley S.W., Hutson J.M. & Auldist A.W. (1996) Appendicitis. In: *Essential Paediatric Surgery*, Arnold, London, pp. 52–7.

Hay S.A. (1998) Laparoscopic versus conventional appendicectomy in children. *Pediatr. Surg. Int.* **13**: 21–3.

Mazziotto M.V., Marley E.F., Winthrop A.L., Fitzgerald P.G., Walton M. & Langer J.C. (1997) Histopathologic analysis of interval appendectomy specimens: support for the role of interval appendectomy. *J. Pediatr. Surg.* **32**: 806–9.

Puri P. (1998) Appendicitis. In: Stringer M.D., Mouriquand P.D.E., Oldham K.T. & Howard E.R. (eds) *Pediatric Surgery and Urology: Long-term Outcomes*, W.B. Saunders, London, pp. 321–8.

— 21 —

Recurrent Abdominal Pain

CASE

A 10-year-old girl presents with recurrent symptoms of abdominal pain.

Q. 1.1 *What underlying fears may the parents have about the nature of the pain?*

Q. 1.2 *How can recurrent abdominal pain syndrome be distinguished from more serious causes of pain on the basis of history and examination?*

Q. 1.3 *Discuss the role of the surgeon in this situation.*

Recurrent abdominal pain syndrome is one of the most common problems seen in paediatric practice. The child usually has frequent short-lived episodes of abdominal colic, which are felt in the periumbilical area. The attacks last only a few minutes, and may be brought on by stress at school or home. Despite these psychological triggers, the pain itself is very real and may be due to gut colic. It can be compared to the psychosomatic stress headaches or gastric problems seen in adults. Constipation and gut upset brought on by 'food allergy' may also cause recurrent abdominal pain. However, the main reason families come to a surgeon with these symptoms is often because of an underlying parental fear of a serious cause for the pain, such as cancer or a 'twisted bowel'. In fact, it is quite unusual to find a serious underlying cause for recurrent abdominal pain. Nevertheless, it is important to exclude these uncommon serious causes for abdominal pain, so the family can then recognise the true nature of the problem that most often is stress-induced. The diagnosis depends on a careful history and physical examination.

HISTORY

The nature, severity and periodicity of the pain is the key to the diagnosis. Recurrent abdominal pain is mild to moderate in severity. The pain comes in short-lived episodes lasting only a few minutes, and is usually situated in the periumbilical region. The episodes of pain are frequent and scarcely a day goes by without pain. On the other hand, pain due to surgical causes such as obstructive hydronephrosis or malrotation with volvulus is severe and prolonged. A child finds it difficult to describe the severity of pain; this is best established by other factors. Severe pain will stop the child from normal activities such as play, or the child may be sent home from school with pain. Severe pain will wake the child from sleep and may make him or her vomit. The vomiting of bile-stained fluid is of particular significance in relation to the possibility of malrotation with volvulus. Surgical pain is prolonged, lasting for some hours, and may be localised in relation to the underlying cause. The pain of an obstructed kidney will be localised to the loin in the older child. Young children find it difficult to localise pain. The periodicity of surgical pain is different from that of recurrent abdominal pain. A child with obstructive hydronephrosis may be well for many months and develop severe prolonged episodes of pain lasting for a week, followed by many pain-free months.

The family and social histories are important. If a relative has recently developed cancer, the parents may have an underlying fear of a tumour in the child. On the other hand, a strong family history of renal anomalies may direct attention to the possibility of hydronephrosis in the child. As stress is a key factor in recurrent abdominal pain the social history is of great importance. Family breakdown, financial distress and moving house are common problems. Occasionally, abdominal pain may be a sign of child abuse. Stress at school may be due to many factors, such as poor student–teacher relations, bullying or unrealistic parental expectations. Sometimes when one asks the question, 'How does your child get on at school?', the parents will answer that there is no problem because the child is always a 'straight A' student. The stress of trying to meet these high parental expectations is often the trigger for recurrent abdominal pain. Many parents spend considerable amounts of time away from home due to work. The stress of separation may manifest itself in the child as recurrent abdominal pain.

PHYSICAL EXAMINATION

In most patients with recurrent abdominal pain the physical examination is normal. The child appears to be perfectly well, and a careful and complete physical examination, including measurement of the child's height and weight on a growth chart, offers a powerful reassurance to the parents. The most common abnormal physical finding is the presence of faecal masses in the left iliac fossa. Although this may not be the complete explanation of the pain, correction of the constipation may be very helpful. A loin

mass due to an enlarged hydronephrotic kidney is an uncommon finding. Weight-loss associated with malaise and lethargy may indicate a serious underlying cause for the pain.

SPECIAL INVESTIGATION

In the majority of children, special investigation is not helpful, although it may be useful to allay specific parental anxieties. Of all investigations the abdominal ultrasonography is the most useful and least invasive: the kidneys, bladder, ovaries, gall bladder, liver, spleen and pancreas can all be examined. Investigation should be reserved for patients with a possible surgical cause of the pain. The return on the investigation of recurrent abdominal pain is not particularly good, but occasionally a child is treated for recurrent abdominal pain for many years before a hydronephrosis is diagnosed on ultrasonography.

TREATMENT

Following the exclusion of significant pathology, recurrent abdominal pain is treated by reassurance, identification of the stress factors (if any) and by helping the family to understand the possible link between the stress and the child's symptoms. It is hard to 'cure' the pain, but if the family understands the pathology they can live with the symptoms.

It is important to uncover any possible hidden fears the family may have, such as the risk of cancer. These underlying fears must be dispelled by demonstrating to the parents' satisfaction that the child is free of these problems. Tranquillisers have been used for children with recurrent abdominal pain, but they do not treat the underlying cause.

Constipation may be a factor aggravating recurrent abdominal pain. It is a simple matter to use laxatives to clear the faecal load, and in some children this may be helpful in reducing the colic.

Some parents worry that their child has 'chronic appendicitis'. While laparotomy or laparoscopy and appendicectomy are performed sometimes in a small, select group of the more severely affected children, the results are variable and if the selection is poor the symptoms are made worse. The best results are obtained in those children who were previously well, who undergo frequent hospitalisation for pain that is typical of acute appendicitis, but settles quickly. This diagnosis of 'chronic appendicitis' is uncommon, and surgical exploration should be a rare event.

The management of children with recurrent abdominal pain is a test of clinical acumen and counselling skills. The cases presenting for surgical opinion are usually more severe and it is important to exclude any underlying 'surgical' cause. A thorough clinical history and physical examination is the basis of diagnosis; extensive, traumatic or invasive investigations are rarely indicated, and ultrasonography examination probably gives the best return.

FURTHER READING

Bloom D.A., Ritchey M.L. & Jordan G.H. (1993) Pediatric peritoneoscopy (laparoscopy). *Clin. Pediatr.* **32**: 100–4.

McCallion W.A., Baillie A.G., Ardill J.E.S., Bamford K.B., Potts S.R. & Boston V.E. (1995) *Helicobacter pylori*, hypergastrinaemia, and recurrent abdominal pain in children. *J. Pediatr. Surg.* **30**: 427–9.

— 22 —

Constipation

CASE 1

A 6-month-old baby presents with pain and rectal bleeding with defaecation.

Q. 1.1 Discuss the management of this common problem.

CASE 2

A 6-year-old boy presents with a long history of faecal impaction and faecal soiling.

Q. 2.1 Discuss the diagnosis and treatment of this condition.

Constipation is a common problem in infancy and childhood. Severe acute constipation presents to the surgeon with abdominal pain or rectal prolapse. Chronic constipation may present with soiling or an abdominal mass.

ACUTE CONSTIPATION

This is mainly seen in babies at the age of 6 months. Dietary problems lead to the passage of a hard stool that tears the sensitive anal lining to cause an acute anal fissure with pain and bleeding. The pain on defaecation makes the baby hold on to stool and a cycle of constipation is established. This problem is easily treated with dietary advice and the reduction of the volume of cow's milk. An excess of cow's milk satisfies the baby's thirst at the expense of other fluids, such as water or juice. Too much cow's milk also suppresses the baby's appetite for other foods. Dietary change is the long-term solution, but relief of the acute problem is obtained by laxatives, such as Maltogen added to the milk and other laxatives, for example, senna or paraffin, to soften the stool. Disposable enemas or suppositories are

useful to clear the initial hard stool from the rectum. Parents also may have an underlying fear that the rectal bleeding is due to cancer, so this subject should be explored and the parents reassured. Acute constipation is sometimes seen in older children following another illness; for example, measles or time in bed after surgery. The results of treatment for acute constipation are excellent. In a child with previously normal bowel habits the rectum maintains its muscle tone and recovers rapidly with treatment, though laxatives should be continued until the precipitating factors are corrected.

CHRONIC CONSTIPATION

This is a common debilitating problem in children and the treatment is difficult and prolonged. In most cases the anorectal mechanism and bowel is normal, but in rare cases there can be an underlying cause, such as Hirschsprung's disease.

Chronic constipation presents with a history of many months or years with soiling, abdominal pain and abdominal distension. The general diagnosis of constipation is made by the presence of hard faecal masses in the abdomen. These are felt along the line of the colon and especially in the sigmoid colon. These masses can be indented with digital pressure. This is a characteristic feature that differentiates faeces from other abdominal masses. Inspection of the anus may reveal faecal soiling with a lax, open anal canal.

It is rare that other features on physical examination may indicate a serious underlying disease. Hirschsprung's disease usually presents with neonatal bowel obstruction (Chapter 7) but occasional cases present at a later age with chronic constipation. These children are usually sick with poor nutrition and marked abdominal distension. The anal canal in Hirschsprung's disease is tight, as against the lax anus seen in other causes of chronic constipation. Intestinal neuronal dysplasia describes a group of conditions with (presumed) congenital defects in bowel motility due to functional anomalies of the neural plexuses of the bowel wall. These children present with chronic unremitting constipation that fails to resolve with normal treatment.

An early clue in both Hirschsprung's disease and intestinal neuronal dysplasia is delayed passage of the first meconium stool beyond 24 hours after birth. Another useful clinical feature is that, despite infrequent bowel actions, the retained stool in patients with intestinal neuronal dysplasia is usually soft. Most patients with intestinal neuronal dysplasia have a deficiency of substance P-immunoreactive staining of the myenteric nerves in the colonic muscle, although a small number have hyperplastic or hypoplastic ganglia.

Congenital anorectal anomalies usually present at birth with an imperforate anus. However, some minor anomalies may present later with anal stenosis. The anus in this situation will be tight and anteriorly placed. Spina bifida anomalies are usually apparent at birth, but some cases of spinal dysraphism are not so obvious, and may present later with constipation. Diastematomyelia, sacral agenesis and spinal cord lipoma may all be diagnosed by careful clinical examination of the spine. Digital examination of the rectum is useful in assessing constipation, but should only be undertaken after discussion with the parents and in their presence.

Special investigations

In most cases of constipation, special investigation is unnecessary. A plain X-ray is sometimes performed to assess the extent of faecal loading. Barium enema studies usually are not indicated.

If, on clinical history and examination, a rare underlying cause is suspected, further tests may be indicated, particularly if standard diet and laxative therapy has failed. Hirschsprung's disease may be diagnosed with suction rectal biopsy showing aganglionosis. Diagnosis of intestinal neural dysplasia is a more complex procedure, entailing nuclear transit study to confirm delayed colonic transit and multiple laparoscopic biopsies taken along the length of the large bowel to assess the level of neuropeptide staining.

Spinal dysraphism is diagnosed on a plain X-ray of the lower spine and anorectal anomalies are best assessed with an examination under anaesthetic.

Treatment

While chronic constipation is easy to diagnose it is difficult to treat: treatment is more prolonged than the parents expect. The essence of treatment is to empty the rectum and to keep it empty as often as possible for weeks or months until colonic and anorectal tone returns (Box 22.1). The normal rectum is empty most of the time except when a mass reflex of the colon conveys faeces into the rectum once or twice a day to stimulate rectal receptors to give the urge to defaecate. This urge is suppressed until socially convenient. If the stool is left too long in the rectum, water resorption makes it hard and more difficult to pass. As more faeces accumulate in the rectum, distension of the smooth muscle reduces its contractility and sensation. Eventually, this process causes faeces to bank up in the colon and stools are only passed by overflow incontinence past a

Box 22.1 Predisposing factors in chronic constipation:

(1) Holding back — behavioural problems with toilet-training.

(2) Dietary factors — low fibre and fluid intake.

(3) Postoperative cause due to bed-rest, inactivity and narcotics.

(4) Intercurrent illness; for example, chicken-pox.

(5) Emotional upset at home or school.

(6) Rare organic causes — Hirschsprung's disease, intestinal neuronal dysplasia, spina bifida, congenital anorectal anomalies.

lax anal sphincter that dilates in response to a chronically distended rectum.

Treatment follows four lines:

(1) Dietary advice with a reduction of cow's milk, and increase of fibre with a normal mix of the main food groups, and increased fluids.

(2) Behavioural training is required to establish normal toileting. This is initially difficult as the child has diminished rectal sensation and motility due to chronic distension.

(3) Laxatives both soften the stool and stimulate the bowel. The child may be quite dependent on continuous laxatives for many weeks.

(4) Enemas are the most invasive form of treatment but are necessary in severe cases. Initially full bowel wash outs in hospital may be required to clear gross faecal impaction. Less severe degrees of constipation respond well to small disposable enemas.

Treatment must be carefully supervised until a normal bowel habit is established. Constipation is often underestimated and undertreated. Soiling and abdominal pain occurs in primary school children; these are all too common as both parents and medical practitioners have an inadequate understanding of the problem.

Rectal prolapse (see Fig. 27.2)

Rectal prolapse is a particularly distressing consequence of constipation. Straining to pass a hard stool leads to a prolapse of the poorly supported rectum in the young child. The rectum may reduce spontaneously leaving blood and mucus around the anus, or the parents may reduce the prolapse. In children, this problem resolves quickly by treating the underlying constipation with laxatives and enemas. It is rare that rectal prolapse may indicate an underlying anomaly such as malabsorption due to coeliac disease or cystic fibrosis. Rectal prolapse is also seen in spina bifida because of paralysis of *levator ani*.

FURTHER READING

Alizai N.K., Batcup G., Dixon M.F. & Stringer M.D. (1998) Rectal biopsy for Hirschsprung's disease: what is the optimum method? *Pediatr. Surg. Int.* **13**: 121–4.

Chait P.G., Shandling B. & Richards H.F. (1997) The cecostomy button. *J. Pediatr. Surg.* **32**: 849–51.

Curry J.I., Osborne A. & Malone P.S.J. (1998) How to achieve a successful Malone antegrade continence enema. *J. Pediatr. Surg.* **33**: 138–41.

Graf J.L., Strear C., Bratton B., Housley H.T., Jennings R.W., Harrison M.R. & Albanese C.T. (1998) The antegrade continence enema procedure: a review of the literature. *J. Pediatr. Surg.* **33**: 1294–6.

Hosie G.P. & Spitz L. (1997) Idiopathic constipation in childhood is associated with thickening of the internal anal sphincter. *J. Pediatr. Surg.* **32**: 1041–4.

Poenaru D., Roblin N., Bird M., Duce S., Groll A., Pietak D., Spry K. & Thompson J. (1997) The pediatric bowel management clinic: initial results of a multidisciplinary approach to functional constipation in children. *J. Pediatr. Surg.* **32**: 843–8.

Puri P. (1997) Variant Hirschsprung's disease. *J. Pediatr. Surg.* **32**: 149–57.

Wheatley J.M., Hutson J.M., Chow C.W., Oliver M. & Hurley M.R. (1999) Slow transit constipation in childhood, *J. Pediatr. Surg.* **34**: 1–6.

— 23 —

Bleeding from the Alimentary Canal

CASE 1

A 2-year-old girl is being toilet-trained by her mother when a small amount of bright blood is seen at the anus.

Q. 1.1   *List the causes of minor rectal bleeding in childhood.*

Q. 1.2   *What is the likely problem in this case?*

Q. 1.3   *Describe the management of a fissure.*

CASE 2

James, an 8-month-old toddler who has enjoyed good health, presents with hypovolaemia after the passage of two very large bowel motions containing dark-red blood.

Q. 2.1   *What causes major rectal bleeding in children?*

Haemorrhage, large or small, can occur from any part of the alimentary canal and at any age. Sometimes the haemorrhage threatens the life of the child; on other occasions it is an important sign of other medical or surgical pathology.

Alimentary tract bleeding may present with a variety of symptoms, according to the level and rate of haemorrhage. It may be 'occult' and present as iron-deficiency anaemia, or it may be seen as blood passed per rectum; in this instance there may be melaena (dark changed blood) or bright red bleeding (Table 23.1).

If bleeding occurs into the oesophagus, stomach or duodenum, it may present as either 'coffee grounds' or frank blood in the vomitus.

'COFFEE GROUNDS' VOMITING

A small amount of blood mixes with the gastric contents, is denatured and changes to a brown colour. When vomited, these flecks of blood may

Table 23.1 Vomiting of blood

'Coffee gounds'	Pyloric stenosis
	Reflux oesophagitis
Frank blood	Oesophageal varices
	Peptic ulcer
Others	Nose bleeds
	Nasogastric tube ulceration
Rare causes	Aneurysm of bed of tonsil
	Foreign body perforation of aorta

have the appearance of coffee grounds. It is seen in a variety of conditions:

Pyloric stenosis

Obstruction of the pylorus results in gastritis and small amounts of blood mix with the gastric contents and may be vomited. Hypertrophic pyloric stenosis, which occurs in approximately 1 : 600 infants, causes vomiting at about 1 month of age. Cardinal clinical features are projectile vomiting, visible gastric peristalsis and a pyloric 'tumour' palpable in the epigastrium (Chapter 18).

Reflux oesophagitis

Acid reflux into the lower oesophagus sometimes causes ulceration of its mucosal surface. Small vomits occur after meals and when lying flat, often with epigastric discomfort. Initial treatment of this common condition includes thickening of the feeds, administration of antacids and posturing the baby prone with the head elevated. Surgical treatment (fundoplication) is sometimes necessary for complications (especially oesophageal stricture) (Chapter 18).

Non-specific gastritis

This condition may be due to a viral infection, and usually responds to non-specific measures.

Mallory–Weiss syndrome

This can occur in any child who vomits or retches continually, and it is thought to be due to the formation of small longitudinal splits in the upper gastric mucosa. Fortunately, it responds to medical treatment if the vomiting can be stopped.

HAEMATEMESIS

The vomiting of frank blood means that there has been significant loss of blood into the stomach.

Oesophageal varices

Oesophageal varices are the result of portal hypertension and, in children, this occurs in two main groups:
(1) Extrahepatic portal hypertension, where thrombosis of the portal vein in the neonate results in 'cavernous malformation' of the portal system.
(2) Intrahepatic portal hypertension due to:
   (i) cirrhosis of the liver, caused by biliary atresia; (ii) inborn errors of metabolism, such as alpha$_1$-antitrypsin deficiency; (iii) chronic viral hepatitis; or (iv) cystic fibrosis.

Oesophageal varices may bleed torrentially, and many require tamponade with a Sengstaken–Blakemore tube followed, if necessary, by surgical treatment. Surgery consists of direct injection of the varices with sclerosants at endoscopy, oversewing the varices, or creating a shunt to join the portal system to the systemic venous system, aiming to lower the pressure in the portal system.

Peptic ulcer

Peptic ulcer disease is rare in children, but a 'stress ulcer' may occur in a child of any age with severe burns, cerebral tumour, head injury or other forms of severe stress. In all these conditions there tends to be an increased production of gastric acid with resultant diffuse ulceration of the gastric lining or more localized ulceration in the duodenum. Peptic ulceration also may occur as a complication of drug treatment; for example, after administration of steroids. In adolescents who develop peptic ulceration the aetiology is the same as in adults (that is, *Helicobacter pylori* infection). There may be a strong family history of ulcer disease.

Treatment

For a bleeding peptic ulcer the treatment is:
(1) To adequately resuscitate the patient with blood replacement.
(2) The treatment of the cause; for example, H$_2$ antagonists and triple antibiotic therapy.
(3) Surgery to the bleeding point that is uncontrolled by other measures.

IRON-DEFICIENCY ANAEMIA

Iron-deficiency anaemia in children is caused by poor dietary intake, but it can be due to reflux oesophagitis or one of the other causes mentioned in Box 23.1.

Box 23.1 Occult bleeding causing iron-deficiency anaemia

Reflux oesophagitis

Haemangioma of bowel

Polyps

Inflammatory bowel disease

Box 23.2 Rectal bleeding in children

Neonatal
  Necrotizing enterocolitis
  Volvulus with ischaemia
  Haemorrhagic disease of the newborn
  Gastroenteritis
  Anal fissure
  Maternal blood

Ill child with an acute abdominal condition
  Intussusception
  Gastroenteritis
  Henoch–Schönlein purpura

Major haemorrhage from the gastrointestinal tract
  Oesophageal varices
  Peptic ulcer — gastric erosions
            — duodenal ulcer
  Meckel's diverticulum
  Tubular duplications

Small amount of bright blood in the well child
  Anal fissure
  Rectal polyps
  Unrecognized prolapse
  Haemorrhoids
  Idiopathic

Chronic illness with diarrhoea
  Crohn's disease
  Ulcerative colitis
  Non-specific colitis

RECTAL BLEEDING

Rectal bleeding in children can be considered under various distinct clinical groups (Box 23.2).

Neonatal bleeding

There are two important surgical conditions and several important medical conditions that lead to rectal bleeding in children.

Necrotizing enterocolitis (Chapter 7)

This is an important condition that has become more common with the advent of the modern neonatal nursery that cares for extremely premature babies. Most babies with necrotizing enterocolitis respond to supportive treatment consisting of adequate ventilatory care, support of their circulation, resting the gastrointestinal tract and the administration of antibiotics. Some patients require surgery for full-thickness necrosis of the intestine, as revealed by free intraperitoneal gas on X-ray or by continued clinical deterioration despite intensive supportive care.

Volvulus neonatorum with ischaemia (Chapter 7)

Volvulus of the mid-gut occurs at any age, but is more likely in the neonatal period. In the presence of malrotation the attachment of the mid-gut to the posterior abdominal wall is via a narrow mesentery that allows easy twisting of the entire mid-gut. The first sign results from obstruction of the lumen of the bowel causing bile-stained vomiting; but the most serious event that may occur is ischaemia of the mid-gut, due to obstruction of the vessels in the twisted mesentery. Bleeding from the bowel is a late sign, and very urgent surgical treatment is necessary at this stage if there is to be any hope for the baby.

Non-surgical causes

Haemorrhagic disease of the newborn is due to Vitamin K deficiency and is prevented by routine administration of Vitamin K_1. Gastroenteritis may occur in the neonatal period, resulting in blood mixed with diarrhoea. An anal fissure may occur at any age, and it is common in the neonate after a rectal examination. The baby may swallow maternal blood, either during delivery or from a cracked nipple.

A small amount of blood in a child who is well

A small amount of fresh blood may be passed in a healthy child. This is by far the most common clinical group, and the cause of the bleeding often may be distinguished on the history alone (Fig. 23.1).

Anal fissure

Anal fissure occurs at any age and is usually due to constipation (Chapters 22 and 27). The child passes a large, hard stool that splits the anus, usually in the midline, either posteriorly or anteriorly. The child complains of pain on defaecation and there is bright blood on the surface of the stool or immediately following it.

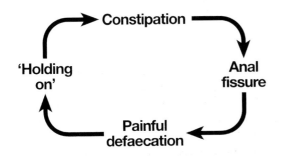

Fig. 23.1 The cycle of anal fissure. The treatment aims to break the cycle

The fissure can be seen by gently parting the anus. Rectal examination causes severe pain and should be avoided. The fissure heals quickly, and even when a fissure is not seen the history may be quite diagnostic. Sometimes, a 'sentinel pile', a mound of oedematous skin just external to the fissure, is visible. Anal fissures in children almost always respond to adequate treatment of the constipation. Local applications of anaesthetic agents achieve little, and surgical operations on the anal sphincter are rarely indicated in children.

Polyps

Juvenile polyps are relatively common in children and should be suspected when there is no constipation or no pain on passage of a stool (Chapter 27).

Rectal prolapse

Prolapse of the rectum is easily diagnosed on the history or by direct observation (Chapter 27). Sometimes the rectal prolapse may become congested or traumatized, bleed and then reduce spontaneously; the parents observe the bleeding without knowing its cause. Rectal prolapse may occur with malabsorption or chronic diarrhoea, straining with constipation, and occasionally, as the presenting symptom of cystic fibrosis.

Haemorrhoids

Symptoms from haemorrhoids are rare in children but do occur. The presence of a venous malformation of the rectum should be considered. In older children, haemorrhoids may cause bleeding and can be treated conservatively. In some children no cause for rectal bleeding can be found.

An ill child with an acute abdominal condition

In these children the symptom of bleeding is not important in its own right, but points to another significant condition.

Intussusception

Intussusception presents with vomiting, colic, pallor and lethargy. In 50 per cent of patients the stools are blood-stained — the typical 'red-currant jelly stool' (see Chapter 19).

Gastroenteritis

Patients with severe gastroenteritis often have vomiting, colic and blood mixed with the stool. The separation of these patients from those with intussusception can be difficult in the child under 2 years (see Chapter 19).

Henoch–Schönlein purpura

This condition causes arthralgia and a typical rash over the extremities and buttocks. Submucosal haemorrhages in the bowel with abdominal pain and passage of blood rectally also occur. Henoch–Schönlein purpura may lead to intussusception: ultrasonography will make the diagnosis.

Chronic illness with diarrhoea

Crohn's disease may occur anywhere in the bowel and should be suspected in a patient with a chronic illness, unexplained fever, weight loss, bowel symptoms and chronic blood loss in the stools (Chapter 24). Many children present with chronic perianal disease. In patients with ulcerative colitis the diarrhoea is more prominent, and again it may contain blood. In non-specific colitis there is usually involvement of only the lower part of the large bowel with less general symptomatology.

Major haemorrhage per rectum

In these patients the haemorrhage is enough to cause anaemia or to require acute transfusion. The causes range from oesophageal varices and peptic ulcer (as discussed under the heading of vomiting) to Meckel's diverticulum and tubular

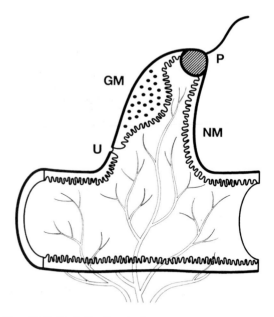

Fig. 23.2 Meckel's diverticulum. A composite diagram showing ectopic pancreas (P) and gastric mucosa (GM). An ulcer (U) lies in the adjacent normal ileal mucosa (NM). The site of attachment of a vitello-intestinal or Meckel's Band is shown at the tip.

duplications (both latter anomalies can contain ectopic gastric mucosa).

Meckel's diverticulum

Meckel's diverticulum occurs in 2 per cent of the population, and in a small proportion of these patients, ectopic gastric mucosa forms part of the lining of the diverticulum (Fig. 23.2). Acid produced by the gastric mucosa causes ulceration of the adjacent ileal mucosa. The bleeding usually presents as painless 'brick-red' stools with associated anaemia. The patient may require transfusion, but the bleeding usually stops spontaneously without the need for emergency surgery. The definitive investigation is surgery, but a technetium scan may show the ectopic gastric mucosa (Fig. 23.3). A Meckel's diverticulum may result in a variety of other complications (Box 23.3).

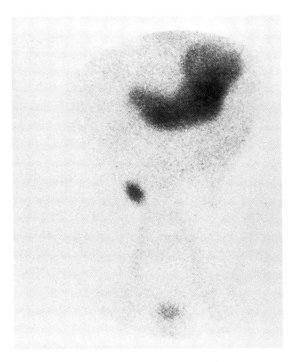

Fig. 23.3 A technetium scan showing ectopic gastric mucosa in a Meckel's diverticulum.

Box 23.3 Complications of Meckel's Diverticulum

(1) Bleeding.

(2) Intussusception from an inverted diverticulum.

(3) An associated fibrous band causing a small bowel obstruction.

(4) Diverticulitis (rare in children).

(5) Peptic ulceration with ileal perforation.

(6) Strangulation of diverticulum by its own band.

(7) Strangulation of diverticulum in an inguinal hernia.

Tubular duplications

These are less common than a Meckel's diverticulum. Tubular duplications of the small bowel occur in the mesenteric side of the bowel and communicate proximally or distally with the bowel. They may be lined by gastric mucosa and cause bleeding when adjacent small bowel mucosa becomes ulcerated. Like a Meckel's diverticulum, they can be demonstrated by a technetium nuclear scan.

FURTHER READING

Arensman R.M. (1998) Gastrointestinal bleeding. In: O'Neill J.A., Rowe M.I., Grosfeld J.L., Fonkalsrud E.W. & Coran A.G. (eds) *Pediatic Surgery*, 5th edn, pp. 1253–6, Mosby, St. Louis.

Beasley S.W., Auldist A.W., Ramanujam T.M. & Campbell N.T. (1986) The surgical management of neonatal necrotising enterocolitis, 1975–1984. *Pediatr. Surg. Int.* **1**: 201–17.

Cull D.L., Rosario V., Lally K.P., Ratner I. & Mahour G.H. (1990) Surgical implications of Henoch–Schönlein purpura. *J. Pediatr. Surg.* **25**: 741–3.

Hutson J.M. & Beasley S.W. (1988) Gastro-intestinal bleeding. In: *The Surgical Examination of Children*, pp. 202–7, Heinemann Medical, Oxford.

Previtera C. & Guglielmi M. (1990) Limitations and dangers of the Sengstaken–Blakemore tube in the treatment of haemorrhage from gastric varices. *Pediatr. Surg. Int.* **5**: 422–4.

Tsang T.-M., Saing H. & Yeung C.K. (1990) Peptic ulcer in children. *J. Pediatr. Surg.* **25**: 744–8.

— 24 —

Inflammatory Bowel Disease

CASE 1

A 6-year-old girl presented with a 1-month history of weight-loss and mild diarrhoea, containing blood and mucus.

> *Q. 1.1   What is the likely diagnosis and how is it confirmed?*

CASE 2

A 12-year-old boy presents with vague pains in the abdomen, some weight loss and a perianal abscess.

> *Q. 2.1   How is the diagnosis made?*
>
> *Q. 2.2   How are the different forms of inflammatory bowel disease distinguished?*

Three categories of inflammatory bowel disease are encountered in childhood:
(1) Crohn's disease
(2) ulcerative colitis
(3) inflammatory bowel disease of indeterminate pathology.

Incidence

Inflammatory bowel disease has been regarded in the past as uncommon in childhood, but there has been a dramatic increase in the incidence of Crohn's disease in Australia since the early 1980s. This increase in incidence mirrors that reported in the northern hemisphere. In contrast, the incidence of ulcerative colitis has remained relatively static.

CROHN'S DISEASE

Crohn's disease is a chronic inflammatory disorder of unknown aetiology that can affect any part of the gastrointestinal tract from the mouth to the anus. It is a transmural inflammatory process that most commonly occurs in the terminal portion of the small intestine and the colon.

Clinical features

Age of onset of symptoms

Most childhood Crohn's disease presents during adolescence, but 30 per cent of patients are aged less than 10 years at commencement of symptoms.

Delay in diagnosis

There is often a delay in the diagnosis of this condition because of the low index of suspicion of medical practitioners concerning its occurrence in childhood, and the variety of non-specific presenting symptoms.

The typical patient is a young adolescent who presents with recurrent abdominal pain, often associated with weight-loss and growth failure.

There may also be a delay in the onset of puberty. In many patients there is no disturbance in bowel habit, but diarrhoea with rectal bleeding may occur.

Perianal inflammation

One-third of paediatric patients with Crohn's disease have perianal inflammation, and this may be the presenting feature, which precedes the onset of abdominal symptoms.

Extra-intestinal manifestations of Crohn's disease

Examples of extra-intestinal manifestations include arthritis and erythema nodosum, which may be presenting symptoms.

Unusual modes of presentation of Crohn's disease

Very occasionally, Crohn's disease may present with acute right-sided abdominal pain and gastrointestinal disturbance, mimicking acute appendicitis. The diagnosis is then made at laparotomy or laparoscopy.

It is rare that the patient may present with chronic inflammation of the oral cavity, including the lips; biopsy reveals features consistent with 'cheilosis', with chronic inflammatory changes, and granulomas consistent with Crohn's disease.

Investigations

Role of endoscopy

Endoscopy has a crucial role in diagnosis, initial evaluation and continuing assessment of children with Crohn's disease.

Upper and lower ('top and tail') gastrointestinal endoscopy with biopsies is the key investigation for achieving a diagnosis and obtaining an initial assessment of the extent and severity of the disease. Colonoscopy has a

high chance of providing the diagnosis as 70 per cent of paediatric patients with Crohn's disease have colonic involvement. Gastroduodenoscopy is performed as well as colonoscopy because involvement of the upper intestinal tract is common. Biopsies of the upper intestinal tract may clinch the diagnosis.

Endoscopy has an important role in assessing the response to treatment and distribution of the disease, and is performed at periodic intervals.

In Crohn's disease the inflammation is typically segmental, and the characteristic appearance is single or multiple ulcers with the intervening mucosa appearing normal ('skip lesions'). In some instances the diagnosis may be made by serial biopsies even when the macroscopic appearances are normal. Histological diagnosis depends on the demonstration of granulomas, in association with other chronic inflammatory changes in the bowel wall.

Barium meal and follow-through

This investigation is performed to assess the small intestine, which is not accessible to endoscopy. It also may provide valuable information concerning disease in the colon. Most commonly, abnormalities are demonstrated in the terminal ileum and often in the colon (Fig. 24.1). Abnormal findings include an irregular bowel contour, longitudinal ulcers and fissures, a narrowing of the lumen by oedema, and separation of loops by mural thickening. There may be evidence of stricture formation associated with dilatation of the proximal bowel. Bowel loops may be displaced by the presence of an inflammatory mass.

Other imaging, including ultrasonography or CT with contrast, may be used to evaluate complicated pelvic Crohn's disease; for example, pararectal abscess.

Other investigations

Full blood examination (FBE) is performed to detect evidence of anaemia, and liver function

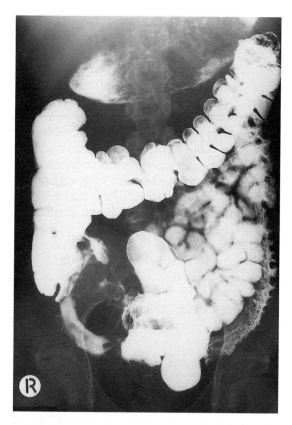

Fig. 24.1 Crohn's disease. Barium meal and follow-through showing irregular inflamed terminal ileum and colon.

tests are performed to exclude associated liver disease.

Stool cultures are performed to rule out chronic infection due to such enteric pathogens as Salmonella, Shigella, Campylobacter and Yersinia.

Medical treatment

High doses of oral steroids are used to produce a remission; for example, Prednisolone, 2 to 3 mg/kg (maximum 60 kg/day) for 4 weeks, with gradual reduction to nil after 8 weeks. Sulphasalazine, or one of its analogues such as mesalamine, which has fewer effects, is introduced when the Prednisolone dose is reduced. It may be necessary to continue low-dose Prednisolone (5 mg/day).

Imuran is occasionally used in resistant cases, and Metronidazole may be helpful for perianal Crohn's disease.

Nutrition

Children with inflammatory bowel disease fail to grow because of the disease, not its treatment, and the reason the disease influences growth is because of its effect on appetite and caloric intake. High caloric dietary supplements, and occasionally enteral tube feeding or parenteral nutrition, all have their place in management.

Surgical treatment

The indications for surgical treatment of Crohn's disease are as follows:
(1) perianal disease
(2) intestinal complications
(3) acute abdomen — possible acute appendicitis.

1 Perianal disease

The most common indication for surgical intervention in Crohn's disease is perianal disease (Fig. 24.2). Perianal inflammation is invariably associated with rectal and colonic Crohn's disease. There may be extensive involvement of the soft tissues of the perineum, scrotum, penis or vulval region.

Skin-tags and anal fissures are very common, and do not require surgical treatment. A perianal abscess requires incision and drainage. A fistula *in ano* may need to be excised.

The aim of surgical treatment is to control infection and promote healing. In perianal Crohn's disease, healing is often delayed and chronic inflammation may be protracted despite appropriate treatment.

Extensive suppuration can occur with development of an ischio-rectal abscess. Appropriate surgical management of this complication includes drainage of the abscess, and faecal diversion in the form of a colostomy or ileostomy may be necessary. Faecal diversion may control infection, but it does not influence the activity of the disease

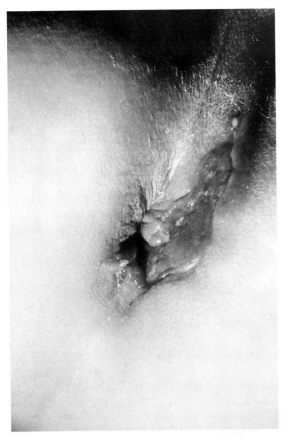

Fig. 24.2 Perianal disease in a child with Crohn's disease.

itself. The potential end result of severe ischio-rectal sepsis is damage to the sphincter muscles.

2 Intestinal complications and acute abdomen

These complications are due to transmural inflammation and include the following:

- localised stricture formation
- localised disease unresponsive to medical treatment
- localised disease associated with growth delay and often a delay in pubertal development
- inflammatory mass
- intestinal fistulae
- rectal stricture.

The aim of surgical treatment for these complications is to preserve as much intestine as possible.

Localised strictures may be treated by simple stricturoplasty (without loss of bowel) or resection. An important role for surgery is the resection of localised disease associated with growth delay or delay in pubertal development, despite maximal medical treatment. In the majority of these patients a sustained remission can be expected, together with 'catch-up' growth and the resumption of normal schooling. The best results can be anticipated with resection of localised ileo-caecal disease before or at the onset of puberty.

Resection may be necessary for inflammatory masses and fistulae.

There is a high incidence of rectal strictures in paediatric Crohn's disease. It is often associated with perineal inflammation.

The management of this complication includes steroid therapy, both systemic (as previously mentioned) and local steroid medication as administered in enema form. The surgery includes regular dilatations of the stricture under GA, usually conducted in association with endoscopic evaluation. The associated perianal inflammation tends to resolve with control of the rectal stricture.

ULCERATIVE COLITIS

Ulcerative colitis is a chronic inflammatory disease of the rectal and colonic mucosa, the aetiology of which is unknown.

Clinical features

The onset is usually insidious, but an acute onset similar to a Salmonella infection can occur. The disease usually begins after 5 years of age, but may occur as early as the first year of life.

The typical features are as follows:

(1) unexplained bloody diarrhoea, with mucus, lasting more than 2 weeks

(2) anaemia

(3) fever

(4) weight-loss.

All degrees of severity are encountered, and the predominant symptom varies from one patient to another.

Perianal complications occur in between 10 and 20 per cent of patients, and include ulcers, abscesses and fistulae. As in Crohn's disease, perianal complications may be the presenting problem, but more commonly the development of this disease is preceded by a period of diarrhoea.

Investigations

1 Colonoscopy

Colonoscopy accurately assesses the extent of macroscopic disease and biopsies taken at this stage achieve the diagnosis. In ulcerative colitis, inflammatory changes are always seen in the rectum and extend for varying distances proximally in the colon. The changes range in severity from loss of the normal mucosal sheen and vascularity with associated mucosal friability to diffuse ulceration with blood and pus in the lumen. Numerous biopsies taken during colonoscopy will confirm the histological diagnosis and indicate the severity of inflammation at various levels. The histology can be reported, at best, as 'consistent with' ulcerative colitis, for there is no pathognomonic lesion.

In some instances, even when macroscopic appearances at endoscopy are normal, multiple biopsies will provide diagnostic histological changes.

2 Barium enema

This investigation may show a 'saw-tooth' or marked irregularities in the mucosa, with deep ulceration. Later, the colon becomes narrow, rigid and devoid of visible peristalsis or haustration (Fig. 24.3). Finally, there may be pseudo-polyps or stenosis due to the development of a fibrous stricture.

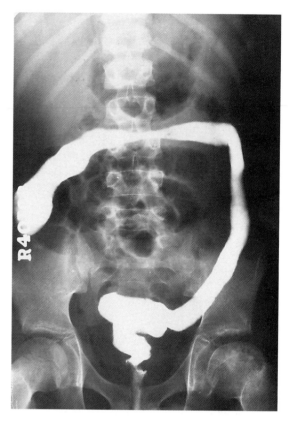

Fig. 24.3 Ulcerative colitis. Featureless colon with 'sawtooth' outline on barium enema.

3 Other tests

Other tests include an FBE to demonstrate anaemia. Bacteriology tests should include a careful search for enteric pathogens, including Salmonella, Shigella, Campylobacter and Yersinia. Blood for Yersinia antibodies should be collected.

Course of the disease

Improvements in medical treatment, with more aggressive use of steroids, have produced better control of the disease. Many children have remissions lasting several years, to the extent that the diagnosis is subsequently questioned. A small proportion continue to have recurrent lapses and may require colectomy.

Risk of malignancy

The incidence of carcinoma is directly proportional to the duration of the disease. The risk in its first 10 years is very low. After 10 years the rate increases by 10 per cent for each subsequent decade.

Surveillance by regular colonoscopy and detection of dysplasia by biopsies as a predictor of potential malignancy is an important component of management of paediatric patients with ulcerative colitis. Colectomy is recommended after 10 years of proven disease.

Medical treatment of ulcerative colitis

The principles of medical treatment are similar to those for Crohn's disease. These principles have been enumerated previously.

Surgical treatment of ulcerative colitis

Procto-colectomy is curative, but other surgical procedures have a place in the treatment of this disease.

The indications for surgical treatment are as follows:
(1) severe inflammation unresponsive to medical treatment
(2) severe disease associated with growth delay and a delay in pubertal development
(3) long-term risk of malignancy (see above)
(4) rare complications
(5) acute haemorrhage
(6) perforation
(7) toxic megacolon.

It is most important to realise that the absence of symptoms should not be taken as evidence of quiescent or inactive disease, or of healing. Surveillance by regular colonoscopy should continue in proven cases of ulcerative colitis.

Surgical options

SUBTOTAL COLECTOMY WITH ILEO-RECTAL ANASTOMOSIS

This procedure may be considered in a situation where there is minimal rectal inflammation, particularly in an adolescent entering young adulthood. This procedure may avoid the need for an ileostomy. However, this option requires continuing endoscopic surveillance, together with biopsies every 6 months. Removal of the rectum will be necessary after 10 years of disease.

PROCTO-COLECTOMY

This procedure may be achieved with a number of techniques as follows:
(1) ileo-anal anastomosis with ileal reservoir
(2) ileo-anal anastomosis without reservoir — Soave pull-through procedure
(3) procto-colectomy with permanent continent ileostomy.

CHRONIC INFLAMMATORY BOWEL DISEASE OF INDETERMINATE PATHOLOGY

In a small number of patients the pathology is uncertain and a diagnostic dilemma arises as to whether the patient has ulcerative colitis or Crohn's disease. The principles of medical treatment are similar to those outlined previously in this chapter. The principles of surgical treatment depend on what is considered to be the most likely condition as judged on clinical, endoscopic and histological evidence.

FURTHER READING

Cywes R., Harmon C.M. & Coran A.G. (1998) Inflammatory bowel disease. In: Stringer M.D., Mouriquand P.D.E., Oldham K.T. & Howard E.R. (eds) *Pediatric Surgery and Urology: Long-term Outcomes*, W.B. Saunders, London, pp. 300–20.

Davidson P.M., McLain B.I., Beasley S.W. & Stokes K.B. (1992) Perianal disease in childhood Crohn's disease; its frequency, characteristics and prognostic significance. *Pediatr. Surg. Int.* **7**: 174–6.

Davidson P.M., McLain B.I., Stokes K.B. & Beasley S.W. (1992) Crohn's disease: the Melbourne experience. *Pediatr. Surg. Int.* **7**: 165–70.

Doig C.M. (1998) Crohn's disease. In: O'Neill J.A., Rowe M.I., Grosfeld J.L., Fonkalsrud E.W. & Coran A.G. (eds) *Pediatric Surgery*, 5th edn, Mosby, St. Louis, pp. 1321–32.

Fonkalsrud E.W. (1998) Ulcerative colitis. In: O'Neill J.A., Rowe M.I., Grosfeld J.L., Fonkalsrud E.W. & Coran A.G. (eds) *Pediatric Surgery*, 5th edn, Mosby, St. Louis, pp. 1333–44.

McLain B.I., Davidson P.M., Stokes K.B. & Beasley S.W. (1990) Growth after gut resection for Crohn's disease. *Arch. Dis. Child.* **65**: 760–2.

Patel H.I., Leichtner A.M., Colodny A.H. & Shamberger R.C. (1997) Surgery for Crohn's disease in infants and children. *J. Pediatr. Surg.* **32**: 1063–8.

— 25 —

The Child with an Abdominal Mass

CASE 1

A 9-year-old boy presents with a 2-week history of intermittent pain in the left loin and flank. Physical examination reveals a large smooth mass in the left side of the abdomen. The mass is firm, but not solid, and is 'ballottable'.

> Q. 1.1   What is the likely diagnosis?
>
> Q. 1.2   What investigations might be needed?

CASE 2

A previously well 4-year-old girl presents with a large, smooth and solid mass in the left side of the abdomen, noted incidentally during examination. The blood pressure is 110/80.

> Q. 2.1   What is the differential diagnosis?
>
> Q. 2.2   What treatment might be needed?

CASE 3

A 5-year-old girl has been 'unwell' and pale in recent weeks. The school nurse finds a large, hard and craggy mass in the upper abdomen.

> Q. 3.1   What investigations should be undertaken and what is the likely diagnosis?
>
> Q. 3.2   What would you tell the parents?

The following points need to be considered for a child with a mass in the abdomen:
(1) The 'site' of the mass and its precise characteristics to determine the probable organ of origin.
(2) The age of the patient and the most likely pathological process arising in that organ at that age.
(3) The length of history and the type of symptoms (for example, fever and tenderness may suggest an infection).

NORMAL AND ABNORMAL MASSES

The most common abdominal masses in infancy and childhood are non-pathological. They are usually accounted for by the liver, which normally extends below the right costal margin until 3 or 4 years of age; faeces in the colon; or a full bladder (Table 25.1). In addition, there are three common pathological conditions that warrant special consideration as a group presenting as a

— 165 —

Table 25.1 The more common normal and abnormal abdominal masses in children

Normal	Abnormal
Liver	Hydronephrosis
Faeces	Wilms' tumour
Bladder	Neuroblastoma
Lower pole of kidneys	

mass in the loin: hydronephrosis, Wilms' tumour of the kidney and abdominal neuroblastoma.

They have certain features in common:

(1) They arise most frequently in infants and toddlers between 1 and 3 years of age.

(2) At this age the abdomen is normally protuberant and tends to conceal the mass, which is often quite large when first detected.

(3) General or local symptoms are frequently minimal or absent. The mass itself is usually the presenting feature, and typically is discovered by the mother while drying the child's abdomen after a bath.

The mass may extend downwards towards the iliac fossa, forwards, across to the other side, or it may straddle the midline. As a general rule it is only slightly tender and is so large that it may not move with respiration. When the mass is centred on the midline in the upper abdomen, a primary neuroblastoma is the most likely cause, particularly if the child is less than 4 years of age. Massive hepatic metastases (from a neuroblastoma) and a primary hepatoblastoma are other possibilities.

Investigations

The basic investigations are a plain abdominal X-ray and abdominal ultrasonography. The plain film of the abdomen may show calcification within the mass, more commonly in neuroblastoma (Fig. 25.1) than in Wilms' tumour, and not at all in hydronephrosis.

Abdominal ultrasonography will determine whether a mass is 'cystic' or 'solid'. Cystic masses include hydronephrosis, polycystic kidneys, multilocular or simple renal cysts and a dilated kidney from severe vesico-ureteric reflux. Ultrasonography indicates the size, position and extent of a solid tumour, and gives an indication of blood vessel involvement (for example, the extension of a Wilms' tumour into the inferior vena cava). Lymph nodes, and even metastases, may be demonstrated. A nuclear scan of the kidneys will demonstrate the function of a hydronephrotic kidney or one involved by tumour, as well as the degree of function of the contralateral kidney. A more extensive assessment may be necessary, including an abdominal computerised tomography (CT) scan or magnetic resonance imaging and, on occasions, angiography, to determine vascular supply. The management of hydronephrosis is described in Chapter 33.

NEUROBLASTOMA

This is one of the common malignant tumours of early childhood. It arises from fetal neural crest cells, and the adrenal gland is the commonest site of origin (Fig. 25.1); the tumour may also arise in the adjacent retroperitoneal sympathetic plexus, the mediastinum, the pelvis and, less commonly, in other sites.

Early metastases are found frequently and may be in the bone marrow, the cortex of long bones, the skull, the regional or distant lymph nodes, or in the liver. The numerous sites of origin and the occurrence of early distant metastases account for the variety of presenting features, including a rubbery lymph node in the neck or in the axilla (lymph node metastases); paraplegia of rapid onset (spinal involvement); a nodule in the skull or proptosis and periorbital-ecchymoses or pain and tenderness in the long bones (bone metastases); fever, lethargy and loss of weight; fleeting pain in the limbs; failure to thrive with or without anaemia (bone marrow involvement); and diarrhoea caused by tumour metabolites.

In view of the highly malignant nature of neuroblastoma, it is a paradox that in a

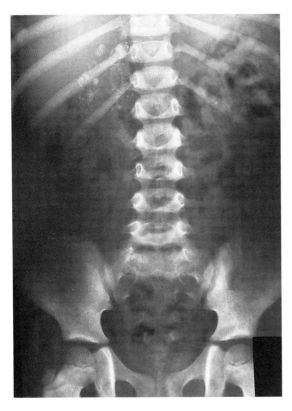

Fig. 25.1 Neuroblastoma showing calcification in the right paravertebral region.

small number of cases the tumour may regress completely with a spontaneous cure. This only occurs if there is a small primary tumour with bone marrow, liver, lymph node or skin metastases; and never if there is cortical bone disease. Almost all children in this group are under 1 year of age. In 65 to 75 per cent of cases, disseminated disease is present already when the diagnosis is made.

Diagnostic criteria

When an abdominal mass is suspected to be a neuroblastoma the diagnosis can be confirmed by:
(1) A marrow biopsy for metastatic neuroblastoma, present at diagnosis in 65 to 75 per cent of patients.
(2) A 24-hour collection of urine for biochemical analysis for tumour catecholamine metabolites

(VMA, MHMA (3-methoxyy-4-hydroxymandelic acid), dopamine, adrenaline, noradrenaline).
(3) Biopsy of either the abdominal tumour or other sites of suspected metastases; for example, lymph nodes.
The diagnosis is confirmed when neuroblastoma cells are identified within the bone marrow or in a biopsy specimen. When tumour metabolites in the urine are elevated significantly and neuroblastoma cells are seen in bone marrow a laparotomy can be avoided. A chest X-ray should be performed pre-operatively to look for paravertebral extension of the tumour and mediastinal involvement. The MIBG nuclear scan highlights active metastases when meta-iodo benzyl guanidine is incorporated into functioning neuroblastoma tissue.

Treatment

Complete surgical excision of an abdominal neuroblastoma is not always possible and non-resectability is indicated by retroperitoneal extension of the tumour encasing the aorta and inferior vena cava. If a small localised tumour is found it should be removed. Treatment for large primary tumours and metastatic neuroblastoma involves an intensive combination of chemotherapy and a reassessment after 3 to 6 months with surgical removal of the residual tumour, if feasible. Finally, high-dose chemotherapy is given with autologous bone marrow rescue. In rare cases, radiotherapy may be used.

In children over one year the prognosis is poor, with less than 25 per cent of children surviving when metastases are present at diagnosis.

WILMS' TUMOUR

Wilms' tumour, or neuroblastoma of the kidney, arises from primitive embryonic cells and produces a mixed histological picture of epithelial structures resembling tubules and a variety of mesenchymal tissues, including striated muscle fibres.

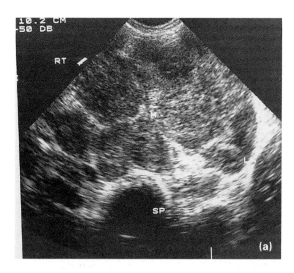 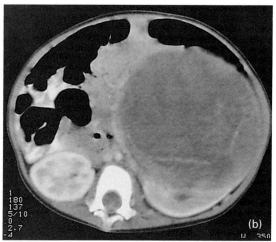

Fig. 25.2 (a) Ultrasonography showing a large Wilms' tumour (M) arising from the left kidney (LK); (b) CT scan showing a child with bilateral Wilms' tumour.

A bilateral Wilms' tumour is often seen in children. Where this is present there may be an underlying genetic defect, and chromosomal analysis should be performed to search for an abnormality on chromosome 11. There may be an increased risk of recurrent primary tumours.

Clinical features

A Wilms' tumour usually presents as a smooth mass in the loin that seldom crosses the midline, but extends downwards into the iliac fossa and upwards, under the costal margin. A right-sided Wilms' tumour may extend behind the liver that, if pushed downwards, can present as hepatomegaly. On the left side, a Wilms' tumour may be mistaken for an enlarged spleen.

Haematuria, often following minor trauma, may present in some children, but it does not indicate a poor prognosis. Clinical examination of the child should always include a blood pressure measurement, as this may be elevated.

Investigation

Ultrasonography provides detailed information of the site, size and extent of the tumour (Fig. 25.2a;

Table 25.2 Staging of Wilms' tumour

Stage	Tumour spread
(1)	Confined to kidney and removed completely
(2)	Microscopic local disease after resection
(3)	Macroscopic residual disease after resection
(4)	Distant metastases

Table 25.2). Ultrasonography also identifies renal vein and inferior vena cava involvement. The liver is examined for the presence of metastases and a chest X-ray excludes the presence of pulmonary metastases. A CT scan is employed on occasions (Fig. 25.2b).

Treatment

If it is possible the kidney is removed. In stage 1 tumours, adjuvant chemotherapy is given for a period of 3 months. In stage 2 tumours, two-agent chemotherapy will be used for 12 to 15 months, and in stage 3 tumours, three-agent chemotherapy is used for 12 to 15 months, with radiotherapy as an occasional adjunct. If the tumour is large, chemotherapy may be used to 'shrink' the tumour prior to surgical removal. In stage 4 tumours, chemotherapy is the mainstay of treatment.

Two rare causes of a renal mass, mesenchymal hamartoma and multilocular cyst of the kidney, cannot be confidentially diagnosed by investigations or on their macroscopic appearance at operation, and are removed with the kidney.

Prognosis

Wilms' tumour, in contrast to neuroblastoma, usually has a good outcome. In stage 1, the cure rate is greater than 95 per cent. Even in unfavourable circumstances, for example, with pulmonary metastases, the results are better than 50 per cent 5 years' survival. Late occurrence locally, or as pulmonary metastasis, is rare after 1 or 2 years, but careful follow-up with abdominal ultrasonography and chest X-ray is required, particularly in the first 12 months of treatment.

LIVER TUMOURS

Hepatobastoma is the most common malignant tumour presenting as a right upper quadrant mass in children less than 1 year of age. Alternative diagnoses include arteriovenous malformation (which may be accompanied by thrombocytopenia) and mesenchymal hamartoma, both of which are benign liver masses. Elevation of serum alpha-fetoprotein — a tumour marker — is highly suggestive of hepatoblastoma with a liver mass. Accurate pre-operative assessment is necessary with imaging techniques including ultrasonography, CT scan and angiography. Surgical resection of the lesion, either locally or by lobectomy, remains the mainstay of treatment for all primary liver tumours. Pre-operative chemotherapy has been shown to improve survival significantly. Liver transplantation occasionally is used if the tumour is unresectable after chemotherapy.

FURTHER READING

Davidson P.M. & Auldist A.W. (1988) Surgical anatomy and operative techniques for elective hepatic resection in children. *Pediatr. Surg. Int.* 4: 7–10.

de Campo J. & Phelan E. (1988) Imaging of liver tumours in childhood. *Pediatr. Surg. Int.* 4: 1–6.

Grosfeld J.L. (1998) Neuroblastoma. In: O'Neill J.A., Rowe M.I., Grosfeld J.L., Fonkalsrud E.W. & Coran A.G. (eds) *Pediatric Surgery*, 5th edn, Mosby, St. Louis, pp. 405–20.

Ikeda H., Suzuki N., Takahashi A., Kuroiva M., Nagashima K., Tsuchida Y. & Natsuyama S. (1998) Surgical treatment of neuroblastomas in infants under 12 months of age. *J. Pediatr. Surg.* **33**: 1246–50.

Otherson H.B., Tagge E.P. & Garvin A.J. (1998) Wilms' tumour. In: O'Neill J.A., Rowe M.I., Grosfeld J.L. Fonkalsrud E.W. & Coran A.G. (eds) *Pediatric Surgery*, 5th edn, Mosby, St. Louis, pp. 291–404.

— 26 —

Spleen, Pancreas and Biliary Tract

CASE 1

A 4-year-old girl presents with a distended epigastrium and paralytic ileus. On physical examination there are several old fractures with callus formation.

Q. 1.1   *What causes pancreatitis?*

Q. 1.2   *How is pancreatitis diagnosed?*

Q. 1.3   *What is a pseudocyst?*

CASE 2

A 3-week-old infant develops gastroenteritis from her older siblings. After resolution of diarrhoea, she is noted to be jaundiced.

Q. 2.1   *How would you determine whether obstructive jaundice was present?*

Q. 2.2   *What differences in management are there between a bile duct stone and biliary atresia?*

THE SPLEEN

Some haematological diseases require splenectomy during the course of their treatment (see below) but splenic trauma is nearly always treated non-operatively (see Chapter 38).

Spherocytosis

In spherocytosis the red cells are abnormally spherical and are destroyed in the spleen. This tends to result in:
(1) chronic anaemia
(2) episodic haemolytic jaundice
(3) a tendency to form pigment gallstones.

These complications can be controlled by splenectomy, but unless they are severe, splenectomy is delayed until at least the age of 7 years of age because of the risk of postsplenectomy sepsis. About 2 weeks before elective splenectomy the patient is immunized with multivalent pneumococcal vaccine and against *Haemophilus influenza* (HiB). After splenectomy, long-term oral penicillin is recommended.

Idiopathic thrombocytopenic purpura

This is a common condition that usually resolves spontaneously. In children with a persistently low platelet count, steroids or gamma-globulin infusions may improve the platelet count. However, in selected patients not responding to this treatment, laparoscopic or open splenectomy is required, and usually improves the platelet count.

Thalassaemia

In thalassaemia major, a homozygous condition, the production of abnormal haemoglobin results in chronic haemolytic anaemia. In the past, chronic anaemia, blood transfusions and subsequent increasing iron stores have resulted in the patient developing a very large spleen, producing the added problem of secondary hypersplenism. The enlarged spleen tends to destroy all cellular elements in the blood.

Transfusions keep the children healthy while regular parenteral desferrioxamine chelates excess iron liberated from haemolysed red cells and maintains normal serum iron levels. Splenectomy is rarely required in this condition.

Sickle cell anaemia

The presence of abnormal haemoglobin S results in an abnormally shaped red cell during hypoxia. These 'sickle cells' tend to flow through small vessels slowly, causing ischaemia in the organ involved. Splenic infarcts can occur.

Splenectomy is usually contra-indicated as a higher haemoglobin tends to be associated with increased 'sickling' of the red cells.

THE PANCREAS

Pancreatitis

Pancreatitis in children is rare, but it may occur following trauma (for example, handle bar injury or a punch to the upper abdomen), mumps, other viral infections or choledocholithiasis. Many cases have no identifiable cause. In the absence of a history of blunt abdominal trauma (beware of child abuse), other underlying causes must be considered; for example, biliary tract stones. Investigations include serum lipase/amylase and imaging, such as CT scan or MRI. Occasionally MRCP or ERCP is required. The treatment is usually conservative, with pain relief, rest of the alimentary tract and intravenous fluids — and treatment of the cause, if applicable.

Pseudocyst

Pancreatic injury and other causes of pancreatitis may result in the accumulation of pancreatic fluid in the lesser sac or adjacent to the pancreas. Treatment is initially non-operative, and change in the size of the 'cyst' can be followed by ultrasonography while the patients and their alimentary tract are rested. After several weeks it may be necessary to drain the pseudocyst into the stomach (or occasionally externally).

Hyperinsulinism (causing hypoglycaemia)

Excessive production of insulin may occur in several situations:
(1) In babies of diabetic mothers as a temporary response to high sugar levels.
(2) Beta-cell hyperplasia, a condition of unknown aetiology in which there is excessive production of insulin, which usually settles down with drug treatment (Diazoxide). Extensive pancreatectomy is only necessary occasionally.
(3) Beckwith–Weidemann syndrome, a condition of newborn babies that is characterised by exomphalos; organomegaly (large tongue and abdominal organs); hemihypertrophy; and transient low blood sugar from excessive insulin production.
(4) Islet cell tumours are a rare cause of hypoglycaemia; they can be cured if the tumour (usually benign) is localised and excised.

THE BILIARY TRACT

Gallstones

In children, gallstones are seen in the following circumstances:
(1) Pigment calculi in babies: in all neonates there is an increased load of pigment associated with the change from a high fetal haemoglobin to a lower, newborn level. Occasionally, this results in pigment stone formation in the gall-bladder.
(2) Pigment calculi in haemolytic anemia: in spherocytosis and thalassaemia the high pigment load may produce gallstones.

(3) Congenital obstructive abnormalities of the bile duct or choledochal cysts are more likely to form stones.

(4) Cholesterol stones in adolescents, in which there is often a family history.

The ways in which a child with gallstones may present are summarized in Box 26.1

Box 26.1 Presentation of the child with gallstones

(1) Biliary colic: pain from a stone in the neck of the gall-bladder or in the common bile-duct.

(2) Cholecystitis: chemical or bacterial inflammation of the gall-bladder usually associated with cystic duct obstruction.

(3) Obstructive jaundice: dark urine and pale stools due to a stone obstructing the common bile-duct.

(4) Pancreatitis.

Treatment

Treatment involves laparoscopic cholecystectomy (and removal of stones in the common bile-duct, if present).

Choledochal cysts

Choledochal cysts have many forms, but usually represent cystic enlargement of the common bile-duct (Fig. 26.1). The presenting symptoms and signs include pain, jaundice, an upper abdominal mass and fever. Occasionally, prenatal ultrasonography reveals a cystic lesion in the abdomen, which can be treated postnatally before symptoms arise. The cause is unknown, but it may be a prenatal infection or inflammation.

Treatment

Treatment is by excision of the cyst and drainage of the proximal bile-duct by a choledocho-jejunostomy anastomosis to a loop of jejunum ('Roux-en-Y').

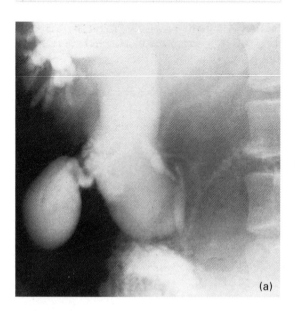
(a)

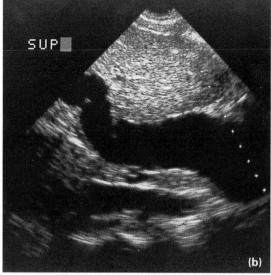
SUP
(b)

Fig. 26.1 Contrast X-ray (a) and ultrasonography (b) of biliary tract showing the massive tubular dilatation of a choledochal cyst.

Biliary atresia

Biliary atresia presents with obstructive jaundice in the first weeks of life. The baby has persisting jaundice, pale stools and dark urine.

The cause of biliary atresia is unknown, but an accepted theory is that there is viral damage to the extrahepatic duct system, often accompanied by damage to the liver itself.

Diagnosis

Diagnosis is by history, clinical examination and liver biopsy (the most helpful test). A nuclear medicine scan (for example, HIDA scan) shows decreased bile flow. The diagnosis is confirmed at laparotomy or laparoscopy where an operative cholangiogram shows an absent or incomplete biliary tree.

The disease must be distinguished from both metabolic disease (for example, galactosaemia and α_1-antitrypsin deficiency) and from neonatal hepatitis caused by viral hepatitis, cytomegalovirus or syphilis.

Treatment

Biliary atresia is treated by porto-enterostomy (Kasai procedure). At operation the remnant of the common hepatic duct is dissected to the porta hepatis where a mass of fibrous tissue is found at the confluence of the hepatic ducts. This area is excised and joined to a jejunal loop ('Roux-en-Y').

Despite the absence of visible ducts this operation is successful in up to 50 per cent of patients. The earlier in life that the porto-enterostomy is performed the better the results. Liver transplantation is required if progressive liver failure develops.

FURTHER READING

Howard E.R. (1998) Biliary atresia. In: Stringer M.D., Mouriquand P.D.E., Oldham K.T. & Howard E.R. (eds) *Pediatric Surgery and Urology: Long-term Outcomes*, pp. 402–16, W.B. Saunders, London.

Idowa O. & Hayes-Jordan A. (1998) Partial splenectomy in children under 4 years of age with hemoglobinopathy. *J. Pediatr. Surg.* **33**: 1251–3.

Miyano T. (1998) The pancreas. In: O'Neill J.A., Rowe M.I., Grosfeld, J.L., Fonkalsrud E.W. & Coran A.G. (eds) *Pediatric Surgery*, 5th edn, pp. 1527–44, Mosby, St. Louis.

Sawyer S.M., Davidson P.M., McMullin N. & Stokes K.B. (1989) Pancreatic pseudocysts in children. *Pediatr. Surg. Int.* **4**: 300–2.

Schiller M. (1998) The spleen. In: O'Neill J.A., Rowe M.I., Grosfeld, J.L., Fonkalsrud E.W. & Coran A.G. (eds) *Pediatric Surgery*, 5th edn, pp. 1545–54, Mosby, St. Louis.

— 27 —

Anus, Perineum and Female Genitalia

CASE 1

Dylan is a 3-month-old who presents with a tender, red, indurated area (2 × 2 cm) adjacent to the anal verge. Twice in recent weeks antibiotics were prescribed for a similar problem that resolved. On palpation and compression of the mass a drop of pus appears at the anus.

    Q. 1.1   *What is the diagnosis and its treatment?*

CASE 2

A worried mother rushes her 18-month-old daughter to the emergency department after noticing that no vaginal opening is visible. She is frightened something serious is wrong with the genitalia.

    Q. 2.1   *What is the diagnosis?*

    Q. 2.2   *How is it treated and recurrence prevented?*

ANAL FISSURES

These are confined mostly to infants and toddlers in whom the passage of a large stool splits the anal mucosa. There is a sharp pain and a few drops of bright blood on the surface of the stool.

When the area is examined the fissure often has already healed, an indication of its superficial nature and its rapid healing. When still present, it is visible usually anteriorly or posteriorly.

Treatment

The condition is of no consequence in itself and treatment is directed to the underlying constipation (see Chapter 22). No local treatment is required since the mucosal tear heals so rapidly.

After the relief of constipation the child may cry on defaecation for several weeks because he or she may associate defaecation with pain and react accordingly. The emotional tension built up around the act is more difficult to treat than the fissure itself and can be the forerunner of the whole vicious circle of constipation (Chapter 22).

PERIANAL ABSCESS

This is fairly common in infants and arises from infection in the anal glands, which open into the crypts of the anal valves. Although the abscess almost always presents superficially, the fistulous tract passes through the lowest fibres of the internal sphincter to open at the level of the anal valves.

Treatment involves identification and laying open of the fistula and drainage of the abscess (Fig. 27.1). Failure to deal with the fistula will result in recurrent infection.

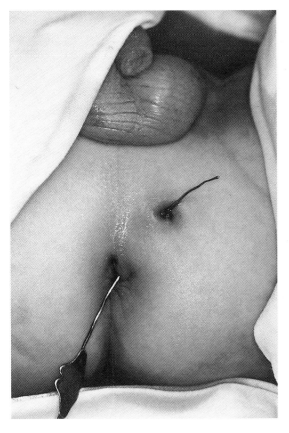

Fig. 27.1 In perianal abscess there is a fistulous tract that runs from the abscess to the anus at the level of the anal valves. The tract is displayed by the lacrimal probe.

Sometimes young children may develop a superficial subcutaneous abscess in the buttock or near the anus, which is often secondary to a nappy rash and involves infection with skin organisms. Simple drainage and antibiotics are curative.

RECTAL PROLAPSE

Rectal prolapse is not uncommon in toddlers and it is an alarming experience for the parents (Fig. 27.2). However, in most cases it disappears spontaneously after a few weeks or months without residual damage.

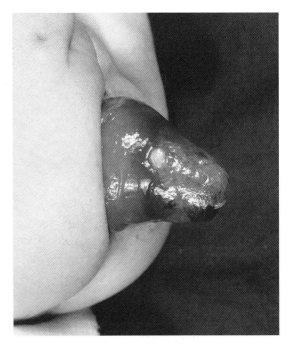

Fig. 27.2 Rectal prolapse. The mucosa is congested and oedematous, and may bleed.

Aetiology

The two common predisposing factors are:
(1) Straining at stool by a child with constipation. Less frequently, diarrhoea as part of a malabsorption syndrome (for example, cystic fibrosis or coeliac disease) may contribute.
(2) Explosive or reluctant defaecation. A healthy child occasionally develops a prolapse because the act is precipitate and little time is permitted for moulding of the stool by the muscles of the pelvic floor. Alternatively, the parents' ill-advised training may demand prolonged attempts to defaecate, producing excessive straining in the absence of constipation.

Rare, organic causes include:
(1) paralysis of anal sphincters (spina bifida)
(2) hypotonia/starvation
(3) ectopia vesicae (abnormal pelvic girdle)
(4) the after-effects of 'pull-through' surgery for an imperforate anus or Hirschsprung's disease.

Clinical features

Most children with prolapse have a normal anatomy. The prolapse rolls out painlessly only during defaecation and usually returns spontaneously; manual replacement is required infrequently. The mucosa may become abraded while it is prolapsed and cause minimal bleeding.

Differential diagnosis

A rectal polyp may prolapse (see below), and this can be identified by observation, digital palpation or proctoscopy. It is rare that the apex of an intussusceptum can appear at the anus. This is accompanied by its own clinical features (Chapter 19).

External haemorrhoids do not occur in childhood, but congestion of the submucosal venous plexus during straining at stool sometimes produces a bluish sessile bulge.

Treatment

Constipation is the commonest cause and treatment for at least several weeks is required (Chapter 22). When there is no constipation the possibility of a malabsorption syndrome should be investigated.

A common error is to squat the child on a pot on the floor, which stretches the pelvic floor and the anal sphincters to the maximum disadvantage. A potty-chair or an insert for an adult seat enables the child to sit with support for the pelvic floor; and a reasonable time limit should be set.

It is rarely necessary to inject a sclerosant into the submucous plane of the rectum to cause fibrosis and contraction of the rectal wall. This is reserved for the few stubborn cases that fail to respond to conservative measures; 0.5 mL of 5 per cent phenol in almond oil is injected into the submucosa at 3 equally spaced points, 2 cm above the anal valves. It is even more rare that a suture need be inserted into the subcutaneous tissues around the anus (Thiersch operation) and

tied while a finger is held in the anus. This is applicable in certain neurogenic lesions and in severe hypotonia, but is contra-indicated in ordinary constipation. The extensive operations for rectal prolapse performed in adults are never justified in infants and children.

RECTAL POLYP

A rectal polyp is a benign hamartomatous lesion and a relatively common cause of rectal bleeding. Bright bleeding is produced painlessly at the end of defaecation and is typically intermittent over long periods. Occasionally, the polyp prolapses through the anus (Fig. 27.3). The polyp is almost always within reach of an examining finger. The diagnosis is discussed in the section on rectal bleeding (Chapter 23).

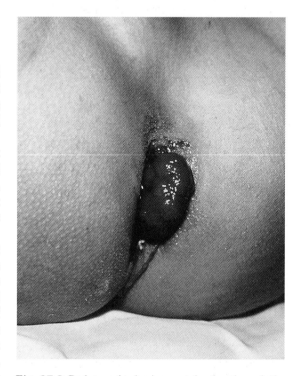

Fig. 27.3 Prolapse of a benign, rectal polyp through the anus.

Treatment

On the rare occasions that the polyp presents through the anus, the base can be ligated without anaesthesia. Otherwise, under general anaesthesia the polyp can be located through the proctoscope and withdrawn to demonstrate its stalk, which is transected with diathermy or transfixed with a suture-ligature. Higher lesions can be similarly removed through a colonoscope. Recurrence is rare and malignancy unknown.

MULTIPLE POLYPOSIS

This is a rare familial condition with malignant potential seen in adults, and even more rarely in children. It should be considered when more than three polyps are identified, and when there is a family history of multiple polyposis. Colonoscopy and a double contrast barium enema are indicated. In children, major fluid and electrolyte losses may ensue and the colon should be removed.

The Peutz–Jegher's syndrome

This is an even rarer condition that has gained prominence because of the external evidence of its existence — the presence of pigmented freckles on the mucocutaneous margins of the lips and the anus. Polyps are found anywhere in the gastrointestinal tract, especially in the jejunum, and give rise to massive bleeding, intussusception or intestinal obstruction. The polyps may become malignant, but this is less common than in familial polyposis of the colon.

POSTANAL DIMPLE (COCCYGEAL DIMPLE)

Many babies have a small shallow pit in the skin over the coccyx that is of no significance. Occasionally it is narrow and deep and may become infected, in which case it should be excised.

A simple benign coccygeal dimple is not to be confused with a sacral sinus that, although rare, is potentially more dangerous. The sacral sinus lies over the sacrum, not the coccyx, and it is associated with an underlying spina bifida occulta (Chapter 9). The depths cannot be seen and there is likely to be a small track that communicates directly with the spinal theca or with an intraspinal dermoid cyst. This track is a source of recurrent meningitis and the child should be referred to a neurosurgeon for treatment.

SACROCOCCYGEAL TERATOMA

A teratoma arising from and attached to the tip of the sacrum or the front of the coccyx occurs in 1 : 40 000 births, and slightly more frequently in females (Fig. 27.4). It is usually obvious at birth and may be so large as to cause obstetric difficulties. Occasionally, the swelling is in the pelvis and does not protrude from the perineum.

The tumour is a mixture of solid and cystic areas arising from all embryonic layers. The incidence of malignancy varies — from 5 to 35 per cent — and it is a type known as an endodermal sinus or yolk-sac tumour. Malignant degeneration is less likely when a teratoma is removed immediately after birth.

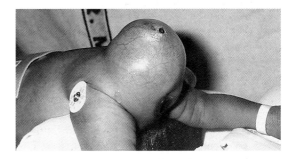

Fig. 27.4 Sacrococcygeal teratoma of medium size; note the distortion of the perineum and anal canal, and a small ulcer on the surface of the tumour. The prognosis for faecal continence after operation, however, is excellent.

Management

Even very small lesions over the coccyx should be referred to a tertiary paediatric centre for excision at birth. Differential diagnosis includes other rare tumours (chordoma or ganglioneuroma) or an anterior sacral meningocele. A computerised tomography scan or magnetic resonance image may be required to determine the extent of the intrapelvic tumour. Excision is undertaken in the first few days of life if the infant has no other developmental anomalies that might take priority. In spite of gross stretching of the pelvic floor, its nerve supply and the anal canal, the structures usually recover completely after careful surgery without any long-term neural deficit or lack of function.

Prognosis

Local malignant recurrence is uncommon, but more likely if:
(1) the tumour is uniformly solid and devoid of cysts
(2) the operation is not undertaken until after the age of 1 month.

The large benign teratoma presents at birth and could hardly be overlooked; it is removed in the neonatal period. However, a small malignant teratoma may escape diagnosis until a rapid increase in size brings it to notice later in the first year of life.

THE FEMALE GENITALIA

Developmental anomalies are rare in girls: the commonest abnormality, adhesion of the labia minora, is caused by ulceration of the labia (nappy rash) with secondary adhesion during re-epithelialisation.

Labial adhesions

This is a common condition, which may cause discomfort during micturition, but is more often discovered on routine examination (Fig. 27.5a and b). There is a delicate midline adhesion of the two labia minora that partially closes the posterior introitus, overlying the opening of the urethra, and may extend as far anteriorly as the clitoris.

Congenital absence of the vagina frequently is diagnosed in error, causing the parents much unnecessary anxiety. Labial adhesions never present at birth.

Treatment

In infants and young children the fused labia can be separated by exerting gentle lateral traction on the labia minora without anaesthesia or by sweeping them apart with the blunt end of a thermometer. In older children the labia may require separation under anaesthesia. Because of the tendency for the adhesions to recur, the mother should separate the labia daily for 2 weeks and apply petroleum jelly to the introitus to help prevent recurrent adhesion.

Imperforate hymen

This is a rare condition, which presents either at birth (the vagina secretes mucus that accumulates beneath the bulging imperforate hymen to form a mucocolpos; Fig. 27.6) or at puberty when apparent primary amenorrhoea, haematocolpos or even haematometrocolpos may be the presenting features, with cyclic attacks of abdominal pain. During childhood the condition is usually symptomless, except for possible urinary symptoms such as 'wetting', or dysuria when the cystic swelling distorts the urethra.

Treatment at birth sees the removal of a circular disc of membrane to provide drainage.

Vaginal discharge

The chief symptom is vulval irritation, but in some cases the discharge itself may be the only complaint. A profuse offensive or blood-stained discharge suggests the presence of a foreign body. Small objects may be successfully removed

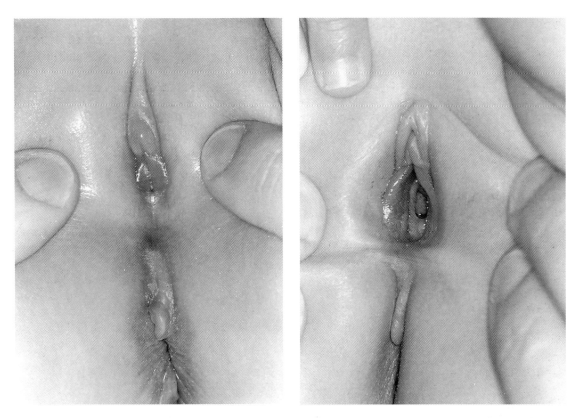

Fig. 27.5 Adherent labia minora (labial adhesions). The normal labia majora have been flattened by lateral traction to display the line of fusion (a). Following the separation the introitus is fully visible (b).

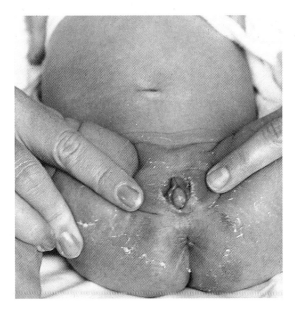

Fig. 27.6 Imperforate hymen causing mucocolpos in a newborn infant.

by irrigation using a soft rubber catheter or instrumental removal under anaesthesia, through a miniature vaginoscope.

The possibility of sexual abuse must be considered, and where suspected, the discharge should be sent for microbiological examination (Chapter 36).

FURTHER READING

Beasley S.W., Hutson J.M. & Auldist A.W. (1996) The anorectum and perineum. In: *Essential Paediatric Surgery,* Arnold, London, pp. 58–66.

Beasley S.W., Hutson J.M. & Auldist A.W. (1996) Labial adhesions. In: *Essential Paediatric Surgery*, Arnold, London, pp. 115–20.

Ein S.H., Mancer K. & Adeyemi S.D. (1985) Malignant sacrococcygeal teratoma-endodermal sinus, yolk sac tumour — in infants and children: a 32-year review. *J. Pediatr. Surg.* **20**: 473–7.

Shilyansky J., Lelli J.L., Drongowski R.A. & Coran A.G. (1997) Efficacy of the straight endorectal pull-through in the management of familial adenomatous polyposis — a 16-year experience. *J. Pediatr. Surg.* **32**: 1139–43.

Stafford P.W. (1998) Other disorders of the anus and rectum, anorectal function. In: O'Neill J.A., Rowe M.I., Grosfeld J.L. Fonkalsrud E.W. & Coran A.G. (eds) *Pediatric Surgery*, 5th edn, Mosby, St. Louis, pp. 1449–60.

Stephens F.D., Smith E.D. & Hutson J.M. (1996) Congenital anomalies of the urinary and genital tracts. Isis Medical Media, Oxford.

— 28 —

Undescended Testes and Varicocele

CASE 1

At birth a baby boy was noted to have only one testis in the scrotum. Re-examination at 3 months showed that both testes were now in the scrotum.

Q. 1.1   *What is the likely natural history of the testis?*

Q. 1.2   *Is treatment required later in childhood?*

CASE 2

No testes were palpable in the scrotum or groin in a baby at the 6-week postnatal check.

Q. 2.1   *What is the differential diagnosis?*

Q. 2.2   *What is the management?*

CASE 3

Unilateral undescended testis is diagnosed at birth and confirmed at the 6-week check in a baby with no other anomalies.

Q. 3.1   *What is the recommended age for surgery?*

Q. 3.2   *What is the prognosis for fertility and cancer risk?*

DEFINITIONS

Congenital undescended testis

A congenital undescended testis is one that has failed to reach the bottom of the scrotum by 3 months post-term. It represents the second most common problem in paediatric surgery after indirect inguinal hernia. At birth 4 to 5 per cent of boys have undescended testes, but postnatal descent may continue for the first 3 months, when the incidence of cryptorchidism falls to 1 to 2 per cent. Further descent after 3 months is rare. Most undescended testes have no recognisable primary abnormality, but become secondarily dysplastic if they do not reside in the scrotum. In the majority of cases the cause of maldescent is unknown, but it is likely to be from a mechanical rather than a hormonal defect. Placental insufficiency may be a factor.

Acquired undescended testis

The concept of acquired undescended testes is controversial, but it explains the high frequency of children presenting later in childhood. The cause may be failure of the processus vaginalis to disappear completely after descent, thereby leaving a remnant in the spermatic cord that prevents normal elongation with age (the length of the spermatic cord increases from about 5 cm in infants to 8 to 10 cm in adolescents).

Retractile testis

A normal retractile testis can be manipulated to the bottom of the scrotum regardless of the position in which it is first located. A retractile testis will remain in the scrotum for some time after manipulation. It is a normal size and there is a history that it is present in the scrotum on some occasions, such as during a warm bath. Testes may retract into an extension of the tunica vaginalis between the external oblique aponeurosis and the superficial abdominal fascia, known as the 'superficial inguinal pouch'. The position of the testis is controlled by the cremaster muscle that regulates testicular temperature by retracting the testis out of the scrotum when cold; it also protects the testis from trauma. Cremasteric contraction is absent in the first few months after birth and is maximal between 2 and 8 years. Retractile testes may be normal, but in severe cases they may represent acquired maldescent.

Ascending testis

An 'ascending' testis is one that is in the scrotum in infancy, but where the spermatic cord fails to elongate at the same rate as body growth. As a result, the testicular position becomes progressively higher during childhood. There is often a history of the testis descending into the scrotum some weeks after birth. This anomaly is thought to be a form of acquired undescended testes.

Impalpable testis

An impalpable testis is uncommon (< 10 per cent) and in about half of these the testis has undergone prenatal or perinatal atrophy. A grossly hypoplastic testis may be impalpable and only identified by exploration.

EXAMINATION

The examination of the testis should take place in warm and relaxed surroundings, and is begun by placing one finger on each side of the neck of the scrotum to pull the scrotum up to the pubis and to prevent the testes from being retracted out of the scrotum by the other examining hand. Each side of the scrotum is then palpated for a testis; if it is not there the fingertips are placed just medial to the anterior superior iliac spine and moved firmly towards the pubic tubercle (Fig. 28.1a), where the other hand waits to capture the testis if it appears (Fig. 28.1b). Its range of movement is determined carefully, for the diagnosis depends on this. The precise diagnosis of a palpable testis is made by determining how far it can be manipulated into the scrotum.

More than two-thirds of undescended testes are located in the 'superficial inguinal pouch' (that is, they are palpable in the groin) (Fig. 28.2). The testes are normal in size and are within the tunica vaginalis, which makes them deceptively mobile. It is rare that the testis will migrate to a truly ectopic position, such as the perineum, the base of the penis (prepubic) and the thigh (femoral).

SEQUELAE OF NON-DESCENT

The higher temperature of the extra-scrotal testis causes failure of postnatal germ cell maturation and poor development of the seminiferous tubules. After puberty there is oligospermia or azoospermia. A testis in the inguinal region is more liable to direct violence and torsion.

The risk of a seminoma arising in an undescended testis in later life is 5 to 10 times greater than in a normal testis after surgery at about 10 years of age. It is expected that orchidopexy early in life may prevent the development of infertility or tumours, but it remains to be proven.

TREATMENT OF UNDESCENDED TESTES

The object of treatment is to preserve normal spermatogenesis and prevent dysplasia, which could lead to malignancy. Hormone function at puberty (that is, testosterone output) is normal

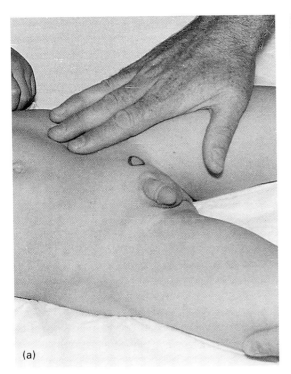 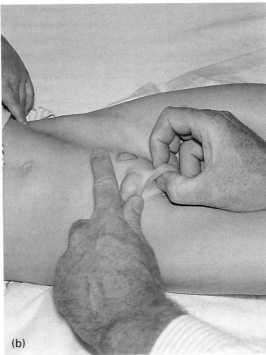

Fig. 28.1 Examination to locate the position of the testis: (a) the fingers of one hand push the testis towards the neck of the scrotum; (b) the other hand 'snares' the testis at the top of the scrotum to see whether it can be pulled right down to the bottom of the scrotum.

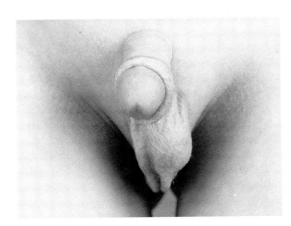

Fig. 28.2 Undescended right testis. Once out of the scrotum the testis often is invisible, even though it is palpable in the groin.

regardless of treatment. The maturation of gonocytes to spermatozoa is adversely affected in undescended testes from the age of 4 to 12 months onwards, and to a degree proportional to the length of time the testis remains undescended beyond this age. Testes with acquired maldescent may descend fully at puberty, but they are poorly developed and spermatogenesis is deficient.

The best time for orchidopexy for congenital cryptorchidism is at about 6 to 12 months of age, as shown by evidence of subsequent biopsies and sperm counts. Orchidopexy usually is performed as a day surgery procedure. Acquired undescended testes should have orchidopexy once they can no longer reside spontaneously in the scrotum.

Laparoscopic exploration for the uncommon impalpable testis is worthwhile, for in about 50 per cent of cases a useful testis can be brought down, and in the other 50 per cent there is either no testis present (testicular agenesis or intrauterine testicular torsion) or a useless and potentially neoplastic testis is removed. Gonadotrophic hormones are ineffective except for borderline retractile testes. A coexistent indirect inguinal hernia is almost universal but usually latent; when it becomes apparent clinically, herniotomy is necessary regardless of the boy's age, at which time orchidopexy is performed.

Absent testes

It is rare that the testis is absent or excised because of torsion (and necrosis), tumours or dysgenesis. These boys may have psychological problems and suffer significant embarrassment in the locker room. The use of prosthetic testes can be considered when psychological problems arise, but ideally insertion of a prosthesis should be delayed until adolescence when adult-sized implants can be accommodated in the scrotum.

VARICOCELE

A varicocele is an enlargement of the veins of the pampiniform plexus in the spermatic cord and usually appears in boys over 12 years of age, at or before the onset of puberty. The mass of veins is visible and palpable when the patient is standing, and feels like 'a bag of worms'. There is sometimes a small secondary hydrocele and the hemiscrotum is redundant. The varicosites empty when the boy lies down, and clinical examination should always include getting the boy to stand up. It is usually on the left side and symptomless, though a dragging ache may develop when the varicocele is large.

The problem of varicocele relates to the effect of the varicocele on spermatogenesis, because a unilateral collection of veins warms both testes and, by raising their temperature several degrees, causes oligospermia.

Treatment

The optimal temperature for spermatogenesis (and the normal scrotal temperature) is 33°C, 4°C below body temperature. Relative infertility

cannot be assessed until late adolescence, but secondary atrophy of the testis is well-recognised and if the affected testis is significantly smaller than the other then early operation is indicated.

High ligation of the spermatic vessels or ligation of the cremasteric veins, which anastomose freely with the spermatic veins, should prevent recurrence in most patients.

It is very rare that a varicocele develops as the result of obstruction of the renal veins by a renal or perirenal tumour (for example, Wilms' tumour or a neuroblastoma) almost always on the left side in a boy less than 5 years of age. The tumour can usually be palpated as an abdominal mass.

FURTHER READING

Clarnette T.D. & Hutson J.M. (1997) Is the ascending testis actually 'stationary'? Normal elongation of the spermatic cord is prevented by a fibrous remnant of the processus vaginalis. *Pediatr. Surg. Int.* **12**: 155–7.

Das S. & Springer A. (1990) Controversies of perinatal torsion of the spermatic cord: a review, survey and recommendations. *J. Urol.* **143**: 231–3.

Fenton E.J.M., Woodward A.A., Hudson I.L. & Marschner I. (1990) The ascending testis. *Pediatr. Surg. Int.* **5**: 6–9.

Hutson J.M. (1998) Undescended testes, torsion and varicocele. In: O'Neill J.A., Rowe M.I., Grosfeld J.L., Fonkalsrud E.W. & Coran A.G. (eds) *Pediatric Surgery*, 5th edn, Mosby, St. Louis, pp. 1087–110.

Hutson J.M. (1998) Undescended testes. In: Stringer M.D., Mouriquand P.D.E., Oldham K.T. & Howard E.R. (eds) *Pediatric Surgery and Urology: Long-term Outcomes*, W.B. Saunders, London, pp. 603–15.

Hutson J.M., Williams M.P.L., Attah A., Larkins S. & Fallat M. (1990) Undescended testes remain a dilemma despite recent advances in research. *Aust. NZ J. Surg.* **60**: 429–39.

Koff W.J. & Scaletscky R. (1990) Malformations of epididymis in undescended testis. *J. Urol.* **143**: 340–3.

Thong M.K., Lim C.T. & Fatimah H. (1998) Undescended testes: incidence in 1002 consecutive male infants and outcomes at 1 year of age. *Pediatr. Surg. Int.* **13**: 37–41.

Thorup J. & Cortes D. (1990) The incidence of maldescended testes in Denmark. *Pediatr. Surg. Int.* **5**: 2–5.

— 29 —

Inguinal Region and Scrotum

CASE 1

A 6-month-old boy presents with an intermittent swelling in the left groin. Both testes are in the scrotum.

    Q. 1.1   *What is the likely diagnosis?*

    Q. 1.2   *What is the treatment?*

CASE 2

A 7-year-old boy complains of pain and swelling in the right scrotum for 6 hours. He had mumps recently.

    Q. 2.1   *What is the differential diagnosis?*

    Q. 2.2   *Could he have mumps orchitis?*

    Q. 2.3   *What is the treatment?*

The inguinoscrotal region is the commonest site for surgical conditions in childhood. Because the area is readily accessible to inspection and palpation, accurate diagnosis is easy, but it depends on knowing the normal anatomy and the many conditions that may occur in the area.

The inguinoscrotal region is not isolated from the rest of the body. Symptoms and signs can arise here in systemic diseases and vice versa; for example, blood or meconium in the tunica vaginalis from intraperitoneal haemorrhage or meconium peritonitis, or torsion of the testis presenting with pain referred to the abdomen. A careful examination of the area, and of the whole patient, is necessary to avoid diagnostic errors.

THE 'ACUTE SCROTUM'

There is a group of conditions that cause a red, swollen and painful scrotum (Box 29.1)(Fig. 29.1).

There are wide variations in the speed of onset, the rate of progression and the local signs, and in the severity of pain.

Torsion of the testis

Testicular torsion is not the most common cause of an acute scrotum, but it is the most important. The spermatic cord undergoes torsion, obstructing the spermatic vessels; this is a surgical emergency because of the high incidence of necrosis of the testis if the cord is not untwisted promptly. The risk of torsion is highest just after the testis enlarges at puberty in 13- to 16-year-olds. Also, the risk is high in unoperated cryptorchid testes.

Two kinds of torsion occur:

(1) Intratunical (or 'intravaginal'), the most common, is made possible by an abnormally long mesenteric attachment of the testis and epididymis within the tunical vaginalis. The predisposing abnormality is almost always

Box 29.1 Causes of acute scrotum in children

(1) Torsion of one of its appendages; that is, the appendix testis (hydatid of Morgagni)   60%

(2) Torsion of the testis   30%

(3) Epididymo-orchitis   <10%

(4) Idiopathic scrotal oedema   <10%

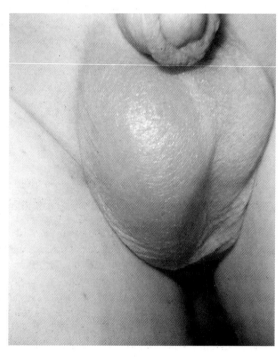

Fig. 29.1 Acutely inflamed right scrotum in a prepubertal boy. The inflammation is confined by the tight tunica vaginalis. Torsion of a testicular appendage or of the testis itself are likely causes.

present on the opposite side as well, and this testis should be fixed to prevent torsion at the time of surgery. It is rare that torsion occurs between the testis and the epididymis,

which are connected by a thin sheet of tissue. Unoperated cryptorchid testes are at risk as their fixation within the tunica is commonly tenuous.

(2) Extratunical (or 'extravaginal') torsion is rare, and confined to the neonate in whom there is a plane of mobility in the areolar tissue outside the tunica after testicular descent, but before the tunica normally becomes fixed to the scrotum. The testis is always necrotic by the time the diagnosis is made.

Clinical signs

The onset is usually sudden, with pain in the testis and/or ipsilateral iliac fossa, nausea and vomiting. Sometimes the onset is more gradual, without severe pain, and the diagnosis will be delayed if only the more acute form is accepted as typical.

A previous history of similar but short-lived, even momentary pain, is suggestive of episodes of incomplete and spontaneously resolving torsion. A horizontal 'lie' of the testes when the child stands indicates the possibility of torsion, and should be taken as an indication for exploration and orchidopexy.

The swollen testis and epididymis are exquisitely tender (unless already necrotic) and may be partially obscured by overlying scrotal oedema and an effusion into the tunica (reactive hydrocele). The amount of swelling depends on the time that has elapsed and the rate of progression. The hydrocele and the exquisite tenderness may make precise palpation of the testis difficult. As the pathology is within one tunica vaginalis, the signs are confined to the ipsilateral hemiscrotum.

Treatment

Urgent exploration of the scrotum is arranged to untwist the testis and epididymis and to anchor ('pex') both it and the contralateral testis to prevent subsequent torsion. If the testis is completely necrotic, it should be removed.

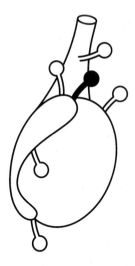

Fig. 29.2 Torsion of a testicular appendage. The hydatid of Morgagni is the commonest (remnant of the cranial Mullerian duct), and is at the upper pole. It is rare that there may be appendages on the spermatic cord and epididymis (upper or lower poles).

Torsion of an appendage

Torsion of an appendage (for example, 'hydatid of Morgagni') is the commonest cause of the acute scrotum in the prepubertal boy. The vestigial remnants are attached to the testis or the epididymis, and are present in about 90 per cent of the male population (Fig. 29.2). Recurrent attacks of pain also occur, sometimes very frequently, and the boy may present with a suggestive history, but few acute signs. A small tender lump at the upper pole of the testis is diagnostic.

Clinical signs

The boy complains of severe pain in his scrotum. A blue-black spot may be seen through the skin of the scrotum near the upper pole of the testis: palpation of it causes extreme pain, whereas palaption of the testis itself causes no discomfort. It may be impossible to distinguish torsion of a testicular appendage from testicular torsion once a secondary hydrocele has developed.

Treatment

Where torsion of the testis cannot be excluded on clinical examination, urgent exploration is mandatory, and at operation the appendix testis is removed. If the tender 'pea' of a twisted testicular appendage is palpable, surgical excision of it provides immediate relief of symptoms and prevents recurrence.

Epididymitis/Epididymo-orchitis

Epididymo-orchitis is rare in childhood, and virtually never occurs between 6 months of age and puberty. It is common practice to refer to inflammatory conditions in the scrotum as 'epididymo-orchitis', even though the epididymis alone is usually affected.

Escherischia coli may be carried by retrograde flow along the vas deferens from the urinary tract. Predisposing factors include abnormalities of the urinary tract or urethral instrumentation.

Clinical signs

The usual findings are acute scrotum in a baby or adolescent. A lax secondary hydrocele is common, and bilateral signs are particularly suggestive of epididymitis. Examination of the urine may show pyobacteriuria. The seminal vesicles and prostate may be tender on rectal examination.

Babies with epididymitis due to urinary organisms should have renal ultrasonography and micturating cysto-urethrogram after the epididymitis has subsided; this is to identify anomalies of the lower urinary tract before irreversible damage to the kidneys has occurred.

Differential diagnosis

The clinical picture can mimic torsion of the testes so closely that in most if not all children, the diagnosis should be made only after exploration of the scrotum. True acute orchitis is very uncommon, but may occur in mumps or septicaemia. Mumps orchitis is extremely rare prior to puberty. The testis is larger and harder than in epididymo-orchitis. Infiltration of the testis is rare also, but it does occur occasionally in leukaemia or with a primary neoplasm (embryonal adenocarcinoma, seminoma or a benign tumour of the interstitial cells of Leydig).

Treatment

Treatment of epididymitis consists of rest, antibiotics (for example, Septrin®, Furadantin®), a high fluid intake and alkalinization of the urine. Severe or repeated infections may lead to an abscess or progressive destruction of the testis, but sterility is rare when only one side is affected.

'Idiopathic' scrotal oedema

In this condition there is rapidly developing oedema of the scrotum that may then spread to the inguinal region, penis and foreskin, or on to the perineum.

The scrotum is symmetrically swollen, pale pink or red, and there is slight discomfort rather than acute pain. The pathology is in the skin (and therefore spreads beyond the tunica vaginalis), and is often allergic inflammation.

Careful palpation reveals non-tender testes that are normal in size and position. The oedema subsides in 1 to 2 days, but may occasionally recur some weeks later. There may be a history of allergy or of playing out of doors at the onset; a bite from an insect or a spider is a probable cause in some, but as a rule the history is inconclusive.

Differential diagnosis

It can be distinguished from other causes of the 'acute scrotum' by the complete absence of tenderness in the epididymis and testis, and by the spread of oedema beyond the confines of the scrotum.

The spread of infection from a pustule in the perineum can produce an area of slightly reddened skin and subcutaneous oedema that extends beside or across one-half of the scrotum. A tender enlarged inguinal node at or near the external inguinal ring assists in the diagnosis of perineal lymphangitis.

A toddler who sustains a straddle injury or sits on a toy with a sharp projection may injure the urethra, causing extravasation of urine. Pain on voiding, blood at the urethral meatus, and progressive oedema of the perineum, scrotum and suprapubic region are suggestive of urethral injury, which is confirmed on urethrography (Chapter 38).

Fat necrosis of the scrotum

This extremely rare condition presents with tender, usually bilateral, comma-shaped lumps in the scrotal wall of stout boys. Trauma may be responsible, but often there is a history of swimming in very cold water, suggesting that cold injury is the cause. Treatment is supportive, as the necrotic fat gradually absorbs. If doubt exists, exploration is required.

Management of the acute scrotum

As a general rule, urgent exploration is required in all cases of acute scrotum in which the possibility of testicular torsion cannot be completely excluded. The diagnosis of epididymitis or orchitis is unlikely, unless there is a history of urinary tract infection, a known developmental anomaly of the renal tract or significant pyobacteriuria.

A midline scrotal incision has advantages: when torsion of the testis is found it can be untwisted and fixed, and exploration and fixation of the opposite testis is done through the same incision.

INGUINAL LYMPHADENITIS

The superficial inguinal lymph nodes drain the lower limbs, the perineum, the buttocks and the perianal region — all common sites of minor skin infections in the 'napkin area' in infants. Infections often reach the inguinal nodes, which become enlarged and may form an abscess after the initial focus has disappeared. Occasionally, MAIS infection in preschool children involves these nodes. The axilla, neck and spleen should be examined for evidence of a generalised lymphadenopathy. In small children an inguinal abscess may be mistaken for a strangulated inguinal hernia. Treatment of an abscess is incision and drainage.

Deep external iliac adenitis

The proximal drainage of the nodes of the femoral canal is a group of deep iliac nodes on the brim of the pelvis around the external iliac artery. For no apparent reason an infection may pass inconspicuously through the more superficial inguinal nodes to form an abscess in these iliac nodes on the front of the external iliac artery and the iliopsoas muscle.

Clinical features

These are vague; general signs of toxaemia and fever are variable, and the hip may be held in slight flexion. The abscess is at first too deep to palpate clearly, and the diagnosis may be delayed until the abscess is large enough to appear above the inguinal ligament.

On the right side it may resemble an appendiceal abscess, but a distinguishing point is that a deep iliac abscess is contiguous with the inguinal ligament, whereas in an appendiceal abscess there is a gap between the two. The absence of vomiting and bowel disturbance is also helpful.

Treatment

Extraperitoneal drainage is required when pus is present, even if fluctuation cannot be detected clinically because of the thickness of the intervening tissues.

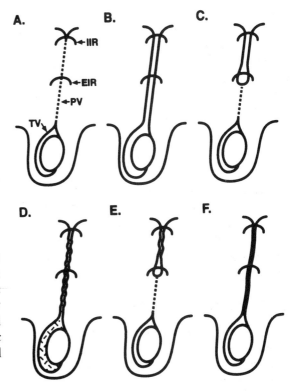

Fig. 29.3 Hernias and hydroceles. (a) The normally obliterated processus vaginalis (PV) between the internal inguinal ring (IIR), external inguinal ring (EIR) and the tunica vaginalis (TV); (b) a completely patent hernia; (c) incomplete hernia; (d) hydrocele with narrow but patent PV; (e) encysted hydrocele with fluid collecting as a 'cyst' in the spermatic cord; (f) residual fibrous remnant of PV that may cause ascending testis (reproduced with permission of Clarnette & Hutson (1997) *Pediatr. Surg. Int.* **12**: 155–7).

INGUINAL HERNIAS

The testis descends into the scrotum during the seventh month *in utero* through a diverticulum of peritoneum, the processus vaginalis. This begins to obliterate shortly before birth and closure is normally completed during the first year of life, leaving only the tunica vaginalis surrounding the testis (Fig. 29.3a)

Failure of obliteration of the processus vaginalis accounts for several clinical conditions in infancy and childhood: hernia, hydrocele and encysted hydrocele of the cord (and also possibly acquired undescended testes).

A hernial sac may extend from the internal inguinal ring to the tunica vaginalis — the so-called inguinoscrotal hernia (Fig. 29.3b). More commonly, there is a so-called 'incomplete sac' proximal to an obliterated segment that intervenes between the sac and the tunica vaginalis (Fig. 29.3c). This accounts for the vast majority of inguinal hernias in children.

A hydrocele in childhood is a collection of the lubricating fluid that is formed by the omentum within the peritoneal cavity; the fluid trickles down a narrow processus and collects in the space between the tunica vaginalis and the testis (Fig. 29.3d).

An encysted hydrocele of the cord develops in the same way; the peritoneal fluid collects in a loculus of the processus at some point along its course in the spermatic cord. This loculus usually retains its communication with the peritoneal cavity (Fig. 29.3e).

Combined abnormalities: multiple spaces or cysts develop along the processus, and it is not uncommon to find a proximal hernial sac communicating through a narrow tract with a distal hydrocele.

The higher incidence of abnormalities on the right side may be because the right testis descends later than the left and the processus on the right side is therefore more likely to remain patent. The higher incidence of hernias in premature babies is because the normally higher postpartum intra-abdominal pressure compared with the fetus makes it more difficult for the processus to close spontaneously.

In girls, the canal of Nuck undergoes the same obliteration as the processus vaginalis in boys. The obliteration is more likely to be complete, with a lower total incidence of hernias but a higher incidence of bilateral hernias.

Indirect inguinal hernia

Nearly all inguinal hernias in children are indirect, with an incidence of 1 in every 50 live male births.

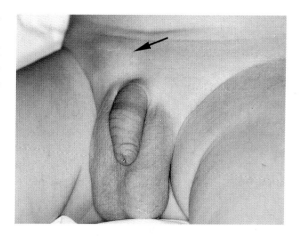

Fig. 29.4 Right indirect inguinal hernia (arrowed) in an infant.

This is the commonest condition requiring surgery during childhood and there is a high familial incidence.

Some 12 per cent of indirect inguinal hernias occur in girls, in whom they appear more evenly throughout childhood than in boys. In boys, the greatest incidence is in the first year of life, especially the first 3 months (Fig. 29.4): 60 per cent are on the right side, 25 per cent on the left and 15 per cent bilateral. The sac usually contains loops of small bowel, and sometimes omentum. In girls, the ovary is often palpable in the sac and may be difficult to reduce.

Diagnosis

The child's mother reports that there is an intermittent swelling overlying the external inguinal ring. It is usually painless but on occasions may cause discomfort. It is often present when there is an episode of crying or straining, and in infants it is seen during nappy changes. It may reach the bottom of the scrotum, as in the case of a 'complete' sac, and there is an impulse on crying or straining.

When the history is suggestive but the hernia is not seen during examination the index finger can be rolled transversely across the spermatic cord at the point where it lies on the pubic crest;

when there is a hernial sac, the spermatic cord is thickened in comparison with the side on which no swelling has been seen, and the 'rustle' of contiguous layers of peritoneum represents the empty hernial sac.

One source of confusion between the history and the clinical signs arises when the parents mistake a testis in the superficial inguinal pouch for a hernia, and the site of the reported swelling should be precisely indicated and the concurrent presence of a testis in the scrotum documented. If doubt still exists, a further examination is made a few days later.

The opposite side should always be examined, and both testes confirmed to be descended in the scrotum.

Differential diagnosis

The primary distinction to be made is between a hernia and a hydrocele; the latter is cystic, brilliantly transilluminable and irreducible, with no impulse on crying or straining, and its upper limit is identifiable distal to the external ring.

Femoral and direct inguinal hernias are rare but should be kept in mind; a retractile or undescended testis may mislead the unwary, and in young children, an inguinal lymph node may be situated close to the external inguinal ring.

Treatment

Surgery is necessary in all cases because of the danger of strangulation, which occurs most commonly in the first 6 months of life. An operation should be performed as soon as practicable, unless there is an intercurrent condition that requires attention; for example, a skin infection or bronchitis.

A herniotomy is performed through an incision in the transverse inguinal skin crease, and is a relatively simple operation in experienced hands, even in the newborn. Recurrence does not occur.

Exploration on the opposite side is usually undertaken in boys under 6 months of age, in whom a significant contralateral sac is present in

more than 50 per cent of cases. In 75 per cent of girls of any age a sac is found on the opposite side.

Strangulated inguinal hernia

Strangulation is the only significant complication of an indirect inguinal hernia; it is common in infancy but somewhat less common in older children. A loop of small bowel becomes trapped in the hernial sac, and although the blood supply is not compromised immediately in most cases, a hernia that is even temporarily irreducible should be considered as being potentially strangulated. The obstruction in the sac is at the external inguinal ring, unlike in adults where the obstruction is often at the internal ring.

Strangulated hernias are seen more often in infants under 6 months of age, such that up to 30 per cent of infants with an inguinal hernia initially present with a strangulated hernia.

Clinical features

The infant cries and cannot be pacified; when the mother changes the nappies a swelling in the groin is noted — perhaps for the very first time. There is a tense, tender swelling at the external inguinal ring and no impulse on crying. There may be generalised colicky abdominal pain, vomiting, abdominal distension and constipation when complete intestinal obstruction supervenes — but this may occur 12 hours after the onset. With delay in diagnosis, there may be redness and induration overlying the lump, or signs of peritonitis, suggesting bowel ischaemia.

Differential diagnosis

The differential diagnosis includes an encysted hydrocele of the cord, which may appear suddenly — but the swelling is not tender, the cyst moves readily with traction on the cord, and abdominal signs and symptoms are lacking.

Absence of a testis in the scrotum on the affected side may point to torsion of an undescended testis or of a descended testis that has been elevated out of the scrotum with torsion.

Lymphadenitis or a local inguinal abscess may be so confusing in young children as to warrant exploration to clarify the diagnosis.

Secondary effects

The testicular vessels can be severely compressed by a tense, strangulated hernia. Some degree of testicular atrophy has been reported in 15 per cent of boys after an episode of irreducibility and strangulation. For this reason early reduction is as important for the testis as for the imprisoned bowel. Occasionally, in infant girls, the ovary can be strangulated inside the sac.

Treatment

A strangulated hernia may reduce spontaneously *en route* to the hospital, but more often than not it persists. The strangulated hernia should be reduced by taxis. The tips of the fingers of one hand are applied to the fundus of the hernia while the fingertips of the other hand are cupped at the external ring. Gentle pressure is exerted initially to disimpact the hernia from the external ring, and then the contents of the hernia are reduced along the line of the inguinal canal. Nothing seems to be accomplished for a minute or two, and then the bowel suddenly gurgles and returns to the abdomen. Taxis is a manipulative trick, not a matter of force, and if necessary it can be attempted several times. A distressed child can be sedated with chloral hydrate 15 mg/kg. There is virtually no chance of producing reduction *en masse*, and in over 90 per cent of cases, taxis is successful. When this is so the patient should not return home until herniotomy has been performed, usually after 24 hours, to give time for the oedema of the sac and its investing tissue to subside.

When taxis is unsuccessful the child should be transferred immediately to a tertiary paediatric surgical centre for operation. The friable sac is difficult to handle and the surgery should always be

performed by a paediatric surgeon. In exceptional cases the bowel is gangrenous and a segmental excision with anastomosis may be necessary. The need for resuscitation before operation will be obvious from the clinical findings.

Direct inguinal hernia

Direct inguinal hernias are rare in paediatric practice, forming less than 1 per cent of inguinal hernias. They are occasionally seen in premature infants who develop bronchopulmonary dysplasia after prolonged ventilation, and in teenage children with cystic fibrosis. Repair of the posterior wall of the inguinal canal medial to the epigastric vessels is required.

Femoral hernia

Femoral hernias are equally rare. The diagnosis is made clinically when the swelling is below the inguinal ligament and lateral to the pubic tubercle.

As in adults, femoral hernias are more common in females, and the diagnosis is usually made between 5 and 10 years of age. The hernia is usually small and irreducible; most of it is composed of a fibro-fatty investment of the fundus. The hernia can be repaired easily from below the inguinal ligament.

HYDROCELES

Almost all hydroceles in infancy and childhood communicate with the peritoneal cavity via a patent processus. Much less common is the development of an 'acute' hydrocele secondary to some affliction of the testis or epididymis; for example, torsion, infection, trauma or tumour.

Clinical signs

A hydrocele is a painless cyst containing peritoneal fluid that has tracked down a narrow but patent processus vaginalis. It is situated in front of the testis, is brightly translucent and cannot be emptied by pressure because of a 'flap valve' at its junction with the processus. When the hydrocele is lax, the testis within it can usually be palpated with ease, or, when the hydrocele is tense, its shadow can be demonstrated by transillumination.

The upper limit of the hydrocele is clearly demonstrable; that is, the palpating finger 'can get above it', except in unusual varieties that extend up to the inguinal canal. There is no impulse on crying or straining.

Hydroceles in infants

Unilateral or bilateral hydroceles are common in the first few months of life. They are often large, lax, nearly always symptomless and have a strong tendency to close and absorb spontaneously. Most will have disappeared by the age of 1 year and surgery is only required if the hydrocele persists beyond about 2 years.

An encysted hydrocele of the cord is a loculus of fluid located above and separate from the tunica vaginalis. It does not require surgery in infancy, and may be considered a variety of the natural process of obliteration. After 2 years of age, or after observation for a year, operation to close the communication with the peritoneal cavity may be required.

Hydroceles in older children

In boys more than 2 years of age, there is often a diurnal variation in its size. It is small or absent in the mornings and at its biggest in the late afternoon, when it may cause a dragging ache.

These changes reflect the narrow communication with the peritoneal cavity along which the fluid returns during recumbency, and re-accumulates by the effect of gravity during the day. Despite the patency of the processus, the fluid can almost never be expelled by pressure.

A hydrocele in this age group rarely disappears spontaneously and surgery is required. The processus is transfixed and divided at the internal inguinal ring (that is, herniotomy).

FURTHER READING

Azmy A.A.F. (1994) Acute penile and scrotal conditions. In: *Surgical Emergencies in Children: A Practical Guide*, Raine P.A.M. & Azmy A.A.F. (eds) Butterworth-Heinemann, Oxford, pp. 256–71.

Beasley S.W., Hutson J.M. & Auldist A.W. (1996) *Essential Paediatric Surgery*, Arnold, London, pp. 67–76, 90–4.

Clift V.L. & Hutson J.M. (1989) The acute scrotum in childhood. *Pediatr. Surg. Int.* **4**: 185–8.

Cox J.A. (1985) Inguinal hernia of childhood. *Surg. Clin. North Am.* **65**: 1331–42.

Das S. & Singer A. (1990) Controversies of perinatal torsion of the spermatic cord: a review, survey and recommendations. *J. Urol.* **143**: 231–3.

Hutson J.M. & Beasley S.W. (1988) Inguinoscrotal lesions. In: *The Surgical Examination of Children*, Heinemann Medical, Oxford, pp. 35–54.

Ong T.H. & Solomon J.R. (1973) Fat necrosis of the scrotum. *J. Pediatr. Surg.* **8**: 919.

Puri P. & Surana R. (1996) Inguinal hernia. In: *Newborn Surgery*, Puri P. (ed.), Butterworth-Heinemann, Oxford, pp. 408–12.

— 30 —

The Penis

CASE 1

A mother brings her 6-week-old son to her general practitioner for advice on the care of the foreskin.

    Q. 1.1   *Should she retract and clean the foreskin?*

    Q. 1.2   *At what age does the foreskin become easily retractable?*

CASE 2

Alex is a 5-year-old boy who has a non-retractable foreskin.

    Q. 2.1   *How do you differentiate between normal preputial adhesions and phimosis?*

    Q. 2.2   *What types of treatment are available for phimosis?*

CASE 3

A mother of a newborn baby boy asks for advice on the pros and cons of circumcision.

    Q. 3.1   *What advice would you give on neonatal circumcision?*

    Q. 3.2   *If circumcision has to be performed, discuss the standards of surgery involved.*

    Q. 3.3   *What are the complications of circumcision?*

CASE 4

A newborn baby presents with hypospadias.

    Q. 4.1   *At what age is corrective surgery performed?*

    Q. 4.2   *What are the aims of surgery for hypospadias?*

    Q. 4.3   *What are the principles of hypospadias surgery?*

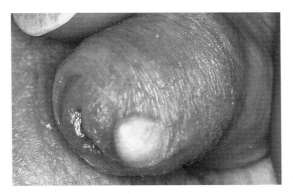

Fig. 30.1 Accumulation of smegma beneath the foreskin appears as a yellowish bulge at the level of the coronal groove.

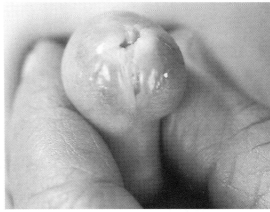

Fig. 30.2 Phimosis. Scarring of the distal foreskin causes stenosis of the opening.

THE PREPUCE AND GLANS PENIS

The prepuce (foreskin) is lightly adherent to the glans in the first few days of life, but becomes more densely adherent during the first year.

The foreskin cannot be retracted until spontaneous separation of these preputial adhesions occur. This is usually in infancy, but it may take 5 years or even longer. The normal process of separation of preputial adhesions is by the build-up of shed skin cells from the inner aspect of the foreskin (smegma). This sebaceous deposit of white cheesy material builds up under the foreskin to lift it off the glans; the discharge of this material is often mistaken for infection.

Accumulation of smegma may produce a yellowish bulge in the preputial skin (Fig. 30.1), and may be mistaken for a sebaceous cyst or even a tumour!

Care of the normal foreskin

The normal foreskin needs no special care in young children. If the foreskin is healthy it need not be retracted and does not have to be more specially cleaned than any other part of the body. After puberty the foreskin should be retracted for cleaning due to hormonal activity in this skin area. Young children do get problems with infection in the foreskin, but this is usually due to phimosis and the foreskin cannot be retracted in this pathological condition. Three abnormal conditions arise in the prepuce.

Phimosis

Phimosis (Fig. 30.2) is stenosis of the preputial orifice, caused by ill-advised forceful retraction, recurrent balanitis or an incomplete circumcision. Ammoniacal dermatitis (nappy rash) also is a common cause of phimosis. Both phimosis and the normal preputial adhesions can present as a non-retractile foreskin. Phimosis is defined clinically by the failure of gentle retraction of the foreskin to allow visualisation of the glans. In the case of normal preputial adhesions, gentle retraction opens out the foreskin to reveal the tip of the glans, but the adhesions prevent further retraction. Phimosis prevents drainage of the space between the foreskin and the glans leading to accumulation of stagnant urine and smegma. This leads to persistent low-grade infection which causes further damage to the foreskin and aggravates the phimosis.

Phimosis may be treated by the local application of steroid cream applied daily to the phimotic skin for two weeks. This steroid treatment is successful in many cases, but

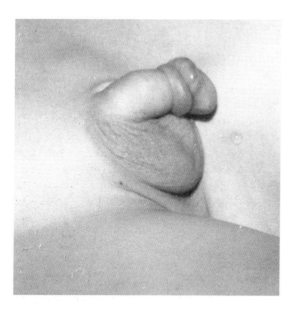

Fig. 30.3 Paraphimosis. The penis is red, swollen and painful. The prepuce has been retracted behind the glans and is compressing the shaft, causing oedema and venous congestion.

circumcision will be necessary if steroid treatment is not successful. It is important to treat phimosis actively. If a child is allowed to grow into adult life with phimosis, he will suffer from pain during intercourse due to the damaged foreskin. Chronic low-grade infection will occur under the foreskin and if this low-grade infection persists for many decades, it can lead to squamous cell carcinoma of the glans in later adult life. Ballooning of the foreskin on micturition is a sign of urinary obstruction requiring circumcision.

Paraphimosis

This occurs when a tight foreskin has been forcibly retracted. The retracted foreskin forms a constricting ring around the coronal groove of the glans, causing venous engorgement and painful swelling of the glans (Fig. 30.3). Retention of urine occurs and the problem demands urgent resolution. Reduction of the paraphimosis often requires general anaesthesia. If there is associated phimosis, this is treated once the swelling has settled.

Balanitis

Balanitis is an infection of the glans and foreskin. It occurs most commonly when infected urine pools under the foreskin due to phimosis. Once the infection is controlled the phimosis will need to be treated. Infection can also occur when the normal preputial adhesions are partially separated. In this circumstance, pockets of urine can be caught under the partially retractile foreskin. This infection responds quickly to topical or systemic antibiotics. Recurrent infection can occur until the preputial adhesions have separated completely.

Circumcision

Phimosis and the complications of phimosis, paraphimosis and balanitis are the medical indications for circumcision. However, the application of steroid cream may cause a rapid resolution of phimosis and this has reduced the need for circumcision (Box 30.1).

Circumcision also may offer some protection against urinary tract infection. This is not of great significance for the normal child but circumcision is often performed in a child with severe urinary tract abnormalities to prevent recurrent urinary tract infection.

Box 30.2 Complications of circumcision

Bleeding

Infection (local/septicaemia)

Ulceration of glans/meatus

Meatal stenosis

Penile deformity

Apart from these medical indications circumcision is also performed for religious and social reasons. The pendulum of opinion has swung back and forth, but circumcision for social reasons is now performed less frequently.

The commonest reason given for circumcision is for cleanliness and convenience, in that the foreskin does not have to be retracted. However, general standards of hygiene are now so high that prophylactic circumcision is not recommended. Carcinoma of the foreskin does occur as a rare tumour in adults with long-standing phimosis; the lesson here is that phimosis should be treated, rather than the normal foreskin removed.

There can be complications after circumcision (Box 30.2). The penis has a very good blood supply and postoperative bleeding may occur. In the neonatal period, any bleeding is of major concern as the blood volume of the average newborn is 80 mL/kg, which is 240 mL for a 3 kg baby. Any blood loss over 25 mL is life-threatening. By the age of 6 months a baby has doubled its birth weight and the safety factor on blood loss is more acceptable. Infection with coliform organisms to the open wound in the napkin area may lead to septicaemia in the neonatal period as the baby's own immunity is poorly developed. By the age of 6 months the baby is better able to cope with infection. The other common complication of circumcision is ulceration of the thin delicate epithelium of the glans. This can occur at any age, and sometimes leads to later meatal stenosis from scar contraction around the meatus. The glans needs to be protected

after circumcision with copious amounts of moisturising cream applied via nappy liner cloths for 2 to 3 weeks after the surgery.

Circumcision for religious reasons will be performed at the age and situation decreed by the religion. Circumcision for medical or social reasons needs to be performed at the optimal time for the best standards of medical practice. The standards of safety and skill expected of surgery and anaesthesia are very high, and the previous methods of circumcision performed in the neonatal period do not meet these standards. Circumcision should be performed after the age of 6 months in an operating theatre under general anaesthesia, with a careful surgical technique. The parents should receive consultation and education, so they can give informed consent. In years gone by the large numbers of babies presenting for social circumcision gave rise to the practice of circumcision in the neonatal period without anaesthesia, with a surgical technique in which speed, rather than meticulous tissue-handling, was the main consideration. The situation today is quite different, and circumcision should be judged by the same standards that apply to any important operation.

Meatal stenosis

This occurs as an acquired lesion caused by ulceration of the glans around the urethral meatus following circumcision. It leads to a thin urinary stream with dysuria and bleeding. The problem can be prevented by protection of the glans with moisturising cream for 2 weeks after circumcision. Scar contracture after meatal ulceration leads to meatal stenosis, and this requires surgical meatoplasty to correct the problem.

HYPOSPADIAS

Hypospadias is caused by the failure of fusion of the inner and outer genital folds that form the urethra, scrotum and the skin on the shaft of the penis. The urethral orifice opens on the ventral

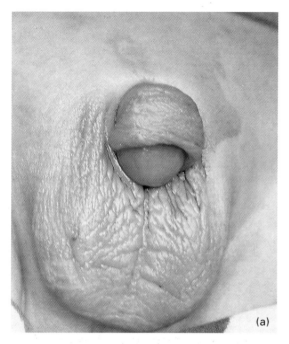

(a)

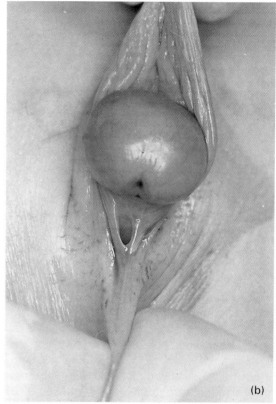

(b)

Fig. 30.4 Hypospadias. Incomplete fusion of the inner genital folds leads to a proximal urethral meatus, a dorsal hooded prepuce and chordee. The penis may look fairly normal (a) until the foreskin (dorsal hood) is pulled upwards, revealing the proximal urethral meatus (b).

surface of the penis and does not reach the end of the glans. In severe cases the urinary meatus may open in the scrotum or perineum. There is deficiency of the ventral foreskin and the skin on the ventral penile shaft (Fig. 30.4). The lack of tissue on the ventral surface of the penis leads to a tight 'bow-string' effect causing a ventral bending of the penis, known as chordee. This chordee deformity is more marked during erection and will cause difficulty with intercourse in later life if it is not corrected.

The malposition of the urinary orifice and the chordee deformity are usually present together, but in some cases severe chordee may be present with an orifice at the end of the penis.

Severe hypospadias with a bifid scrotum and undescended testicles is a presentation of intersex with ambiguous genitalia (Chapter 10).

The clinical findings in hypospadias are:
(1) Downward deflection of the urinary stream from the ventrally placed meatus.
(2) The penis is bent ventrally with the chordee, which causes pain on erection.
(3) The foreskin forms a dorsal hood and is deficient ventrally, which gives an abnormal cosmetic appearance to the penis.

These disabilities are functional: the affected boy finds it difficult to direct his urinary stream, and in later life, intercourse is difficult due to the chordee. The disabilities are also psychological, as severe anomalies of the penis may interfere with the development of the normal male body image. Therefore, the age for correction of hypospadias has been made younger, and now the recommended age for commencement of surgery is 6 months.

Investigation

Hypospadias is associated with some increase in other anomalies of the urinary tract and investigation with renal ultrasonography is recommended. Severe hypospadias with bifid scrotum and/or undescended testes (ambiguous genitalia) requires full investigation for intersex.

Treatment

The four aims of treatment are:
(1) To correct the chordee.
(2) To bring the urinary meatus to the tip of the penis.
(3) To provide a good cosmetic appearance.
(4) To achieve the above aims with the minimum complications.

Hypospadias surgery is one of the most difficult areas of surgery in children. As the primary defect is failure of tissue fusion, there is tissue missing from the ventral surface of the penis and any simple attempt at closing the defect has a high failure rate. There are over 250 different operations described for hypospadias because there have been problems in past years with hypospadias surgery. However, with modern surgical techniques the results of surgery are quite good and the success rate should be 95 per cent. The principles of surgery are as follows:
(1) The skin of the penis is mobilised extensively to correct the chordee deformity.
(2) The dorsal foreskin is advanced on to the ventral surface of the penis to replace the missing tissue on the undersurface of the penis. This new tissue is important for the correction of chordee.
(3) The skin advanced on to the ventral surface is used to make a new urethra up to the end of the penis.
(4) The new urethra is made with a 4-layer complex repair to provide adequate healing.
(5) Postoperative urinary drainage is usually aided by a urinary catheter or a urethral stent.
(6) In most cases of hypospadias the surgery is performed in a single stage; however, in severe cases the surgeon may elect to correct the chordee first and go on to do the urethroplasty at a later operation to reduce the complication rate.

Complications

Failure of healing with complete breakdown, or a partial breakdown with urinary fistula formation, is a distressing problem. Strictures may occur in the neourethra, and poorly corrected chordee will lead to troubles in adult life. These complications used to be common, but the standards of surgery for hypospadias are now quite high and one should expect good results.

EPISPADIAS

In this condition the urethra opens at the base of the penis, on its dorsal aspect. It is part of the spectrum of lower abdominal wall defects in which ectopia vesicae is the most severe form (Chapter 8). Most boys with epispadias are incontinent of urine because the bladder neck is deficient; epispadias as an isolated abnormality in a continent child is exceptionally rare, even rarer than ectopia vesicae itself, which occurs in 1 in 30 000 live births.

Apart from the problem of the repair of the urethra, using the same type of urethroplasty as in hypospadias, there are many of the same major difficulties that arise in ectopia vesicae.

FURTHER READING

Beasley S.W., Hutson J.M. & Auldist A.W. (1996) The penis. In: *Essential Paediatric Surgery*, Arnold, London, pp. 98–106.

Chatterjee S. (1989) Circumcision in India. Letter to the editor. *Pediatr. Surg. Int.* 4: 236–7.

Coran A.G. (1989) Circumcision in the United States: medical and non-medical attitudes. *Pediatr. Surg. Int.* 4: 229–30.

Cuckow P.M. (1998) Circumcision. In: Stringer M.D., Mouriquand P.D.E., Oldham K.T. & Howard E.R.

(eds) *Pediatric Surgery and Urology: Long-term Outcomes*, W.B. Saunders, London, pp. 616–24.

Cywes S. (1989) Circumcision in South Africa. *Pediatr. Surg. Int.* **4**: 233–5.

Ellis D.G. & Mann C.M. Jr (1998) Abnormalities of the urethra, penis and scrotum. In: O'Neill J.A., Rowe M.I., Grosfeld J.L., Fonkalsrud E.W. & Coran A.G. (eds) *Pediatric Surgery*, 5th edn, Mosby, St. Louis, pp. 1783–96.

Hofmann V. & Kap-herr S. (1989) Circumcision in Germany. *Pediatr. Surg. Int.* **4**: 227–8.

King P.A., Caddy G.M., Cohen S.H. & Pacca L.E. (1989) Circumcision — Maternal attitudes. *Pediatr. Surg. Int.* **4**: 222–6.

Rickwood A.M.K. (1989) Circumcision of boys in England: current practice. *Pediatr. Surg. Int.* **4**: 231–2.

— 31 —

Urinary Tract Infection

CASE 1

Stacey is a 5-year-old girl who presents with dysuria, pyrexia and haematuria. There is no relevant past history.

> Q. 1.1   What investigations should be done?
>
> Q. 1.2   What is the likelihood of an underlying urinary tract anomaly?
>
> Q. 1.3   If there is no urinary tract anomaly why has the infection occurred?

CASE 2

Thomas is 6 months old and presents with fever, lethargy and smelly, turbid urine. He is not gaining weight.

> Q. 2.1   How would a UTI be confirmed?
>
> Q. 2.2   What tests are needed to document a possible urinary tract anomaly?

Urinary tract infections (UTI) are misdiagnosed commonly in children. Dysuria and the passage of cloudy urine are common symptoms in children with a febrile illness and do not necessarily reflect UTI. On the other hand, many children with a UTI are symptomless, or have unexplained fever, vomiting, or even failure to thrive: in these patients, the diagnosis may be overlooked.

DIAGNOSIS

In the presence of pyuria the definite diagnosis of a UTI can be made from a pure culture of a urinary pathogen grown from an appropriately collected specimen. A high index of suspicion of a UTI is needed in any unwell child.

There are considerable difficulties in collecting a mid-stream specimen of urine (MSSU) in infants

and toddlers, but it should be possible to collect a clean mid-stream specimen in the older child.

A sample reagent strip to detect nitrites in the urine largely excludes UTI when negative. However, the presence of urinary nitrites does not prove UTI.

Suprapubic aspiration of urine

The most reliable technique of collecting urine is by suprapubic aspiration, which is the method of choice in infants up to about 18 months. This is because the bladder in infants is an intra-abdominal organ, making suprapubic needle aspiration of urine simple, quick and reliable. A 'bladder tap' should be performed in any sick infant to exclude UTI, particularly if a urine specimen obtained by other means is inadequate. In a 'septic work-up' it is important to do the suprapubic aspiration first, as infants will void

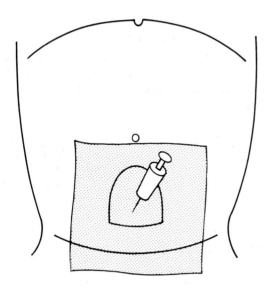

Fig. 31.1 The method of suprapubic aspiration for urine culture. The shaded area is the area of aseptic skin preparation.

during painful procedures such as venepuncture or lumbar puncture.

A 10 mL syringe with a 23-gauge 4 cm needle is used for the procedure (Fig. 31.1). The child is nursed supine and restrained by an assistant. The suprapubic area is swabbed with skin disinfectant and the needle introduced in the midline, 1 cm above the upper margin of the symphysis pubis. The needle should be introduced by aiming perpendicular to the floor: in the neonate insert the needle about 2 cm; further in older infants. The needle is then withdrawn while aspirating on the syringe, until urine is drawn into it. If the child starts passing urine, the urethra should be gently occluded. It is sent for culture in a sterile container. Any pure culture is significant if collected by suprapubic aspiration.

Bag specimen of urine

With the neonate and infant one sometimes has to rely on a bag specimen of urine, which may be contaminated by organisms from the surrounding skin or prepuce in the male, and from retrograde flow of urine into the vagina in the female. A pure culture of a urinary pathogen with a colony of $> 10^5$ organisms, and with more than 100 white blood cells per high-power field, is highly suggestive of a UTI in a bag specimen.

Mid-stream specimen of urine

In a continent male child the foreskin should be retracted until the urethral meatus is exposed, and the glans cleaned with soap and water using a soft flannel. The urine is collected mid-stream during continuous voiding, while keeping the foreskin retracted. The foreskin must be returned to its unretracted state following this procedure.

Similarly, in the older female child the labia should be parted, cleansed with a flannel, soap and water from the front to the back three times, and the child asked to void while holding the labia parted. The urine is collected in mid-stream during continuous voiding. Alcoholic preparations should not be used, as these cause intense pain on delicate mucosa.

Pitfalls in diagnosis

The urine specimen may be clear in a child with early pyelonephritis, especially in the presence of upper tract obstruction. In this instance the child should be treated empirically for pyelonephritis, and further specimens of urine should be taken during the course of treatment, as it is common for bacteriuria to be detected on the second or third day.

The child with an infected urinary calculus may have more than one urinary pathogen cultured from the urine specimen.

Cloudy urine does not always signify UTI. In many instances the cause of the cloudiness is simply precipitation of phosphate crystals when urine cools rapidly.

CLINICAL PRESENTATION

UTI can present with a wide variety of features. Table 31.1 emphasizes the fact that UTI may

Table 31.1 Presentation of urinary tract infection

Infants	Older children
Pyuria of unknown origin	Abdominal pain
Septicaemia	Dysuria
Listlessness and lethargy	Pyrexia
Haematuria	Haematuria
Vomiting	Pyelonephritis
Failure to thrive	Dysfunctional voiding
Persistent neonatal jaundice	

present with vague symptomatology, and hence one must have a high index of suspicion for UTI in any child who is unwell, with no obvious cause.

The purpose of evaluating a child with UTI is to exclude any underlying anatomical abnormality.

History

Previous episodes of UTI may not have been diagnosed. A careful history should be taken, particularly in relation to previous episodes of unexplained fever. Bed-wetting or voiding disorders do not necessarily indicate a urinary tract abnormality, except in a child who has been previously continent, although bladder instability may often present with recurrent UTIs. On the other hand, a history of constant dribbling of urine is abnormal; it requires investigation to exclude an ectopic insertion of a ureter. The family history is pertinent, as vesicoureteric reflux and duplex kidneys are known to be common among siblings.

Clinical examination

Many abnormalities can be diagnosed from the history and physical examination of the infant prior to organ imaging. Radiological investigations often confirm clinical suspicions.

After a general physical examination the abdomen should be examined carefully for a renal mass or an overdistended or expressible bladder, which in a neonate is indicative of a neurogenic bladder. The perineum should be inspected carefully, and perianal sensation and anal tone assessed.

Labial adhesions, phimosis, meatal stenosis (and even rarities such as prolapsing ureterocele in a female) can be diagnosed on inspection. A urological examination includes a neurological examination, as a neurogenic bladder is an important cause of UTI. The lower limbs are examined for signs of muscle-wasting, sensory loss and orthopaedic deformities (for example, talipes) that suggest the possibility of a neurological abnormality. The bony spine is inspected and palpated for occult forms of spina bifida or sacral agenesis. An overlying patch of abnormal skin (for example, pigmented naevus, hair, haemangioma, lipoma or sinus) may indicate the presence of a serious spinal lesion. Measurement of the blood pressure is essential because hypertension in a child with a UTI indicates significant renal pathology.

INVESTIGATIONS

The incidence of urinary tract abnormality in children with one proven UTI is at least 30 per cent, and higher in the first year of life. It is mandatory to investigate all children under 5 after one documented UTI. It cannot be over-stated that adequate documentation of UTI is important, and a clinical diagnosis of 'UTI' without urine culture is inadequate.

A micturating cystourethrogram and renal ultrasonography are the primary investigations, although there are a number of additional investigations that may be indicated in certain circumstances. For example, a plain abdominal X-ray may identify a renal or ureteric calculus (as most urinary calculi in children are radio-opaque).

Micturating cystourethrogram

A micturating cystourethrogram (MCU) is performed by the insertion of a small catheter into the bladder, filling the bladder and screening the patient during voiding to detect abnormalities. While a nuclear cystogram is an excellent investigation to exclude vesicoureteric reflux, it is not appropriate as a first investigation because it will not demonstrate abnormal anatomy such as urethral obstruction, para-ureteric diverticula and trabeculation of a neurogenic bladder.

The only investigation that can exclude local anatomical abnormalities is a radiological MCU. In the male child it is mandatory to examine the urethra during voiding to exclude outlet urethral obstruction.

All children under 1 year should be investigated early in the illness, as urinary obstruction is a common cause of UTI in this age-group. It is appropriate to perform an MCU immediately on these children, provided there is adequate antibiotic cover.

Renal ultrasonography

This is an accepted preliminary investigation to exclude urinary obstruction. It can be presumed that any significant obstruction will produce proximal dilatation, which is manifested as hydronephrosis, hydroureter or both. A good ultrasonography investigation should detect any dilatation within the collecting system. It must be remembered, however, that an ultrasonography examination gives no information on the function of the kidneys, and cannot exclude or diagnose obstruction.

If ultrasonography shows severe hydronephrosis suggestive of obstruction with pyonephrosis, an emergency percutaneous nephrostomy should be considered to drain the infected urine. This is minimally invasive, similar to draining an abscess, provides immediate relief of symptoms and may save the kidney.

Ultrasonography is valuable in the diagnosis of double systems and ureteroceles. Renal size and the status of the renal parenchyma are also measured. Ultrasonography is a good study for children as there is no ionising radiation involved and there is no need for painful injections.

Nuclear isotope imaging

Nuclear imaging of the renal tracts is useful for assessment of renal function, but does not give good anatomical information. The main renal isotope scans available are the 'MAG 3', the 'DTPA' and the 'DMSA'.

The MAG 3 and DTPA are excretory scans that measure differential renal function. The DTPA also measures the glomerular filtration rate. They also indicate obstruction when the clearance after the administration of lasix is measured, as this causes a delay in excretion. The DTPA scan is unreliable in the neonate up to about 6 weeks post-term, due to the immaturity of the neonatal kidney, and for this reason the MAG 3 is used in these patients. Dehydration may interfere with the assessment of obstruction, as low urine flow causes delayed excretion.

The DMSA scan is a more useful test in the neonatal period. DMSA is taken up by functioning renal cortical tissue, but does not give any indication of the excreting or concentrating ability of the kidney. It is useful in determining renal damage in reflux-associated nephropathy, and whether there is any functioning renal tissue in the neonate with gross hydronephrosis.

Intravenous pyelogram

This is a good investigation for delineating anatomy and overall function, but is only infrequently used in children. In specific circumstances, where knowledge of the ureteric and calyceal anatomy is essential (for example, in the management of urinary calculi, duplex systems and ureteroceles), it is the investigation of choice. An intravenous pyelogram not only outlines the renal anatomy and position of the calculus, but also shows obstruction caused by it. It is of limited usefulness in the neonate because of the poor concentrating ability of the immature neonatal kidney. Likewise, in the poorly functioning or very dilated system, dilution of the contrast medium will lead to poor definition of the anatomy. Other disadvantages include the high radiation dose and the lack of quantitation.

Antegrade and retrograde pyelograms

These are invasive investigations and are reserved

for those conditions in which it is essential to define the anatomy. General anaesthesia is needed in most children. An antegrade pyelogram can be performed in conjunction with a percutaneous nephrostomy when drainage of an obstructed system is required.

In general, the choice of 'second-line investigation' is best left to the attending urologist or paediatrician to decide.

THE MANAGEMENT OF URINARY TRACT INFECTION

In the child who is not toxic it is reasonable to obtain a urine specimen and to wait for cultures before commencing antibiotics. If the child is unwell a suprapubic aspirate is performed and treatment started while waiting for the results of the urine culture. It is best to admit these children to hospital. Any child under 1 year of age with UTI is likely to have pyelonephritis and must be treated with intravenous antibiotics.

Choice of antibiotics

The choice of antibiotics is governed by the sensitivities of the urinary pathogen. The commonest causative organism is *Escherichia coli*. For this reason cotrimoxazole or amoxycillin with clavuronic acid are suitable first-line oral antibiotics. Amoxycillin alone is not suitable because of the high numbers of resistant strains of *E. coli*. Nitrofurantoin and nalidixic acid are poor antibiotics in the ill child, as they do not achieve adequate tissue levels. Similarly, the new quinalones, although highly effective for treating adult UTI, are not suitable for children, as they may cause erosion of articular cartilage. Aminoglycosides are useful in serious upper UTI, but need careful monitoring in the child with poor renal function because of nephrotoxicity and ototoxity.

FURTHER READING

Brindle M.J. (1990) Children with urinary tract infection: a critical diagnostic pathway. *Clin. Radiol.* **41**: 95–7.

Hansson S., Hjalmas K., Jodal U. & Sixt R. (1990) Lower urinary tract dysfunction in girls with untreated asymptomatic or covert bacteriuria. *J. Urol.* **143**: 333–5.

Koff S.A. (1991) A practical approach to evaluating urinary tract infection in children. *Pediatr. Nephrol.* **5**: 398–400.

Rickwood A.M.K., Carty H.M., McKendrick T., Williams M.P.L., Jackson M., Pilling D.W. & Sprigg A. (1992) Current imaging of childhood urinary infections: prospective study. *BMJ* **304**: 664–5.

— 32 —

Vesicoureteric Reflux

CASE 1

Melanie is a 5-year-old girl who presents with a history of recurrent urinary tract infection.

Q. 1.1   *Which further investigations should be performed?*

Q. 1.2   *What are the pros and cons of the micturating cystourethrogram?*

Q. 1.3   *Are there any alternatives to the micturating cystourethrogram?*

CASE 2

A 1-year-old child with severe right-sided vesicoureteric reflux and recurrent urinary tract infection is found to have reflux nephropathy with defects in the upper and lower poles of the right kidney.

Q. 2.1   *Is reflux nephropathy congenital or acquired?*

Q. 2.2   *If the recurrent urinary tract infections are kept under control will further renal damage occur?*

Q. 2.3   *What are the indications for corrective surgery?*

Vesicoureteric reflux (VUR) is the most common underlying anomaly in children with urinary tract infections (UTI). Reflux allows transfer of bacteria from the bladder into the kidney with the risk of pyelonephritis and renal scars.

PATHOGENESIS

The normal ureter runs between the bladder muscle and the bladder epithelium for some distance before opening into the bladder cavity. This part of the ureter, known as the submucosal tunnel, allows the increased pressure of the bladder filling or micturition to compress the ureter against the bladder muscle and occlude its lumen. If the submucosal tunnel is short the ureter is not occluded by bladder filling and urine refluxes up the ureter into the kidney.

The urinary tract abnormalities seen in vesicoureteric reflux are due to two main causes:

(1) Congenital malformation: malformation of the ureteric bud during embryonic development of the urinary tract is the cause of VUR. If the abnormality is severe there will be a dilated megaureter and this megaureter will induce poorly developed renal parenchyma from the mesenchyme of the nephrogenic ridge. Thus reflux nephropathy has an important congenital element. This can be demonstrated soon after birth on nuclear medicine scans in babies who have never had a urinary tract infection. Other malformations of the ureteric bud that are associated with VUR include

paraureteric diverticulum and duplication of the ureter.

(2) Pyelonephritic scars: the second element of the renal damage seen in VUR is due to pyelonephritis. Pyelonephritis may cause acquired renal scars and recurrent episodes of pyelonephritis will cause progressive scars. Infants under the age of 1 year are particularly susceptible to pyelonephritis and renal scars.

In severe cases the combination of major renal parenchymal defects due to congenital malformation and subsequent damage from pyelonephritis may lead to renal failure. However, the spectrum of severity of VUR is broad and most cases in fact are mild. These mild cases show no ureteric dilation, the renal parenchyma is normal and nearly all these mild cases resolve spontaneously with normal growth of the bladder wall muscle over time.

PRESENTATION

Urinary tract infection

VUR is the commonest underlying congenital anomaly seen in cases of UTI proven by microscopy and culture of the urine. This is especially so if the UTI involves pyelonephritis or if there are recurrent infections. Many girls have distressing symptoms of UTI, but the urinary culture is negative though there may be pyuria. These symptoms may be caused by vulvovaginitis with coliform organisms, rather than UTI with VUR. A careful urine microscopy and culture on children with symptoms will distinguish vulvovaginitis from UTI.

Antenatal diagnosis

Antenatal ultrasonography is a very sensitive method to detect hydronephrosis and thus will identify the presence of significant VUR that causes upper tract dilatation. The micturating cystourethrogram (MCU) is an important part of the postnatal assessment of antenatally diagnosed hydronephrosis. This early diagnosis means that prophylactic antibiotics can be commenced at birth and now many children with severe reflux can go through life without ever having a UTI.

Associated defects

VUR is associated with other urinary tract abnormalities such as ureteric duplication and ureterocele, urethral valves, pelviureteric obstruction, vesicoureteric obstruction, and neuropathic bladder. A bladder diverticulum due to a muscular defect at the insertion of the ureter is particularly common with reflux. When one abnormality of the urinary tract is diagnosed it is important to investigate the whole of the urinary tract to exclude associated anomalies.

Family history

Some families have a strong history of urinary tract anomalies and particularly VUR. If an index case is diagnosed it is reasonable to perform renal ultrasonography on the siblings, but the MCU is unnecessarily invasive unless there is an additional indication such as UTI or an abnormality detected on ultrasonography.

DIAGNOSIS

There are no clinical symptoms or signs specific to VUR; it can be diagnosed only by special investigations.

Lower tract studies

The MCU is the key test for VUR. The bladder is catheterised and filled with X-ray contrast. The child passes urine under X-ray screening and the status of the urethra, the bladder and any refluxing ureter is documented. The severity of the reflux is graded by its extent and the degree of dilatation of the ureter and collecting system (Box 32.1). The MCU is an invasive, uncomfortable

Box 32.1 Grading of VUR

Grade 1   Reflux up normal calibre ureter without pelvicalyceal filling.

Grade 2   Reflux up normal calibre ureter with pelvicalyceal filling.

Grade 3   Reflux up dilated ureter into the dilated pelvicalyceal system.

Grade 4   Reflux up markedly dilated ureter and collecting system.

test because of the need for urethral catheterisation. However, this test is the most reliable way to diagnose VUR. One of the most difficult decisions in the management of UTI is whether to order an MCU. The following are some of the factors to take into account when ordering the MCU:

(1) Age: Young babies under the age of 15 months tolerate catheterisation and MCU better than older children who may struggle vigorously during attempts at catheterisation. As a result they may need restraint. Before ordering an MCU on an older child one should discuss the nature of the test with the parents and make a clinical assessment of the child's temperament by examining the genital area. If the child vigorously resists any attempt at clinical examination the MCU will be fraught with difficulty.

(2) Recurrent UTI: A child with repeated UTIs proven on urine culture must have an MCU to check for VUR and any associated abnormalities.

(3) First UTI: A child who has had a single infection will require an MCU if: (i) under the age of 15 months; (ii) the severity of the episode indicates pyelonephritis; (iii) there are abnormalities on renal ultrasonography; and (iv) there is a family history of urinary tract anomalies.

In some cases after a single UTI the need for an MCU is a borderline decision. If there is resistance by the parent and child it is wise to delay the MCU until a further infection develops.

There are alternatives to the standard MCU. If an MCU is indicated but the child is older and the parents are hesitant, the catheter for the MCU may be passed under anaesthesia in combination with cystoscopy.

The direct nuclear medicine cystogram also involves catheterisation of the bladder but the radiation dose is lower and the process of screening is easier. However, the demonstration of anatomical detail is poor and any associated defects in the bladder or urethra will not be seen. As a result, the direct nuclear medicine cystogram is not good for the initial assessment of VUR, but it is recommended for the follow-up of previously documented cases of VUR.

The indirect nuclear cystogram does not involve catheterisation. DTPA isotope is given intravenously and washed from the kidneys into the bladder with a diuretic. The child then passes urine and reflux is documented by the reappearance of isotope in the kidney. The other test that does not involve catheterisation is ultrasonography of the bladder and kidneys. Sometimes the ureter and collecting system will dilate during micturition and reflux will be suspected. However, neither the indirect nuclear medicine cystogram nor ultrasonography are reliable enough to assess VUR in the first instance.

The future development of a non-invasive test for VUR will be a great advance in diagnosis. In the meantime one must balance the need to diagnose VUR against the nature of the tests involved.

Upper tract studies

These studies are much less controversial. Renal ultrasonography is well tolerated and gives a good overall evaluation of the renal parenchyma and collecting system. Renal ultrasonography may be repeated periodically to assess renal growth.

Severe parenchymal defects will be detected on renal ultrasonography, but a more accurate measure of renal parenchymal defects is given by the renal isotope DMSA scan. This is, however, a more invasive and expensive test. Intravenous pyelography is rarely used in paediatric practice for the assessment of VUR.

NATURAL HISTORY

There is a strong tendency for VUR to resolve spontaneously in the preschool years with the normal growth of the bladder muscle offering better support to the intravesical ureter. Nearly all mild cases of VUR without ureteric dilatation (Fig. 32.1) resolve spontaneously. More severe cases of VUR with dilatation of the ureter (Fig. 32.2) have a lower rate of spontaneous resolution and may require surgical correction. Many of the renal parenchymal defects seen in VUR are congenital.

Poorly treated episodes of pyelonephritis may cause further acquired scars.

MANAGEMENT

Medical management

The initial management of vesicoureteric reflux is medical. Infection is prevented by using long-term low dose antibiotics given as a single night time dose at one-quarter of the daily therapeutic dosage level. The parents are instructed in the

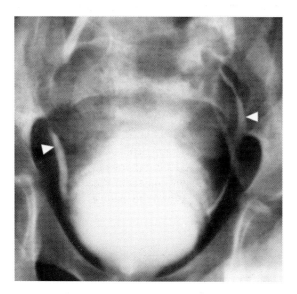

Fig. 32.1 Bilateral Grade 1 vesicoureteric reflux shown on MCU. The contrast in the lower ureters is arrowed. There is a good chance that reflux of this grade will resolve spontaneously.

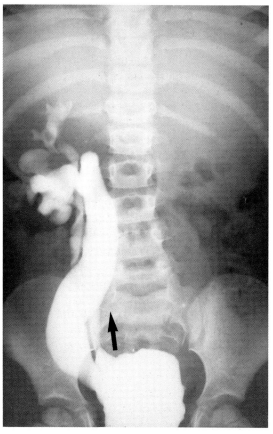

Fig. 32.2 MCU showing gross right-sided vesicoureteric reflux (arrow) up both ureters in a duplex system. There is no reflux on the left.

features of UTI in infants and children (for example, malaise, vomiting, anorexia, pyrexia, irritability), and any breakthrough infections are detected quickly and treated promptly. In most cases of reflux, infection is controlled by prophylactic antibiotics and spontaneous resolution will occur. However, medical management requires close follow-up by the doctor and conscientious care by the parents. Anything short of these high standards leaves the child at risk of repeated episodes of pyelonephritis and subsequent renal parenchymal damage.

Surgical management

Surgical management with reimplantation of the ureter has an important place in the correction of severe VUR. The standard surgical treatment of VUR is open reimplantation of the ureter. The ureter is dissected free from its short subepithelial tunnel and a longer subepithelial tunnel is fashioned. Recent endoscopic treatment with injectable substances has offered a less invasive surgical approach but the nature of the injectable substances is still too controversial to recommend as a standard treatment.

Correction of structural defects

VUR associated with other major abnormalities of the urinary tract such as paraureteric diverticulum, duplication of the ureter, ureterocele, neuropathic bladder, pelviureteric junction or vesicoureteric junction obstruction or urethral valves will usually come to surgical correction.

Failure of medical management

Medical management is not always successful. Breakthrough infections in the presence of reflux may cause pyelonephritis. If prophylactic antibiotics do not control UTI, reflux can be corrected surgically. Infection may still occur after surgical correction of reflux but these infections are usually due to cystitis and do not threaten the kidneys; they are thus less significant. The other problem seen with medical treatment is failure of spontaneous resolution of the reflux. This is often the case with the more severe degrees of reflux where there is gross dilatation of the ureter and pelvicalyceal systems.

Prepubertal girls with persisting VUR form a special group. It is generally recommended that VUR should be corrected in this circumstance because of the problems of pyelonephritis in any future pregnancy and the risk of miscarriage.

Whether vesicoureteric reflux is treated medically or surgically, a prolonged and careful follow-up of cases into adulthood is required. If there is renal parenchymal damage lifelong medical supervision is important because of the risk of hypertension.

FURTHER READING

Cass D.T. (1990) Surgical aspects of primary vesico-ureteric reflux. *J. Paediatr. Child Health* **26**: 180–3.

Ewalt D.H. (1998) Renal infection, abscess, vesicoureteral reflux, urinary lithiasis, and renal vein thrombosis. In O'Neill J.A., Rowe M.I., Grosfeld J.L., Fonkalsrud E.W. & Corun A.G. (eds) *Pediatric Surgery*, 5th edn, Mosby, St. Louis, pp. 1609–22.

— 33 —

Obstructive Lesions of the Urinary Tract

CASE 1

Antenatal ultrasonography at 18 weeks shows bilateral hydronephrosis in the fetus, which is still present in the third trimester, when oligohydramnios develops.

> Q. 1.1   *What is the natural history of antenatal hydronephrosis?*
>
> Q. 1.2   *What conditions cause antenatal hydronephrosis?*
>
> Q. 1.3   *What treatment is required at birth?*

CASE 2

Jamie, an 18-month-old, presents with fever and dysuria. Urine culture shows an infection and ultrasonography shows hydronephrosis and hydroureter (bilateral).

> Q. 2.1   *What causes 'hydroureter'?*
>
> Q. 2.2   *What investigations are needed for UTI?*

Hydronephrosis is an abnormal pelvicalyceal dilatation, due either to obstruction of the urinary tract or dilatation secondary to dysplasia of the urinary tract.

The patient with hydronephrosis presents an investigative challenge, because obstructive and non-obstructive lesions can be difficult to distinguish, and pathology in the ureter or bladder may mimic pelvi-ureteric obstruction.

AETIOLOGIC FACTORS

Pelvi-ureteric obstruction

Partial obstruction of the pelvi-ureteric junction is caused by stenosis, congenital kinking or a lower pole vessel crossing the ureter as it joins the renal pelvis. If the obstruction is intermittent, there is good preservation of renal function in the early stages (Fig. 33.1). Infection and progressive obstruction lead to the loss of renal function unless the blockage is relieved surgically. Occasionally, if progressive deterioration has been identified prenatally, early intervention is necessary after birth. However, less severe degrees of hydronephrosis in the newborn may resolve spontaneously.

Vesico-ureteric obstruction

Stenosis or valve formation in the lower ureter causes partial ureteric obstruction with marked dilatation of the ureter (Fig. 33.2). Mild cases may resolve spontaneously, leaving a persistently dilated ureter that is no longer obstructed. More severe cases require surgical correction.

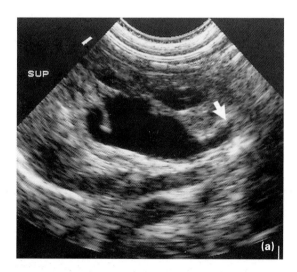

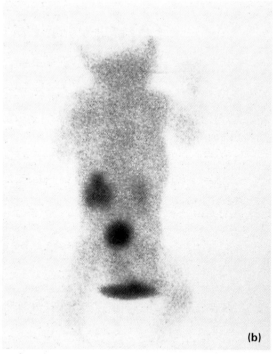

Fig. 33.1 Postnatal ultrasonography examination in an infant with antenatal hydronephrosis, showing (a) pelviureteric junction obstruction (arrow) with pelvicalyceal dilatation, but good preservation of renal parenchyma; (b) nuclear renal scan (DTPA) showing hold-up at the pelvi-ureteric junction at 45 minutes.

Posterior urethral obstruction

In males, two thin epithelial folds running down from the verumontanum on each side of the posterior urethra form a membrane or 'valve' that impedes the flow of urine with back pressure on the bladder, ureters and kidneys. When the obstruction they cause is severe, intrauterine renal failure occurs with fetal death *in utero*, or death soon after birth from Potter syndrome (respiratory insufficiency secondary to oligohydramnios). Less severe obstruction allows the fetus to survive, but if the problem is not detected early, septic complications from urinary tract infection (UTI) and metabolic abnormalities caused by renal failure soon occur. Mostly the diagnosis is made by detecting hydronephrosis on antenatal ultrasonography. The postnatal features include a thick-walled, palpable bladder and a poor urinary stream in a newborn male infant. The diagnosis is confirmed on MCU (Fig. 33.3). Fetal intervention is often considered but seldom appropriate.

Vesico-ureteric reflux

Massive reflux with associated hydroureter also can produce gross hydronephrosis when the upper tract distends with reflux. Secondary obstruction may also occur.

Neurogenic (neuropathic) bladder

Neurogenic bladder causes hydronephrosis in a number of ways. Patients may have a functional bladder neck obstruction from sphincter dysfunction with upper tract dilatation secondary to high intravesical pressure. Many patients with neurogenic bladder have reflux secondary to the neuropathy, which further exacerbates the upper tract dilatation.

Double ureters and kidneys (duplex system)

Congenital duplex kidneys may cause hydroneph-

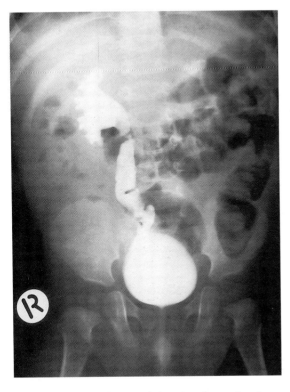

Fig. 33.2 Right vesic-oureteric junction obstruction shown in intravenous pyelogram.

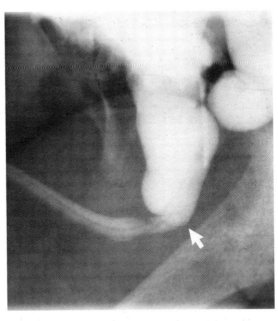

Fig. 33.3 Posterior urethral valves (membrane) seen on a lateral view of the urethra on MCU (arrow). Note reflux into megaureter, massive dilatation of posterior urethra and urethral catheter.

rosis of either part of the duplex system. The upper moiety is usually the more abnormal (Fig. 33.4), and the dilatation is caused by dysplasia or distal obstruction (from the ureterocele; Fig. 33.5), or an ectopic position of the ureteric orifice (for example, in the bladder neck). Ectopic ureteric insertion is often associated with dysplasia in a very poorly functioning subservient upper renal moiety. Dilatation of the more normal lower moiety may be caused by PUJ obstruction, or be associated with high grade VUR.

Stones (urolithiasis)

It is rare that in children a renal or ureteric calculus may cause an acute obstruction resulting in hydronephrosis.

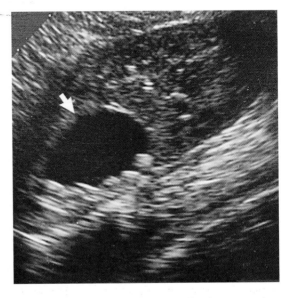

Fig. 33.4 Duplex kidney with a dilated upper moiety (arrow).

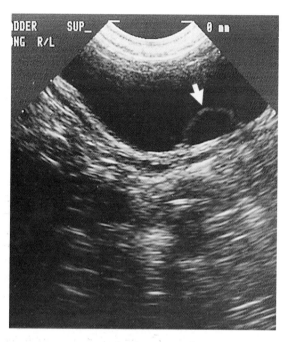

Fig. 33.5 Ultrasonography of bladder showing ureterocele (arrow) in the same patient as Fig. 33.4.

Table 33.1 Clinical presentation of urinary tract obstruction

Child	Infant/neonate
Pain	Antenatal hydronephrosis on ultrasonography
Infection	Incidental finding
Haematuria	Infection
Loin mass	Loin mass
Incidental finding	Haematuria
	Pain
	Septicaemia
	Failure to thrive
	Poor urinary stream (secondary to posterior urethral valves)

CLINICAL PRESENTATION

The clinical presentations of urinary tract obstruction are shown in Table 33.1

Pain is the most common presenting feature in the older child, and it may be accompanied by infection or haematuria, especially after minor trauma. A distinguishing clinical feature is lateralisation of the pain to the loin, and accompanying nausea or vomiting. Symptoms are exacerbated by a fluid load and sometimes by position.

Prior antenatal hydronephrosis on ultrasonography, and UTI, are the most common presentations in infants and neonates. Hydronephrosis may be detected in the neonate as a palpable abdominal mass. Presentation as a loin mass is unusual except in the neonate, in whom 50 per cent of all abdominal masses are renal in origin. The incidence of antenatal hydronephrosis is about 1.5 : 1000 live births.

Another mode of presentation is where renal investigations are performed for suspected abnormalities in children with known multiple anomalies in their siblings.

INVESTIGATIONS

Investigation aims to:
(1) prove obstruction
(2) assess renal function (on both sides)
(3) demonstrate the abnormal anatomy.

Ultrasonography

Ultrasonography is the first investigation performed on children with suspected obstruction. Good quality ultrasonography will not only demonstrate any abnormal anatomy, but it also may determine the likely cause of the problem. However, it will not prove that a dilated system is obstructed, nor will it demonstrate function in the dilated system.

Micturating cystourethrogram

A micturating cystourethrogram (MCU) is essential in the investigation of children with dilated upper tracts, to exclude associated vesico-ureteric reflux and to exclude distal obstruction; for example, posterior urethral valves in boys, or ureterocele.

Renal isotope scan

Renal isotope scans determine if there is obstruction and provide an estimate of the differential and total function of the kidneys. There are several different types of renal scan: an excretory (DTPA) scan for demonstrating overall function and obstruction and a parenchymal (DMSA) scan to demonstrate the amount of functional renal cortical tissue. The interpretation of renal scans is aided by computer analysis. A MAG3 scan can be used in the first few months of life when renal function is low (and DTPA scan is ineffective).

Intravenous pyelogram

Intravenous pyelography is used rarely today for the demonstration of renal function, but it is still an excellent investigation where it is essential to demonstrate the anatomy, particularly in duplex systems where both moieties are functioning.

Retrograde and antegrade pyelography

Both techniques are employed to demonstrate anatomy or obstruction where this is essential to the management of the patient and where it has been difficult to confirm with other tests. An antegrade pyelogram may be combined with a Whitaker test, where fluid is perfused through the upper collecting system while the pressure is measured. This is a dynamic test aimed at demonstrating functional obstruction at high fluid loads.

Pitfalls of investigations

The immaturity of the neonatal kidney presents difficulties in the interpretation of functional tests in the first month of life. As the concentrating ability and total renal function is low in the neonate, functional studies may give misleading results. For this reason it is best to defer functional studies for at least 6 weeks post-term, although a MAG3 scan can be used earlier than this time.

MANAGEMENT OF OBSTRUCTIVE LESIONS

It is best to divide the investigation and management of hydronephrosis into two age-groups: those presenting in the neonatal period and those presenting later.

Antenatal hydronephrosis

Not all hydronephroses demonstrated on antenatal examination turn out to be significant. However, when hydronephrosis is detected, it should be followed throughout pregnancy. If other urinary tract abnormalities are detected on antenatal ultrasonography, the hydronephrosis is likely to be pathological. Increasing hydronephrosis with oligohydramnios suggests low urine output with posterior urethral valves.

Neonates with antenatally diagnosed hydronephrosis should be commenced on antibiotics from birth while awaiting full evaluation, to reduce the risk of a severe UTI developing.

Clinical evaluation includes examination of the abdomen to exclude abdominal masses, and inspection of the perineum to detect clinically obvious abnormalities, such as a prolapsing ureterocele.

Children with antenatally diagnosed hydronephrosis should undergo postnatal ultrasonography to confirm the degree of hydronephrosis (Fig. 33.1), and a micturating cystogram to exclude distal obstruction or vesic-oureteric reflux within the first month. Functional evaluation is of limited value at birth because of the relative immaturity of the kidney; it is best to defer a renal DTPA scan until the baby is at least 6 weeks post-term. Occasionally, a DMSA of MAG3 nuclear scan is useful in this period to demonstrate any functioning renal tissue.

Apart from posterior urethral valves, definitive treatment is deferred usually until completion of the evaluation of the degree of obstruction. Many apparent neonatal pelvi-ureteric junction obstructions improve spontaneously. However, severe obstruction in the neonatal period will require early surgery. Children with severe obstruction usually have gross hydronephrosis on postnatal ultrasonography. The kidney is tense and usually palpable. A DTPA scan may show a non-functioning kidney, but if the DMSA scan shows an appreciable amount of renal cortical tissue, early repair will lead to significant recovery of renal function.

The metabolic and septic complications of posterior urethral valves are treated before endoscopic resection of the valves is performed.

Management of older children with obstructive lesions

In the older child the preliminary investigations should always include renal ultrasonography and MCU. These should be followed by a DTPA scan. Unless renal function is severely impaired (< 10 per cent), surgical relief of the obstruction should be undertaken. Where there is minimal function, the kidney is best removed (Fig. 33.6), and this can be done laparoscopically.

Percutaneous nephrostomy

This is a useful emergency measure to drain an obstructed kidney, particularly in the presence of infection. It leads to rapid clinical improvement in the sick child with pyelonephritis, as well as allowing significant improvement in renal function. Percutaneous nephrostomy enables evaluation of overall renal function and delineation of the anatomy by antegrade pyelography.

Open pyeloplasty

The standard operative procedure to relieve a pelvi-ureteric obstruction is an Hynes–Anderson pyeloplasty. This requires excision of the narrowed pelvi-ureteric junction and anastomosis of the spatulated ureter to the renal pelvis. The functional results of this operation are good, but these kidneys may retain their dilated appearance permanently. Endoscopic pyeloplasty is gaining popularity but the long-term results are not yet known. A

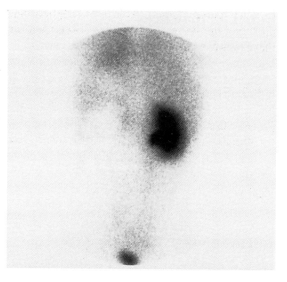

Fig. 33.6 Nuclear renal scan showing no function on left side at 5 minutes (view taken from behind).

nephroscope is inserted into the kidney through a small incision to divide the stricture, which is then stented for 6 weeks while healing occurs.

Total nephrectomy

Nephrectomy may be considered where back pressure from obstruction has destroyed the kidney; the dilated, poorly functioning kidney is a potential source of serious infection. Nephrectomy may be performed laparoscopically.

Partial nephrectomy

Duplex kidneys draining into an ectopic ureter or ureterocele (secondary to ureteric stenosis) may be poorly functioning and a potential source of recurrent infection. Non-functioning upper poles are treated by partial nephrectomy and excision of the ectopic duplicated ureter.

Obstructed megaureters

Excision of the stenotic segment and reimplantation of the ureter into the bladder is accepted treatment for obstruction at the ureterovesical junction and it gives good results. Balloon disruption and dilatation of the segment has also been tried but the results are still to be evaluated.

FURTHER READING

Jorgensen C. & Kullendorff C.-M. (1989) Ultrasonography diagnosis of fetal hydronephrosis: fetal renal pelvic size correlated to postnatal outcome. *Pediatr. Surg. Int.* **4**: 114–17.

Peters C.A., Bolkier M., Bauer S.B. *et al.* (1990) Urodynamic consequences of posterior urethral valves. *J. Urol.* **144**: 122–6.

Webb D.R., Tan H.L., Kelly J.H. *et al.* (1990) Management of urinary calculi using endourology and extracorporeal shockwave lithotripsy (ESWL). *Pediatr. Surg. Int.* **5**: 451–3.

— 34 —

The Child with Wetting

CASE 1

A 6-year-old girl presents with severe day and night wetting and urinary tract infections. She can have dry days, and her symptoms are worse with infection.

> Q. 1.1   *What is the relationship between UTIs and wetting?*
>
> Q. 1.2   *How would you investigate this case?*
>
> Q. 1.3   *Discuss further treatment.*

CASE 2

A 7-year-old girl presents with continuous mild wetting (a few drops leak out every few minutes) every day without fail and there are no other symptoms.

> Q. 2.1   *Of what condition is this a classic history?*
>
> Q. 2.2   *How is the diagnosis confirmed by investigation?*
>
> Q. 2.3   *What treatment is required?*

CASE 3

A 4-year-old boy presents with severe wetting day and night. When his doctor examines the lumbosacral spine, he finds a previously undiagnosed anomaly.

> Q. 3.1   *What are the 'hidden' variants of spinal dysraphism that may be missed in the neonatal physical examination and present at a later age with wetting?*
>
> Q. 3.2   *Why does the further investigation of these anomalies become much more difficult and costly if not performed in the first few months of life?*
>
> Q. 3.3   *How does the management of major neuropathic incontinence differ from dysfunctional wetting?*

Wetting is a very common childhood problem that causes distress to the child and their family and often perplexes the treating doctor. If the wetting is confined to night time only, almost by definition the bladder and its nerve control will be normal as the child has full bladder control except when asleep. Although bed-wetting is distressing, there will be no underlying problem with the bladder or

> ### Box 34.1 Causes of wetting in children
>
> **Bladder dysfunction**   Detrusor instability
> Wetting, UTI, VU reflux syndrome
> Inadequate emptying with overflow incontinence
>
> **Structural anomalies**   Ectopic ureter (females)
> Posterior urethral valve/membrane (males)
>
> **Neuropathy**   Spina bifida
> Spinal trauma
> Spinal tumour/congenital cyst
> Occult spina bifida
> Sacral agenesis

its nerve supply, and it does not pose a 'surgical' problem. Of interest to the surgeon is the more severe pattern of wetting occurring both day and night. The normal development of urinary continence is often called 'toilet training' as if it was a learned behaviour. In fact, the bladder in the young baby empties by frequent automatic detrusor contractions in response to it being filled by urine or sudden increases in bladder pressure because of crying. As the central nervous system develops, a message is sent from the frontal lobe down the spinal cord and along the nervi erigentes (S 3,4 segments) to the bladder muscle to stop any detrusor activity. This allows the achievement of urinary continence by conscious control.

Wetting (Box 34.1) may be classified as:
(1) bladder dysfunction
(2) structural anomalies of the urinary tract; for example, ectopic ureter and urethral valves
(3) neuropathic incontinence.

BLADDER DYSFUNCTION

Bladder dysfunction is expressed in three main forms:
(1) bladder instability
(2) wetting, urinary tract infection and vesico-ureteric reflux syndrome

(3) defective bladder emptying with overflow incontinence.

Detrusor instability

Detrusor instability occurs when there is delayed development of the normal central nervous suppression of bladder detrusor activity. Stimuli such as bladder filling, sudden pressure increase or exposure to cold will trigger detrusor contractions with wetting. Surprisingly, this pattern of wetting is often worse by day and better by night, as there is less activity while the child is asleep to set off detrusor contractions. When children feel the contraction coming on, they may drop into a squat, jamming the heel against the urethra to control the wetting until the detrusor spasm settles. Contraction of the detrusor against a closed bladder outlet leads to work hypertrophy of the detrusor muscle, and makes the wetting worse.

The combination of wetting, UTI and vesico-ureteric reflux

This combination is a syndrome that poses special problems as high pressure detrusor contractions may force infected urine under pressure up the refluxing ureter into the kidney (Fig. 34.1).

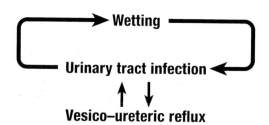

Fig. 34.1 The UTI–VUR-wetting syndrome.

Defective bladder emptying with overflow incontinence

This condition is diagnosed in children with infrequent and incomplete bladder emptying; for example, 2 to 3 times daily and large residual urine volumes. Bladder sensation is poor and the bladder is often palpable.

STRUCTURAL ANOMALIES OF THE URINARY TRACT

These anomalies include:

Ectopic ureter

Ectopic ureter in the female will open into the vagina outside the bladder sphincters with a characteristic pattern of mild but continuous wetting without any periodicity. The patch test is a simple clinical test whereby the young girl sits on a dry sheet during the consultation and a wet patch will be found. This form of wetting is not seen in males as the ectopic ureter opens above the external sphincter. The ectopic ureter drains the upper part of a duplicated collecting system. The upper renal segment is often poorly formed with defective renal function.

Urethral valves (Posterior urethral membrane)

Urethral valves are a male problem, related to an obstructive anomaly in the formation of the prostatic urethra. Most cases present at birth, but some less severe cases are diagnosed at a later age with wetting.

NEUROPATHIC INCONTINENCE

Neuropathic incontinence is usually an obvious diagnosis with spina bifida, spinal trauma or spinal tumour. In some cases, however, the nature of the spinal dysraphism is not immediately apparent unless one examines the lumbo-sacral spine carefully. Thus, in any case of wetting, it is important to turn the child over and examine the back. A dermal sinus will have a skin-opening over the sacrum that tracks to the spine and communicates with an intraspinal dermoid cyst. These lesions are rare, but should be diagnosed before infection occurs, to avoid the disastrous sequelae of abscess formation in the lower spine and spreading meningitis. Spinal cord lipoma shows the external manifestation of a diffuse fatty swelling over the sacrum with skin pigmentation and abnormal sacral hair growth. Diastematomyelia has an abnormal peg of bone growing from the vertebral body through a split spinal cord to the dorsal arch. This is marked externally by a dark skin pigmentation, abnormal hair growth over the affected segment, or duplication of the dorsal spines.

Investigation

Investigation will always start with a voiding chart compiled by the family over a 1- to 2-day period. This chart will record the time and volume of voiding, along with episodes of wetting. This voiding chart, along with the clinical findings, will often be enough to establish the likely diagnosis and plan of treatment in most cases. However, in some cases further investigations will be required. Renal ultrasonography will show damage from infection or may demonstrate an ectopic ureter. A plain X-ray of the lower spine may show a hidden anomaly, and during the first few months of life the spinal cord itself may be imaged simply with ultrasonography. In older children, ultrasonographic images are blocked by the density of the developing bone and a magnetic resonance imaging study would be required.

Urodynamic studies are necessary in all children with neuropathic incontinence and the loss of sensation in these cases means the study is well tolerated. However, these studies are difficult to perform in children with dysfunctional wetting as the study is painful and invasive. General anaesthesia may be necessary and urodynamic studies are only performed for severe and persistent cases of dysfunctional wetting.

In children with recurrent UTIs associated with wetting, a micturating cystourethrogram may detect vesico ureteric reflux or demonstrate urethral valves in males.

Treatment of wetting

Bed-wetting may be treated in a number of ways:
(1) Bladder training encourages the child to void frequently; that is, every 3 hours, with complete bladder emptying sometimes requiring double micturition. This is the basis of treatment for most forms of bladder dysfunction and it is usually managed by a nurse practitioner with paediatric incontinence expertise.
(2) Medication with an anticholinergic drug, for example, oxybutinin, may suppress detrusor instability. Antibiotic treatment will be required for urinary tract infection, but the wetting may persist once the infection has settled, as the underlying bladder dysfunction usually causes the infection.
(3) Clean intermittent catheterisation 5 to 6 times per day is the basis of treatment for neuropathic bladder incontinence.
(4) Surgery is only 'curative' in one condition: ectopic ureter in the female. Excision of the poorly functioning upper pole of the kidney and its draining ureter will cure the incontinence. Surgery for lower spinal problems, such as spinal cord lipoma, will usually arrest the deterioration of bladder function, but the bladder is unlikely to return to normal.

FURTHER READING

Khoury A.E., Hendrik E.B., McLorie G.A., Kulkarni A. & Churchill B.M. (1990) Occult spinal dysraphism: clinical and urodynamic outcome after division of filum terminale. *J. Urol.* **144**: 426–9.

Schulman S.L. & Duckett J.W. (1998) Disorders of bladder function. In: O'Neill J.A., Rowe M.I., Grosfeld J.L., Fonkalsrud E.W. & Coran A.G. (eds) *Pediatric Surgery*, 5th edn, Mosby, St. Louis, pp. 1671–84.

Yannakoyorgos K., Ioannides E., Zahariou A., Anagnostopoulos D., Kasselas V. & Kalinderis A. (1998) Management of nocturnal enuresis in children with desmopressin and bladder physiotherapy. *Pediatr. Surg. Int.* **13**: 281–4.

— 35 —

The Child with Haematuria

CASE 1

A recently circumcised baby is noted to have a spot of blood on the tip of the penis after micturition.

Q. 1.1   *What is the likely problem?*

Q. 1.2   *How is it treated or prevented?*

CASE 2

'Red water' is passed after a 3-year-old falls off a chair on to the side of a toy box. Physical examination reveals a fullness in the upper abdomen on the left.

Q. 2.1   *What is the differential diagnosis?*

Q. 2.2   *What is your plan of management?*

Haematuria usually causes such alarm that the child is brought early for medical attention. Confirmation of the presence of red blood cells should be obtained because haemoglobinuria, ingested dyes and plant pigments occasionally can be misleading.

Unfortunately, haematuria has often ceased by the time the child is examined, and the decision to investigate the child may be based solely on the observations of the parents or colleagues.

The causes are many, and in some the diagnosis is readily made (Box 35.1). In addition to generalised haemorrhagic disorders, haematuria can be due to inflammation, trauma, neoplasia or calculi in almost any part of the urinary tract.

Hydronephrosis and other malformations of the upper urinary tract often present with haematuria. It is seldom the sole presenting feature, and the clinical findings, examination of the urine and renal ultrasonography or nuclear scan, usually make a diagnosis possible.

HISTORY

A history of a recent streptococcal infection will be present in most of those with glomerulonephritis.

Frequency, dysuria, abdominal pains and fever point to an infection in the urinary tract; and injuries severe enough to damage the kidneys, ureter or lower urinary tract nearly always will present with an obvious history of trauma.

Haematuria sometimes has a familial background, and may be associated with familial deafness (Alport's disease) or related to exercise.

Pain on micturition and a few drops of blood at the end suggest urethral abnormality or meatal ulcer.

CLINICAL EXAMINATION

In boys who have been circumcised recently, the first thing to look for is a meatal ulcer. In these

Box 35.1 Plan of investigation of a patient with haematuria

(1) Cause obvious or readily determined

Renal mass	Overt glomerulonephritis
Bleeding disorders	Urinary tract infection
Hereditary haematuria	Meatal ulcer

(2) Cause apparent on simple radiological investigation

(a) Plain film	Urinary calculi
(b) Renal ultrasonography	Hydronephrosis and hydroureter
	Cystic or malformed kidneys
(c) MCU	Vesicoureteric reflux
	Vesical diverticulum
	Urethral polyp

(3) Cause obscure without resort to more extensive investigation

(a) Endoscopy	Urethral membrane
	Vesical diverticulum
	Vascular anomalies
	Small benign neoplasms of ureter or pelvis
(b) Retrograde pyelography	Atypical nephritis
(c) Renal biopsy	Vascular anomaly
(d) Selective renal arteriography	

boys, appropriate local measures will prevent unnecessary investigation. Occasionally it is seen in boys with phimosis after attempted forceful retraction of the foreskin.

Hypertension may point to chronic glomerulonephritis, and a palpable mass in the loin will focus attention on three conditions — hydronephrosis, Wilms' tumour and neuroblastoma — which are examined in greater detail in Chapter 25.

INVESTIGATIONS

Microscopy and culture of a mid-stream or catheter specimen of urine is the basis of diagnosis. Granular and cellular casts or persistent proteinuria in addition to 'Glomerular' red cells will lead to the diagnosis of glomerulonephritis, while pyuria and bacteriuria indicate infection as the cause of bleeding.

Phase contrast microscopy may show crenated and dysmorphic red cells to distinguish atypical focal glomerular lesions from lesions elsewhere in the urinary tract, which tend to give rise to more uniform red cell patterns.

Sterile pyuria accompanied by haematuria raises the possibility of a tuberculous infection.

Renal ultrasonography

Except in children with meatal stenosis or readily demonstrable glomerulonephritis, renal ultrasonography is necessary in every case.

A non-functioning kidney accompanied by a palpable mass may be due to hydronephrosis or a tumour, and renal ultrasonography will differentiate between the two.

Micturating cystourethrogram

A micturating cystourethrogram (MCU) will exclude

vesical or urethral diverticula or urethral polyps. A plain X-ray prior to the MCU may show a calculus.

Endoscopy

In some patients with haematuria all investigations so far are normal. Cystoscopy may be undertaken next, preferably while haematuria is present, although this may be difficult in children, for bleeding is often of short duration. Occasionally, cystoscopy reveals a vesical cause; for example, a small haemangioma or a diverticulum not shown in an MCU, or a urethral cause. An example of this is urethral membrane.

Renal biopsy

Most children with 'idiopathic' or 'essential' haematuria have histological evidence of a focal type of glomerulonephritis in which haematuria is precipitated by physical effort or by an intercurrent infection. Biopsy is not required routinely, but does have a place when haematuria is persistent or severe.

Arteriography/MRI

When haematuria is too persistent and severe to be explained by atypical focal glomerulonephritis, and renal ultrasonography, MCU, cystoscopy and renal biopsy are all normal, renal arteriography or MRI may be needed occasionally to exclude the exceptionally rare vascular anomalies of the renal or ureteric vessels.

TREATMENT

Haematuria is a symptom that leads to a variety of diagnoses, and the treatment of these conditions depends on the diagnosis (see related chapters).

FURTHER READING

Boineau F.G. *et al.* (1989) Evaluation of haematuria in children and adolescents. *Pediatr. Rev.* **11**: 101–8.

Leading article (1970) Haematuria in childhood. *Br. Med. J.* **2**: 678.

— 36 —

Trauma in Childhood

CASE 1

A 10-year-old boy is brought to the emergency department 35 minutes after being knocked off his bicycle at an intersection. Eye witnesses saw the child bounce off the car on to the road. The boy was unconscious on arrival, cyanosed and shocked.

> *Q. 1.1   What are the priorities in initial assessment and management?*
>
> *Q. 1.2   What is a secondary survey?*
>
> *Q. 1.3   Could there be a simple explanation for the loss of consciousness?*

CASE 2

Ian is a 4-year-old who fell over in the backyard (there were no adult witnesses); he has a jagged puncture wound in the palm of his right hand.

> *Q. 2.1   How would a deep visceral (nerve, tendon, arterial) injury be excluded?*
>
> *Q. 2.2   What management is required to prevent anaerobic infection?*

Despite most paediatric trauma being of a minor nature, it still accounts for a significant proportion of paediatric fatalities after the first year of life. Over the last decade there has been a dramatic reduction in the number of children dying of unintentional injury, and most of these reductions have been achieved by a significant reduction in the number of deaths secondary to motor vehicle accidents. The causes of accidents in children are different from those in adults (Table 36.1).

Death from trauma occurs in three well-defined periods:
(1) Early (< 1 hour post-injury): 50 per cent of deaths, secondary to disruption of the brain or major blood vessels.
(2) 'Golden Hour' (1 to 2 hours post-injury): 35 per cent of deaths, most of which are secondary to

extradural haematomas, massive haemothorax or haemo-peritoneum.
(3) Late (> 2 days): 15 per cent of deaths, from brain death, multi-organ failure and/or overwhelming sepsis.

The prevention of these injuries offers the best opportunity to reduce the mortality of childhood trauma.

Table 36.1 The causes of accidents in children

Accident	%
Falls	62
Bicycle accidents	12
Traffic accidents as pedestrians	9
Traffic accidents as passengers of motor vehicles	7
Other	10

INJURY PREVENTION

There are three ways to lessen or prevent childhood injury:
(1) To educate the parents and children about potential accident situations.
(2) To minimize injury in an actual accident; for example, the use of car restraints or cycling helmets.
(3) To limit injuries sustained after the accident; for example, by first-aid techniques. This requires an effective transport system that allows early, accurate assessment of injuries by trained personnel and rapid resuscitation prior to transport to an appropriate institution.

TRAUMA SCORES AND INJURY SEVERITY SCORES

Injury severity determination enables the quantification of the magnitude of single or multiple injuries. Scores based on physiological data can be applied prospectively to determine triage destination and likely outcome; for example, Champion Trauma Score and Paediatric Trauma Score. The Injury Severity Score (ISS) is based on the extent of tissue injury, which changes little following the initial insult. It is determined after physical examination, investigations, surgical intervention and/or post-mortem assessment, and it cannot be used as triage tool.

Glasgow Coma Scale

This was introduced to quantify the central nervous system function. It documents three different brain functions — eye-opening, verbal response and best motor response — after different and graded stimuli (Table 36.2). The Glasgow Coma Scale (GCS) is used widely and enables rapid assessment of neurological injury.

Champion Trauma Score

To quantify the severity of trauma of different types, a numerical value is assigned to five physiological parameters: systolic blood pressure, respiratory rate, respiratory effort, capillary refill and GCS. The sum of the assigned values is the trauma score. On a 0 to 16 range (where 16 is the least injured) (Table 36.3), a trauma score of less than 13 is an indication for transfer to a major trauma centre.

Paediatric Trauma Score

This quantifies the severity of multiple injuries in children to enable a speedy triage and dispatch to an appropriate institution. It measures six different parameters: patient weight, patency of the airways, systolic blood pressure, neurological state, cutaneous wounds and the extent of bony injury. Each parameter is scored minus 1, 1 or 2, with low scores indicating severe trauma (Table 36.4).

Table 36.2 Glasgow Coma Scale

Score	Eye opening	Verbal response	Motor response
6	—	—	Obeys commands
5	—	Oriented	Localises pain
4	Spontaneous	Confused	Withdraws (to pain)
3	To voice	Inappropriate	Flexes (to pain)
2	To pain	Incomprehensible Words	Extends (to pain)
1	None	None	None

Table 36.3 Champion Trauma Score

Score	Respiratory rate (breaths/min.)	Respiratory effort	Systolic BP (mm/Hg)	Capillary return(s)	Glasgow Coma Scale
5	—	—	—	—	14–15
4	10–24	—	> 90	—	11–13
3	25–35	—	70–89	—	8–10
2	> 35	—	50–69	< 2	5–7
1	< 10	Normal	< 50	> 2	3–4
0	None	Shallow/retraction	No pulse	Nil	—

Table 36.4 Paediatric Trauma Score

Score	Body weight (kg)	Airway	Systolic BP (mm/Hg)	CNS	Skeleton	Skin
+2	> 20	Normal	> 90	Awake	None	None
+1	10–20	Controlled	50–90	Obtunded/LOC	Closed fracture	Minor wound
−1	< 10	Unmaintainable	> 507	Coma/decerebrate	Open/multiple fracture	Major/penetrating

There are three categories of mortality risk: Paediatric Trauma Score (PTS) greater than 8 should have no mortality, PTS 8–0 has increasing mortality and PTS less than 0 has 100 per cent mortality.

The Abbreviated Injury Scale and the Injury Severity Score

The Abbreviated Injury Scale (AIS) grades severity of injury from 1 (minor) to 6 (non-survivable) in six different body regions: head and neck, face, chest, abdomen, extremities, and external. The Injury Severity Score (ISS) calculates overall severity by determining the AIS value for each of the three most severely traumatized regions, squaring the scores derived from each and totalling the results. The ISS indicates increasing severity of injury on a scale from 0 to 75. Severe injury is defined by an ISS greater than 15.

Initial assessment and management

In assessing the injured child, many steps are accomplished simultaneously; for example, while conducting a rapid assessment of a patient's respiratory, circulatory and neurological status, the history and the events relating to the injury are obtained. There is often no adult witness to the accident present in the hospital, and it is the ambulance personnel who provide valuable information relating to the time and mechanism of the accident.

Mechanism of injury

The mechanism of injury may suggest that the severity of injury is greater than appears from the physiological state of the patient and the overt injuries. Factors that may indicate severe injury vary in different types of accidents, and are discussed below:

(1) Motor vehicle accidents: important factors are high speed injury (> 60 km/hr), ejection of the patient from the car, death of another person in the same accident and of the child being trapped in a fire.

(2) Falls: important factors include the height of the fall (> 3 metres being significant), the part of the body that first struck the surface and the type of surface; for example, grass or pavement.

(3) Vehicle and pedestrian/cyclist accidents: the speed at which the vehicle was travelling and whether the child was wearing protective head apparatus are also important facts to be documented.

These factors predict that a child may have a major, but as yet undetected, injury and this must be taken into account during assessment.

Establishing priorities

The Early Management of Severe Trauma course (as instituted by the Royal Australasian College of Surgeons) has developed a set of priorities that apply to adults and children. It is important that patients are assessed and treated according to the nature of their injuries, the stability of the vital signs and the mechanism of injury. In general, patient management consists of a rapid primary evaluation, resuscitation of vital functions, followed by a more detailed secondary assessment — and when this has been done, definitive care is initiated.

The primary survey: 'A, B, Cs'

During the primary survey, life-threatening conditions are identified and management is begun simultaneously.

(1) A — Airway maintenance with cervical spine control.

(2) B — Breathing and ventilation.

(3) C — Circulation with haemorrhage control.

(4) D — Disability: neurological status.

Resuscitation phase

Shock management is initiated, patient oxygenation is reassessed and haemorrhage control is re-evaluated. The life-threatening conditions identified in the primary survey are reviewed constantly as management continues. Tissue aerobic metabolism is assured by perfusion of all tissues with well-oxygenated blood. Replacement of lost blood volume with warmed crystalloid, colloid and blood is commenced, as are other modalities of shock therapy.

Secondary survey

The secondary survey begins after the primary survey (A, B, C) has been completed, and the resuscitation phase (management of other life-threatening conditions) has begun. Each region — head, neck, chest, abdomen, extremities — is examined individually and in detail. A careful neurological examination, including the GCS, is an integral part of the secondary survey. An assessment of the eyes, ears, nose, mouth, rectum and pelvis should not be neglected.

Definitive care phase

This phase involves the co-ordinated management of all the child's injuries, including fracture stabilization and any necessary operative intervention. It may also involve stabilization of the child in preparation for transfer to a trauma referral centre.

Triage

Triage is the sorting of patients based on the need for treatment. This is particularly important where the severity of injury may exceed the capability of the hospital and its personnel to treat, and is a reason for transfer to a more specialised institution.

SUPERFICIAL SOFT-TISSUE INJURIES

The extent and severity of soft-tissue injuries tend to be underestimated. It is ill-advised to attempt to explore and suture wounds under local anaesthesia. Most wounds require general anaesthesia for assessment of severity, debridement of contaminated and devitalised tissue, repair of important deep structures (for example, tendons and nerves) and careful suturing of the skin. In small children it may be impossible to examine the external wound edges adequately without anaesthesia, let alone its deeper extensions. Lacerations through the deep fascia (where tendon or nerve damage cannot be excluded definitely) and those on the face (where a good cosmetic result is paramount) require surgical repair under anaesthesia, as do puncture wounds and those containing foreign bodies.

Debridement of wounds

The wound is explored aseptically to determine which structures are damaged and to remove foreign and devitalised tissue. Washing with soap and water, Savlon or chlorhexidine® removes dirt and grass. Where gravel has been ground into the wound, a scrubbing-brush may be needed. Failure to remove dirt from an abrasion may leave the child with a 'tattoo'. Once the wound is clean and free of foreign material the tissues are examined for capillary bleeding. If no bleeding occurs after cleansing, the tissue is likely to be avascular, and needs to be excised surgically. Devitalised tissue is removed until fresh bleeding occurs.

Special soft-tissue injuries

Some injuries and lacerations need special treatment because of their anatomical site.

The face

Facial lacerations can rarely be sutured under local anaesthesia because the child is often too frightened to lie still and the cosmetic result will be compromised. All except trivial lacerations should be referred to a paediatric or plastic surgeon.

The lip

Lacerations that cross the vermilion margin always need an experienced surgeon because failure to align the margin, even by a millimetre, will leave an ugly 'step'. Where the laceration is completely within the mucosa, exact apposition of the wound edges is unnecessary; here, the more important feature is to repair the underlying orbicularis oris muscle to avoid a 'dent' in the lip.

The tongue

Despite initially vigorous bleeding and major deformity of the tongue contour, suture of the tongue is rarely needed. Most lacerations should be left to heal and remodel naturally. Infection of intra-oral lacerations is rare.

The forearm, wrist, hand and foot

These are the sites where even a superficial laceration can sever subcutaneous tendons or nerves. These injuries should be presumed serious by the site and size of the laceration, and not on the presence of clinical signs of nerve or tendon injury, which in small children are extremely difficult to elicit. All these regions need exploration by an experienced surgeon under general anaesthesia. Further details of hand and fingertip lacerations are provided in Chapter 46.

The straddle injury

A slip on to the edge of the bath, bicycle bars or a fence may cause injury to the perineum. In females this causes a tear in the posterior fourchette, often with significant bleeding. Where adequate assessment is not possible in the emergency room the girl should be admitted for examination under anaesthesia. Minor splits do not require sutures. Injuries through the hymen need careful repair.

Where a laceration has penetrated the rectum, a colostomy for faecal diversion is required. Straddle injuries need careful assessment to exclude any possibility of sexual abuse (see below).

In boys a straddle injury may tear the bulbar urethra and cause extravasation of urine into the scrotum and lower abdominal wall. A urethrogram demonstrates leakage of contrast and the need for catheter drainage of urine or primary urethral repair.

TETANUS AND GANGRENE

Successful prophylaxis against clostridial infections rests on the triad of: (i) immunization; (ii) antibiotics; and (iii) adequate surgical cleansing of wounds as described above.

Active immunization

Tetanus immunization should be part of routine childhood immunization. Primary immunization of infants is achieved with three doses of triple antigen (diphtheria, tetanus, pertussis) and a booster at 18 months. Primary immunization of children between 2 and 8 years involves three doses of CDT (diphtheria and tetanus) and beyond this age, with three doses of CDT at not less than 2-month intervals.

Booster doses

Although immunity following complete vaccination is long-lasting, it is considered reasonable to maintain immunity with booster doses at 10-year intervals. With a tetanus-prone injury a booster dose of tetanus toxoid should be given if two or more years have elapsed since the previous dose. Active immunization against clostridial gas-producing organisms is not available.

Passive immunization

Tetanus immunoglobulin is available for the passive protection of individuals who have sustained a tetanus-prone wound, and those who have either not been immunized actively against tetanus or whose immunization history is doubtful. It should also be given to the fully immunized patient with a tetanus-prone wound when more than 10 years have elapsed since the last dose of tetanus toxoid. In all the above instances, active immunization should be commenced at the same time. Although tetanus immunoglobulin and vaccine can be given simultaneously, they should be administered in opposite limbs using separate syringes. The minimum routine prophylactic dose for adults and children is 250 IU given by intramuscular injection.

ANTIBIOTICS

Antibiotics should be used when wounds are contaminated, but antibiotics are ineffective in the presence of dead tissue or foreign matter, and should never be relied on to prevent infection in contaminated wounds.

CHILD ABUSE AND NEGLECT (BATTERED BABY SYNDROME)

Certain clinical signs and other features may raise the index of suspicion of abuse and point to the need for a closer examination of the psychosocial climate of the patient and family. The social and psychiatric aspects are often more important than the trauma itself, but lie outside the scope of this book.

General features

The incidence of intentional injury is difficult to determine, but it is probably far higher than is generally realised, and has been estimated to be from 0.3 to 3.0 per cent of all injuries in childhood. Infants and children less than 3 years of age are particularly vulnerable.

Clinical features

The history of the supposed accident is variable but it may be quite reasonable and acceptable; on other occasions it is conflicting or inconsistent, and sometimes utterly implausible. Information about previous injuries may be denied, distorted or difficult to obtain because the injuries were treated by a different doctor on each occasion.

The modes of presentation are diverse, but include:
(1) Unexplained fractures of limbs, especially when multiple.
(2) Multiple bruises, soft tissue swellings and/or lacerations.
(3) Subdural haematomas, particularly when bilateral.
(4) Failure to thrive, with spectacular gains in weight when admitted for investigation.

Other patients present with features that suggest an obscure, non-traumatic disease of the central nervous system, or a blood dyscrasia with haemorrhages, anaemia and ecchymoses. Accompanying findings that should arouse suspicion are listed in Box 36.1.

Investigation

A full blood investigation and clotting studies will exclude a blood dyscrasia as the cause of spontaneous haemorrhages, ecchymoses or anaemia. A bone scan will identify 'hot spots' that may suggest underlying fractures (Fig. 43.5). These 'hot spots' are X-rayed for evidence of old or new fractures. In children less than 1 year of age a skull X-ray should be taken because the bone scan may be unreliable in determining a skull fracture.

Social history

An inquiry into the family's circumstances, the parents' personalities and the health of the siblings may well provide the grounds for diagnosis. While poverty, hardship and social inadequacy are found commonly, they are not present invariably; and

Box 36.1 Observations suggestive of child abuse

(1) Bizarre scars, scabs, weals, circumferential abrasions on the limbs and hemispherical bite marks.

(2) Multiple retinal haemorrhages.

(3) Periosteal thickening of long bones in unusual areas.

(4) Symmetrical burns or scalds in unusual areas.

(5) Multiple insect bites and/or infestations; for example, pediculosis.

(6) Abnormal behaviour of the child in hospital; for example, withdrawal or stark terror alternating with effusive affection.

(7) An abnormal attitude of the parents to the injury. This varies considerably; for example, lack of affect, indifference, panic, guilt or belligerence. Their reactions may conceal an appeal for help.

(8) An apparently unrelated developmental abnormality: handicaps, both physical and neurological, that make the child 'different' can be associated with them becoming objects of abuse.

cases in well-to-do, sophisticated families are by no means unknown. There is a high incidence of psychiatric disturbance in the parents, as well as alcohol- and drug-dependence.

Diagnosis

This depends to a large degree on an awareness of the possibility that serious injuries in young children may not be accidental. Thus it is important that where there is some suspicion of non-accidental injury the child is admitted to hospital for assessment by the Child Protection Unit or equivalent.

Management

The treatment of injuries is almost the least of the problems and is conducted along the lines described elsewhere.

A plan of management for the individual patient and family is required urgently, bearing in mind that indignation and a punitive attitude towards the person inflicting the injuries, though natural, is unfruitful. The following measures should be instituted:

(1) Immediate protection of the patient.
(2) The assistance of a co-ordinating team composed of a paediatrician (to provide general care and advice), psychiatrist (to assess and treat) and medical social worker (to investigate the home and family, to supply social assistance and to aid rehabilitation of the family as a whole). The members of the team should be notified as soon as possible, ideally before the patient reaches the ward. Psychiatric assistance is rarely refused.
(3) Mandatory reporting of the case to local governments.

Prognosis

The long-term prognosis of children suffering from abuse and/or neglect is unknown, although there is some anecdotal concern that it is an inter-generation problem.

FURTHER READING

Beaver B.L., More V.L., Preclet M.H., Haller A. Jr, Smialek J. & Hill J.L. (1990) Characteristics of pediatric firearm fatalities. *J. Pediatr. Surg.* **36**: 97–100.

Johnson C.F. (1990) Inflicted injury versus accidental injury. In: Reece R.M. (ed.) Child abuse. *Pediatr. Clin. Nth Amer.*, **37**: 791–814.

Lafferty P.M., Lawson G.M., Orr J.D. & Scobie M.G. (1990) The role of the paediatric surgeon in alleged child abuse. *J. Pediatr. Surg.* **25**: 434–7.

O'Neill J.A., Rowe M.I., Grosfeld J.L., Fonkalsrud E.W. & Coran A.G. (eds) (1998) *Pediatric Surgery*, 5th edn, Mosby, St. Louis, Vol. 1, Part II. Trauma. pp. 235–66.

Peclet M.H., Newman K.D., Eichelberger M.R. *et al.* (1990) Patterns of injury in children. *J. Pediatr. Surg.* **25**: 85–91.

Schetky D.H. & Green A.H. (1988) *Child Sexual Abuse. A Handbook for Health Care and Legal Professionals.* Brunner/Mazel, New York.

Tepas J.J. III, Di Scala C., Ramenofksy M.L. & Barlow B. (1990) Mortality and head injury: the paediatric perspective. *J. Pediatr. Surg.* **25**: 92–6.

— 37 —

Head Injuries

CASE 1

An anxious mother brings her 6-year-old son to the emergency department after he fell off the fence.

Q. 1.1 *Which children require admission to hospital after a head injury?*

Q. 1.2 *Is there any indication for skull X-rays after head injury, and which children should have a computer tomographic (CT) scan?*

Q. 1.3 *Which children should be referred to a neurosurgeon after a head injury?*

CASE 2

The air ambulance brings a 4-year-old boy who was hit by a car at 70 km/hour when he ran on to a busy street. He has been unconscious since the accident (20 minutes).

Q. 2.1 *What are the principles of management of a child with a severe head injury?*

CASE 3

A 4-year-old child falls 2 metres out of a tree, striking his head on the ground. There is a 5-minute period of loss of consciousness. There is a boggy scalp haematoma on the left side and the child is pale, drowsy and confused. He has a thready, rapid pulse, complains of headache and has a sluggish dilated left pupil and right-sided limb weakness.

Q. 3.1 *You are the medical officer who receives the child. What is your diagnosis?*

Q. 3.2 *What urgency do you place on the child?*

Q. 3.3 *What management do you propose?*

CASE 4

A 6-month-old baby presents with a history of falling out of a pram. Skull X-rays show a large fracture.

Q. 4.1 *What would lead you to suspect that a head injury was non-accidental?*

CASE 5

A 6-year-old boy falls over at school, hitting his head on concrete. He cannot remember the accident.

Q. 5.1   What is concussion?

Head injuries are a major cause of morbidity and mortality in children. Children show remarkable powers of survival, but too often there are residual changes in behaviour, impaired intellectual performance and post-traumatic epilepsy. Careful neurological assessment, assiduous ongoing observation, vigorous resuscitative therapy with prevention of secondary brain injury and early referral to a neurosurgeon are vital if the many reversible aspects of head injury are to be treated and the outcome maximized.

DETERMINANTS OF INJURY

The pattern of head injuries in childhood is similar to that in adults, but there are some important differences related to the nature of the injury and the physical characteristics of the child's skull and brain.

The nature of the injury

Falls cause a high proportion (40 to 50 per cent) of injuries, with traffic accidents next in frequency. More children are struck while running across the road than are injured as passengers, compared with adults.

The nature of children's play also causes some characteristic injuries, for example, small, localized, depressed and compound fractures, which result from blows by stones, sticks and other weapons.

The physical characteristics of the skull

The vault of the skull is thin and elastic and capable of much greater deformation than in adults. The increased elasticity permits more energy to be absorbed by the skull. This dampens the acceleration or deceleration of the head after impact and reduces the concussive effects. Children can tolerate blows of considerable severity without immediate loss of consciousness, although the conscious state is subsequently depressed by brain swelling and haemorrhage.

The skull elasticity also causes more local brain damage at the point of impact than in adults. In the child, local indentation is often severe enough to produce a significant haematoma in the underlying brain. A child's skull can sustain considerable distortion without fracture, but when the limit is reached the fracture that results is often extensive and frequently of the 'bursting' type. The skull sutures do not close until the fourth year, so that marked diastasis of the sutures may follow bursting injuries.

At the moment of maximal distortion a fracture line may open widely, causing the underlying dura to tear and separate, pushing brain tissue out through the fracture. As the distortion decreases in the next few milliseconds, brain or arachnoid membrane may be nipped by the closing fracture line, so that brain or CSF may be found outside the skull beneath the scalp (Fig. 37.1). These fractures may widen progressively, resulting in the *growing fracture of childhood* that requires operative repair.

The physical characteristics of the brain

A child's brain is more prone to acute focal or general swelling than the brain of the adult. This is due to a cerebral vasculature that may undergo *vasoparalysis* with resultant secondary

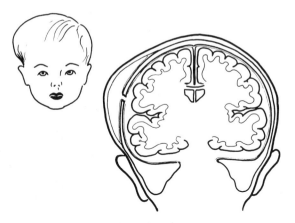

Fig. 37.1 Fractured skull. Cephalohydrocele, an accumulation of CSF beneath the scalp, following a laceration of the dura and arachnoid.

brain engorgement. This may occur acutely, even following minor trauma.

Early epileptic seizures are not uncommon in the first hour following head injury in children, but these do not usually continue.

General factors

The child is more susceptible to haemorrhagic shock than the adult because of the small *blood volume*. Thus, even a large scalp or intracranial haematoma in an infant may cause hypovolaemic shock.

GENERAL MANAGEMENT OF HEAD INJURY

The management of a child with a head injury includes initial triage into those who are observed and those who need admission to hospital (Box 37.1). Some children with minor concussion or its sequelae can be observed in the surgical department, while those with more severe injuries require neurosurgical assessment (Box 37.2). In certain cases, skull X-ray or CT scan may be needed (Box 37.3). Children who suffer major injuries need emergency management for their severe head injury (Box 37.4). Some types of head injury raise suspicion of child abuse (Box 37.5).

Box 37.1 Indications for hospital admission after head injury

(1) Loss of consciousness > 1 minute.
(2) Symptoms or signs of concussion after 4 hours of observation.
(3) Epileptic seizure.
(4) Suspected depressed skull fracture.
(5) Skull fracture on X-ray or CT scan.
(6) CSF leak from ear or nose.
(7) Associated multiple injuries.
(8) Suspicion of non-accidental injury.

Box 37.2 Indications for neurosurgical referral after head injury

(1) Depressed or compound skull fracture.
(2) Penetrating head injury.
(3) A drop of > 2 points in the GCS.
(4) Severe head injury (GCS less than 9).
(5) Persisting symptoms after 2 hours.
(6) CSF leak.
(7) Intracranial bleeding/swelling on CT scan.
(8) Focal neurological signs.

Box 37.3

(A) Indications for skull X-ray after head injury in children

(1) If there is a possible fracture and the child needs GA for CT scan to assess brain injury.
(2) There is a possible depressed fracture.

(B) Indications for CT scan after head injury

(1) Suspected severe brain injury.
(2) Depressed fracture.
(3) Suspected intracranial haemorrhage.

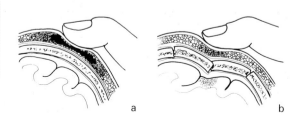

Fig. 37.2 Depressed fracture of the skull. Diagrams illustrate the similarity between (a) a haematoma with peripheral clot, and (b) a depressed fracture.

CHARACTERISTIC INJURIES IN CHILDHOOD

Depressed fractures

These are one of the commonest injuries in childhood and follow a blow with a small object or a fall on to a stone or sharp object.

Clinical findings simulating a depressed fracture (Fig. 37.2) can be caused by a scalp haematoma with a soft compressible centre. These findings are misleading and may cause one mistakenly to dismiss the possibility of a depressed fracture. Radiography offers the only method of determining the presence of a depressed

facture, or of a haematoma, with or without a simple fracture (Fig. 37.3, Box 37.3).

A compound fracture with penetration of the brain and dura is not difficult to diagnose, but a small compound depressed fracture is often missed. The small superficial laceration is sutured or left to heal spontaneously, only to reveal an unsightly depression when the swelling subsides. When the story suggests a blow with a sharp

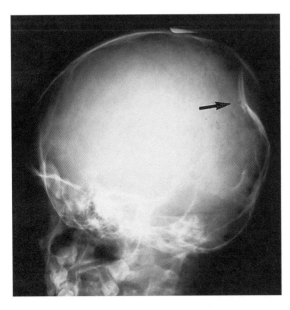

Fig. 37.3 Tangential skull X-ray is the best way to show a localised depressed fracture (arrow).

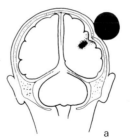 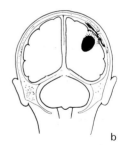

Fig. 37.4 Cortical laceration caused by (a) denting localized trauma and associated with (b) an intra-cerebral haematoma.

object, skull X-rays with oblique views must be taken to determine if there is an underlying depressed fracture. CT scan is an alternative, but may require general anaesthesia.

Penetrating wounds

Small penetrating wounds in the scalp or penetration through the nose or orbit into the anterior cranial fossa caused by sharp objects are not uncommon. The point penetrates the skull and brain with little general disturbance, and the incident may be dismissed as trivial until infection or other complications ensue. Skull X-rays with oblique views are helpful and a CT scan may indicate the degree of penetration; it also shows the extent of haemorrhage along the track.

All compound depressed fractures and penetrating injuries will require exploration, surgical debridement, dural repair and elevation of the fractures, particularly to stop haemorrhage and prevent sepsis. A fracture that is depressed greater than the thickness of the skull will require elevation.

Intracranial haemorrhage

Intracerebral haemorrhage

Intracerebral haemorrhage is common in childhood because the elastic skull is readily indented, thus causing oedema or haemorrhage that may extend deeply into the brain. This type of injury is most common where an indentation is most easily produced; that is, in the posterior parietal region (Fig 37.4), producing sensory and visual field defects on the opposite side.

These haematomas may require evacuation if they are large enough to compromise the child's condition, especially if progressive deterioration occurs.

Subarachnoid haemorrhage

A subarachnoid haemorrhage can occur in the child as a result of a minor head injury. For example, the child falls, strikes his or her head and cries for a while; later headache, vomiting and drowsiness occur, often with fever and neck stiffness, all of which may suggest meningitis. A lumbar puncture excludes infection.

Sometimes deterioration of the conscious state is the main feature, and a subdural or extradural haemorrhage should be considered. Subarachnoid haemorrhage also follows severe brain injury and may occur with an acute subdural haematoma. The subarachnoid haemorrhage is identified on CT scan.

Subdural haemorrhage

Acute subdural haematoma occurs when there is active bleeding in the subdural space, resulting from 3 types of injury:

(1) Sudden deceleration in a motor vehicle accident (passenger, pedestrian or bicycle rider) causes a severe head injury (diffuse axonal injury). A cortical laceration or bursting injury is frequently present, especially when the brain has struck, or been penetrated by, the sharp edge of the lesser sphenoid wing. There is often significant cerebral hemisphere swelling that may be unilateral or bilateral.

(2) The haematoma develops several hours after a fall (Fig. 37.5). There are contralateral pyramidal signs and pupillary inequality (as seen in the adult), but there is also marked pallor from the blood lost into the subdural space, and the haemoglobin may drop significantly.

(3) Non-accidental—shaking injury. There is a shallow subdural haemorrhage, frequently in the midline along the fax, and associated often with significant irritability, unilateral or bilateral brain swelling and retinal haemorrhages.

The acute subdural haematoma after a fall or deceleration requires urgent evacuation and has a high mortality because of the associated severe brain injury. The haematoma following a shaking injury may require evacuation, depending on its size and any other treatment required to relieve the brain swelling.

Chronic subdural haematoma occurs in infants and is discussed in the section on intracranial birth injuries. It is rare in older children.

Extradural haemorrhage

This is not as common in children as in young adults. A direct blow on the side of the head is the common cause. The clinical pattern is the same as in adults, but the volume of haematoma may account for more than half the circulating blood volume in the infant. The resulting pallor

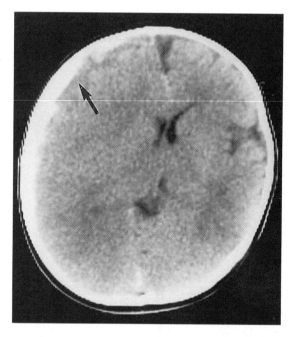

Fig. 37.5 Subdural haematoma on CT scan (arrow). Note the deviation of the midline in large part due to intracerebral swelling.

and hypovolaemic shock can well be appreciated. CT scan confirms the diagnosis and treatment involves urgent craniotomy and evacuation of the haematoma (Fig. 37.6). The operation is life-saving and the results are usually excellent.

Haemorrhagic diatheses

In some children excessive haemorrhage following a mild injury may be the first sign of a blood disease such as acute leukaemia, thrombocytopenic purpura or haemophilia.

Intracranial birth injuries

Most birth injuries of the skull and brain come from excessive or rapid deformation of the skull as it passes through the birth canal, or from compression by obstetrical forceps. Distortion may produce surface lacerations of the brain or tearing of superficial vessels, the large veins or dural

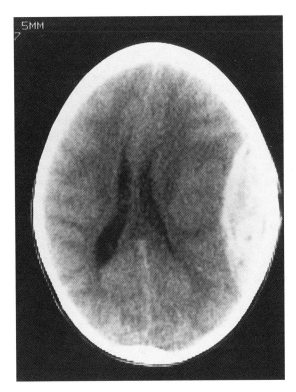

Fig. 37.6 Extradural haematoma on CT scan.

sinuses. The subsequent haemorrhage, as well as cyanosis and anoxia from respiratory depression, may be catastrophic for the developing brain.

Depressed fractures of the skull during birth may be due to 'natural causes', but most result from incorrect placement of obstetrical forceps. The large 'pond-shaped' depression rarely produces neurological signs, but the fracture should be elevated without delay, because it is easiest and safest (to treat) in the first 2 days of life. The bone is easily snapped back into position when the central area is elevated from below via a small opening in the skull at the edge of the fracture line.

Intracranial haematoma

Bleeding into the subdural space or brain is uncommon in the newborn and the clinical picture varies according to the rate of bleeding, site and volume (Fig. 37.5). The typical sites are the middle fossa, parasagittal region and the posterior fossa. The infant will show signs of obtundation, with a tense fontanelle and anaemia. There will also be signs of local pressure; for example, lack of movement or weakness of the contralateral limbs, or depression of respiration and opisthotonus with a posterior fossa bleed.

Chronic subdural haematoma

This type of haematoma may arise from birth trauma or a head injury during infancy. It is rare in older children. The collection develops slowly, giving the brain and skull time to adjust. If the lesion expands there is further compression of the brain and distension of the calvarium. The subdural fluid is watery, yellow or burgundy in colour and is often under high pressure. The clinical signs are an enlarging and sometimes asymmetrical head, delay in reaching the normal milestones, irritability, developmental delay, failure to thrive and occasionally convulsions.

The diagnosis is confirmed by ultrasonography or CT scan or by needle aspiration of the fontanelle. Repeated aspiration may be sufficient, but persistent reaccumulation will require either open drainage via small burr holes, or internal drainage by means of a shunt (subdural to peritoneal).

SEQUELAE OF HEAD INJURIES IN CHILDREN

Neurological

Although children show a surprising capacity for recovery after head injuries, they may suffer permanent disabilities as a result of the more severe injuries. Brain injury in the younger child may disrupt the development of intellectual and physical milestones. A posterior parietal haematoma affecting the dominant hemisphere may cause a permanent defect in the contralateral visual field and, perhaps more importantly, defective visuomotor co-ordination, which makes reading and writing difficult and results in reduced intellectual performance and psychopathological sequelae.

The severe deceleration injury, so common in children involved in automobile accidents, affects the whole brain. This may result in disturbances of behaviour, personality and intellect, but more obviously in spasticity, tremor and dysarthria from damage to the brain-stem, which is often the major manifestation of this injury. The cranial nerves may also be permanently damaged. Cognitive deficits particularly affecting memory disrupt learning ability and produce enormous educational difficulties.

Post-traumatic epilepsy is common after birth injuries, especially those that affect the temporal lobe. In older children it occurs after compound depressed fractures of the vault associated with a laceration of the cortex, or following intracerebral haematomas.

CSF leak

CSF rhinorrhoea may result from a fracture of the base of the skull involving the frontal, ethmoid or sphenoid sinuses, whereas a fracture of the temporal bone may cause CSF otorrhoea The communication with the exterior through a mucosal space is a potential source of meningitis. Prophylactic antibiotics are not recommended because resistant organisms may develop and meningitis may still occur. If the communication persists, meningitis may occur months or years later and a skull defect should be suspected when meningitis is recurrent.

To identify the leaking point the following techniques are all used: CT with fine direct cuts in a coronal plane, CT contrast cisternography (contrast administered via lumbar puncture) or radionuclide cisternography with cotton wool pledgets in the nose to quantify the amount of isotope that has leaked into the pledgets and MRI. Continuous leakage of CSF will require an operative repair using a fascial graft.

FURTHER READING

Cooper P.R. (ed.) (1993) *Head injury*, 3rd edn, Williams and Wilkins, Baltimore.

Narayan R.K., Wilberger J.E. & Povlishock J.T. (eds) (1996) *Neurotrauma*, McGraw Hill, New York.

Reilly P. & Bullock R. (eds) (1997) *Head Injury: Pathophysiology and Management of Severe Closed Head Injury*, Chapman and Hall, London.

Teasdale G.M. (1995) Head injury: neurological management. *J. Neurol. Neurosurg. Psychiatr.* **58**: 526–39.

— 38 —

Abdominal and Thoracic Injuries

CASE 1

Jayden is a 7-year-old who fell off his bike. He was winded initially, but recovered within a few minutes. Several hours later he became pale and developed abdominal and shoulder pain.

> Q. 1.1   *What is the likely diagnosis?*
>
> Q. 1.2   *What is the management strategy?*

CASE 2

A 3-year-old girl stepped on to the road and was hit by a car travelling at moderate speed. On arrival at the emergency department her femur appeared bent. Vital signs suggested hypovolaemic shock and central cyanosis.

> Q. 2.1   *What is your approach to the management?*

INTRA-ABDOMINAL INJURIES

The majority of abdominal injuries in children are due to blunt trauma; penetrating trauma is rare. The commonest organs affected are the kidneys, spleen and liver. When the spleen and liver are torn, intraperitoneal bleeding occurs (haemoperitoneum). The injured kidney bleeds into the retroperitoneal space, and if the urothelium is disrupted, urine may extravasate into the retroperitoneal tissues as well.

A careful history of the accident will help predict the likely injuries. Knowledge of the mechanism of injury will provide clues as to the likely organ(s) injured. For example, a bicycle handlebar injury to the left upper quadrant of the abdomen or to the lower chest is often associated with splenic trauma (Fig. 38.1).

Haemoperitoneum

Haemoperitoneum presents with signs of peritoneal irritation such as tenderness (often widespread) and a variable degree of reflex muscular rigidity (guarding). Abdominal distension results both from the volume of blood in the peritoneal cavity and the swallowed air and ileus that develops rapidly. The clinical evaluation of the abdomen is made easier and more reliable if a nasogastric tube is inserted to decompress the stomach. Also, this is important first aid to prevent aspiration of gastric contents (Mendelsohn syndrome) and acute gastric dilatation. There may be accompanying signs of blood loss and shock.

Variations in posture and the time elapsed since injury result in wide variations in the distribution of the signs of haemoperitoneum and the site of maximum tenderness. When the spleen is ruptured the signs are usually maximal in the left upper quadrant, but it is not unusual for the signs, including pain at the shoulder tip, to be more marked on the right side before the left — this is suggestive of a ruptured liver. Of course, both the liver and spleen may be ruptured.

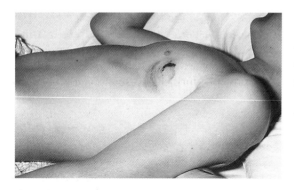

Fig. 38.1 Handle-bar injury with bruising over the lower ribs, which are so elastic the underlying spleen is torn without the ribs themselves being broken.

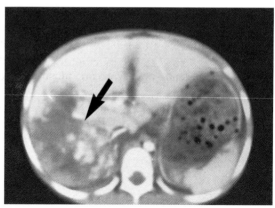

Fig. 38.3 CT scan of upper abdomen showing a ruptured liver (arrow).

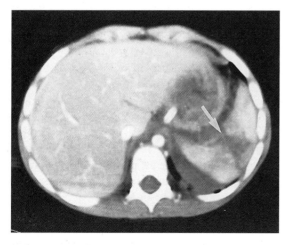

Fig. 38.2 CT scan of upper abdomen showing a ruptured spleen (arrow).

The recognition of haemoperitoneum is far more important initially than the diagnosis of injury to a particular organ.

Radiological investigation

Many children with minor blunt trauma to the abdomen require no specific radiological investigation. Computerised tomography (CT) with contrast is useful for unconscious patients with multiple injuries, or where a serious injury is suspected (for example, ruptured spleen: Fig. 38.2;

ruptured liver: Fig. 38.3; or kidney). Nuclear scans for splenic or hepatic trauma and an intravenous pyelogram for renal injury are useful in some patients.

Recognition of hypovolaemic shock

Shock is recognised in the child by tachycardia, poor peripheral perfusion, cool extremities and a systolic pressure less than 70 mmHg (although this is age-dependent). Familiarity with the age-dependent normal levels of pulse and blood pressure in children will lessen the chance of missing hypovolaemic shock, either initially, or if it develops after primary assessment.

The normal blood pressure in children is not only lower than in adults, but also it remains stable for longer despite hypovolaemia. However, decompensation then occurs quickly. Normotension, therefore, does not exclude major blood loss in a child. The accurate measurement of blood pressure requires the correct-sized cuff. As a general rule the cuff width ought to be at least two-thirds the length of the upper arm.

Non-operative management

Non-operative management is appropriate for most solid visceral injuries in children, provided they are kept under close supervision and are reassessed at frequent and regular intervals.

They are best managed in a facility with intensive care capabilities and an experienced paediatric surgeon. Intensive care must include continuous nursing staff coverage, monitoring of vital signs at frequent intervals, and immediate availability of surgical personnel and operating theatres should they be required. Nearly always the bleeding stops and surgery is not needed.

Indications for surgery

Indications for surgical intervention for blunt abdominal trauma, where injury to the spleen or liver is suspected, include:

(1) Persistent or continued major bleeding, requiring more than 40 mL/kg of intravenous fluid resuscitation in the first 12 hours to maintain cardiovascular stability.

(2) Persistent unstable circulation and hypotension despite appropriate resuscitation.

(3) A proven or suspected gut perforation on clinical or radiological examination.

(4) Severe, concomitant head injury in which an unstable circulation cannot be tolerated, and where significant or ongoing intraperitoneal bleeding is suspected.

In splenic injuries requiring surgery the spleen can be preserved by oversewing the tear ('splenorrhaphy') or by performing partial splenectomy, avoiding the significant risk of post-splenectomy sepsis that can occur when the entire spleen is removed. If the spleen has to be removed completely the child should be given Pneumovax vaccine and commenced on long-term prophylactic antibiotics.

Diagnostic peritoneal lavage is not indicated in children because free blood in the peritoneal cavity is not an indication for surgery.

Haematuria

In all suspected intra-abdominal injuries the presence or absence of blood in the urine must be established. Absence of haematuria virtually excludes a significant urinary-tract injury, except in the rare instance of a transected ureter, which is diagnosed by intravenous pyelogram or a CT scan showing extravasation in the flank or loin that prompts further investigation or operative exploration.

Urethral injury should be suspected in pelvic fractures and straddle injuries with (i) frank blood appearing at the external urethral meatus; (ii) inability to void spontaneously (particularly in the presence of a palpable bladder); and (iii) urine extravasation into the perineum. In these patients a urethral catheter must not be inserted blindly into the urethra, as this may convert a partial tear of the urethra into a complete transection. A carefully performed urethrogram must be obtained first, to delineate the injury. Depending on the type of urethral injury, either primary surgical repair of the urethra or temporary urinary diversion — for example, suprapubic catheter — will be indicated.

Haematuria following relatively minor trauma suggests a predisposing factor, such as hydronephrosis or Wilms' tumour. All children with haematuria, even after trivial injury, need renal ultrasonography or intravenous pyelography to exclude these underlying lesions (Chapter 35).

Extraperitoneal extravasation

The signs of extravasation of blood or urine usually develop more slowly and less dramatically than those of intraperitoneal haemorrhage; they are also more consistently localised and less variable.

Renal injuries

Because the kidney is involved frequently, tenderness and muscular rigidity should be sought in the loin, but a perirenal haematoma may cause localised tenderness and sometimes a mass that is palpable through the anterior abdominal wall.

When haematuria accompanies tenderness and rigidity in the loin, a CT scan with contrast should be performed. This will distinguish between a contusion, which can be managed conservatively, and a rupture of the kidney with urine extravasation, which requires surgical exploration. Ultrasonography enables the renal injury to be monitored subsequently.

Early exploration — that is, within 3 days of injury — is advocated in major renal injuries, rather than a non-operative approach. Delay in the recognition and management of injuries to the renal pelvis or parenchyma, which results in urine extravasation, is followed by severe inflammatory changes that prejudice attempts at conservation and later repair.

Bladder injuries

In extraperitoneal rupture of the bladder or membranous urethra there are signs of extravasation of urine into the perineum, scrotum and suprapubic region.

When haematuria or urethral bleeding accompany signs of intraperitoneal or extraperitoneal haemorrhage or extravasation in the lower part of the abdomen, a cystogram will establish whether the bladder is intact. However, if blood, as opposed to blood-stained urine, is seen at the urethral meatus, the catheter should be passed only after a carefully performed urethrogram has demonstrated that the urethra is intact.

Ill-defined intra-abdominal injuries

Apart from those patients with intraperitoneal haemorrhage, extraperitoneal extravasation or haematuria, there is a difficult group with ill-defined symptoms and signs that may persist for several days after the injury.

Many probably have minor contusions of the abdominal wall or the intestine or its mesentery. Non-operative management usually is justified in these cases. Sometimes, lap-belt deceleration injuries may cause severe trauma to the bowel wall when it is crushed against the sacral promontory. The injuries only become apparent after several days when the bowel perforates and then peritonitis develops suddenly. The same type of trauma may also cause a periduodenal haematoma and pancreatic injuries, some of which may require surgical intervention. Severe lap-belt injuries with abdominal wall bruising ± lumbar bruise (hyperextension tear of lumbar ligaments/ vertebral fracture) need immediate specialist referral.

Children who are comatose from concomitant head injuries require a high index of suspicion of intra-abdominal injuries, and need head and abdominal CT with contrast. The indications for further investigation, which may involve laparotomy, include persistent or increasing pain, severe localized tenderness, the appearance of a localised abdominal mass, and generalised abdominal distension with vomiting.

Emergency diagnostic laparotomy is required occasionally for continued major blood loss despite appropriate resuscitation. As abdominal injuries are frequently multiple rather than single, a systematic examination of all the viscera is mandatory at laparotomy.

THORACIC INJURIES

In contrast to their comparative frequency in adults, major thoracic injuries are not common in children. Most chest trauma in children is blunt; penetrating thoracic injuries are extremely rare. Blunt thoracic trauma tends to form part of a composite picture of multiple injuries that may include cerebral, abdominal and peripheral trauma, any of which may be the predominant threat to life.

The child's chest wall is very compliant and allows energy transfer to the intrathoracic structures, frequently without any external evidence of injury and without fracture to the ribs. The elastic chest wall increases the frequency of pulmonary contusions and direct intrapulmonary haemorrhage. Consequently, pulmonary contusion is the most common significant thoracic injury in children. Tension pneumothorax or haemopneumothorax are less common, but potentially lethal unless recognized and the tension relieved using intercostal drainage. Diaphragmatic rupture is extremely rare and may result from a crushing of the torso and pelvis. Injury to the great vessels is less common than in adults, and reflects a lack of pre-existing vascular disease and fewer high-speed injuries.

The diagnostic and therapeutic approach to chest trauma is the same for children as adults. Significant thoracic injuries rarely occur alone and are often a component of major multisystem trauma. Contusion of the lung and traumatic rupture of the diaphragm are unlikely to be recognised in the presence of multiple injuries unless a chest X-ray is taken. Pneumothorax, with or without haemothorax, may result from pulmonary contusion, and when of significant volume, should be relieved by an intercostal tube with an underwater seal.

Multiple fractures of the ribs are not common because of the elasticity of the thorax in children and, as a consequence, flail chest is rare. When the flail area is large enough to cause respiratory embarrassment, internal splinting by positive pressure ventilation is preferable.

When penetrating injuries occur they may involve the heart and lungs, and the possibility of cardiac tamponade must be kept in mind.

Investigation and treatment

An X-ray of the chest should be taken in all cases of trauma with multiple injuries, in all thoracic injuries and in all patients with respiratory insufficiency.

A penetrating injury should be assumed to have caused injury to underlying viscera until the contrary is proven. The possibility of combined thoraco-abdominal injury should always be kept in mind.

Respiratory symptoms demand investigation and treatment that may include intercostal drainage, thoracotomy or tracheostomy.

FURTHER READING

Akel S.R., Haddah F.F., Hashim H.A., Soubra M.R. & Mounala N. (1998) Traumatic injuries of the alimentary tract in children. *Pediatr. Surg. Int.* **13**: 104–7.

Bass D.H., Mann M.D., Cremin B.J. & Cywes S. (1990) A comparison between scintigraphy and computer abdominal tomography in blunt liver and spleen injuries in children. *Pediatr. Surg. Int.* **5**: 443–5.

Beasley S.W. & Auldist A.W. (1985) Management of splenic trauma in childhood. *Aust. NZ J. Surg.* **55**: 199–202.

Ciftci A.O., Tanyel F.C., Salman A.B., Buyukpamakcu N. & Hicsonmez A. (1998) Gastrointestinal tract perforation due to blunt abdominal trauma. *Pediatr. Surg. Int.* **13**: 259–64.

Cosentino C.M., Luck S.R., Barthel M.J., Reynolds M. & Raffensperger J.G. (1990) Transfusion requirements in conservative nonoperative management of blunt splenic and hepatic injuries during childhood. *J. Pediatr. Surg.* **25**: 950–4.

Eichelberger M.R. & Moront M. (1998) Abdominal trauma. In: O'Neill J.A., Rowe M.I., Grosfeld J.L., Fonkalsrud E.W. & Coran A.G. (eds) *Pediatric Surgery*, 5th edn, Mosby, St. Louis, pp. 261–84.

Hardacre J.M.H., West K.W., Rescorla F.R., Vane D.W. & Grosfeld J.L. (1990) Delayed onset of intestinal obstruction in children after unrecognised seat belt injury. *J. Pediatr. Surg.* **25**: 967–9.

Hutson J.M. & Beasley S.W. (1988) Trauma. In: *The Surgical Examination of Children.* pp. 127–59, Heinemann Medical Publishers, London.

Ildstad S.T., Tollerud D.J., Weiss R.G., Cox J.A. & Martin L.W. (1990) Cardiac contusion in pediatric patients with blunt thoracic trauma. *J. Pediatr. Surg.* **25**: 287–9.

Jerby B.L., Attorri R.J. & Morton D. Jr (1997) Blunt intestinal injury in children: the role of the physical examination. *J. Pediatr. Surg.* **32**: 580–4.

Lally K.P., Rosario V., Mahour G.H. *et al.* (1990) Evolution in the management of splenic injury in children. *Surg. Gynecol. Obstet.* **170**: 245–8.

Lynch J.M., Meza M.P., Newman B., Gardner M.J. & Albaneses C.T. (1997) Computed tomography grade of splenic injury is predictive of the time required for radiographic healing. *J. Pediatr. Surg.* **32**: 1093–6.

Peclet M.H., Newman K.D., Eichelberger M.R., Gotschall C.S., Garcia V.F. & Bowman I.M. (1990) Thoracic trauma in children: an indicator of increased mortality. *J. Pediatr. Surg.* **25**: 961–6.

Shilyansky J., Pearl R.H., Kreller M., Sena L.M. & Babyn P.S. (1997) Diagnosis and management of duodenal injuries in children. *J. Pediatr. Surg.* **32**: 880–6.

Wesson D.E. (1998) Thoracic injuries. In: O'Neill J.A., Rowe M.I., Grosfeld J.L., Fonkalsrud E.W. & Coran A.G. (eds) *Pediatric Surgery*, 5th edn, Mosby, St. Louis, pp. 245–60.

— 39 —

Foreign Bodies

CASE 1

A mother notices that her 12-month-old child put a safety pin in his mouth and swallowed it. An X-ray shows it to be in the stomach. He is asymptomatic.

> Q. 1.1   *Are any further investigations required?*
>
> Q. 1.2   *Is surgery to remove the pin indicated?*

CASE 2

A barefooted 8-year-old girl has trodden on a needle that has broken, part of it in the sole of her foot. A small puncture wound is seen but the needle cannot be felt. It hurts her to walk on it.

> Q. 2.1   *How is it best removed?*

The infant's instinctive exploration of his or her environment and the spirit of experiment in the toddler and older child result in a wide variety of foreign bodies lodging in the oddest places. Most are found in the alimentary tract; others may enter the aural or nasal cavities, the bronchial tree, or they can be accidentally driven into the soft tissues.

SWALLOWED FOREIGN BODIES

In infants, oral exploration of the environment may lead to the accidental swallowing of a variety of objects. Older siblings may feed the 'new baby' inappropriate hardware. Accidental swallowing may be precipitated by a fall or a slap on the back. At any age a bone hidden in food may be swallowed; for example, a chop or fish-bone. Ingestion of a foreign body occurs most commonly during the first year of life.

The vast majority of swallowed foreign bodies pass through the alimentary tract without a problem. If a foreign body becomes lodged in the oesophagus, however, it usually does so just below the cricopharyngeus muscle. With rare exceptions, objects that are first located below the diaphragm will pass naturally without hazard to the child.

The size of coins (the objects that are swallowed most often) determines whether they are likely to become impacted. When a coin or other foreign body becomes lodged in the oesophagus, it should be removed by endoscopy under general anaesthesia. Safety-pins may stick in the oesophagus, but if they enter the stomach they will almost always be excreted without difficulty, even if open.

Broken plastic toys are more dangerous, because they may be jagged or angular, and their radiolucency may lead to a delay in diagnosis. Ulceration, mediastinitis and even acquired tracheo-oesophageal fistulae may occur. A plastic bread-bag clip may cause bowel perforation. Bobby pins and 'Kirby-grips' pass easily as far as the duodenojejunal flexure, but may be too long and rigid to negotiate this flexure in children less than 7 years of age, and require laparotomy for their removal. In children more than 6 or 7 years of age, observation for up to 1 week is justified, although impaction at the duodenojejunal flexure should not be allowed to continue for more than 10 to 12 days.

'Button' or 'disc' batteries used in microelectronic toys, cameras and calculators are particularly hazardous when swallowed. Their small size ensures their passage into the stomach, and the great majority pass through the alimentary canal uneventfully. However, if any hold-up occurs, for example, in the stomach, the nickel-cadmium shell can be eroded with release of strong alkali and cause local necrosis and perforation. Heavy-metal poisoning (mercury, cadmium, nickel, zinc or magnesium) also has been reported. Complications from button batteries can occur in less than 36 hours; if recently ingested in the absence of abdominal signs, a cathartic will facilitate its rapid transit through the alimentary tract.

Clinical features

There may be no symptoms, and it is likely that innumerable small foreign bodies are passed uneventfully and unnoticed. In some cases an attack of gagging, coughing or retching is reported or the incident has been observed.

When the symptoms and history suggest lodgement in the mouth or throat, the oropharynx should be examined carefully. Oesophageal obstruction may present as excessive drooling and dysphagia.

If the accident has not been reported or observed the first symptoms may be due to complications; for example, progressive dysphagia or dyspnoea caused by pressure of the swollen oesophagus on the trachea.

Pain, swelling in the neck and fever are the signs of mediastinitis, and rarely a pneumothorax or pleuritic pain may be the first indication of perforation of the thoracic oesophagus by a foreign body.

Investigation

Radiographs of the head, neck, thorax and abdomen are required because a radio-opaque object may be located anywhere from the base of the skull to the pelvic floor.

A radiograph will distinguish tracheal from oesophageal lodgement, for the maximum dimension of the trachea is in the sagittal plane, and that of the oesophagus is in the coronal plane (Fig. 39.1).

Radiolucent foreign bodies are more difficult to detect radiologically, except on barium swallow.

Management

The vast majority of ingested foreign bodies do not need to be removed.

Endoscopic removal is required for all objects impacted in the oesophagus.

Foreign bodies first located beyond the oesophagus have a good chance of being excreted without incident (Fig. 39.2). Blunt objects small enough to enter the stomach will almost always be passed; the patient should return only if abdominal pain or vomiting occurs. Further radiographs are not usually indicated, but will show that the object has been passed, often unrecognised.

In general, when a blunt foreign body has been impacted without progress for 6 weeks, removal at laparotomy or endoscopy may be considered, even in the absence of symptoms.

Lead poisoning from objects that yield soluble lead salts is now very rare, particularly where legislation has banned lead fillers in paints. However, there have been instances of lead poisoning occurring within 10 days from the absorption of lead salts derived from thin lead foil retained in the stomach. Gastric lavage and analysis of the washings will indicate whether significant absorption is likely.

Multiple, minute, scattered opacities found in incidental X-rays of the abdomen suggest bizarre appetites or oral habits (pica) and also raise the possibility of lead poisoning, such as from ingestion

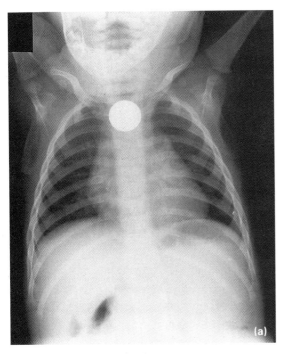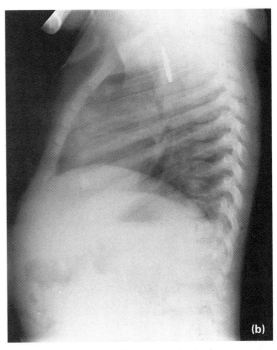

Fig. 39.1 The orientation of a foreign body (for example, coin) will distinguish tracheal from oesophageal lodgement. Here a chest X-ray shows a coin in the coronal plane characteristic of the oesophagus: (a) the AP view and (b) the lateral view. Normally, only the AP view is required.

of flakes of paint gnawed from toys or other accessible articles. X-rays of the long bones showing a 'lead line' in the metaphysis, punctate basophilia in the erythrocytes, and a high content of lead salts in the blood or urine, will confirm this possibility.

Most sharp objects pass uneventfully and should be managed conservatively to begin with, although arrest and failure to progress through the bowel may raise concerns of impending impaction, ulceration and perforation.

A bezoar is a conglomeration of hair (trichobezoar) or vegetable material (phytobezoar) swallowed by emotionally disturbed or handicapped children with bizarre appetites or habits (pica). The mass forms in the stomach or proximal gut and causes pain, vomiting or anorexia, malnutrition or unexplained anaemia. Less commonly, obstruction or perforation occurs.

When X-ray studies indicate a mass of this kind, laparotomy and enterotomy are required.

Prevention

The area on which an infant crawls should be cleared of small objects, and articles should not be pinned to the clothing. Coins and buttons are unsuitable play materials for children of less than 5 years of age.

FOREIGN BODIES IN THE TRACHEA AND BRONCHI

Sudden onset of coughing, spluttering and gagging with a residual wheeze are suggestive of inhalation of a foreign body. The exact clinical picture varies with the size of the object, the

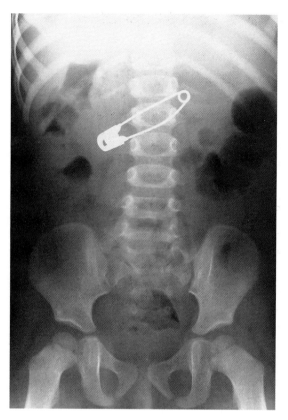

Fig. 39.2 Abdominal X-ray showing a safety-pin in the stomach. This should pass spontaneously.

objects. Films taken in expiration and inspiration show air trapping and assist in localising the presence and size of small radiolucent objects in the lungs; for example, a peanut.

In infants, respiratory symptoms can occur when the object is impacted in the oesophagus; for example acute dyspnoea or progressive stridor, a cough and wheeze. The orientation of the object by X-rays will identify the site of lodgement because the maximum diameter of the trachea is in the anteroposterior plane, compared with the transverse plane in the oesophagus (Fig. 39.1).

Removal at endoscopy under general anaesthesia is required. Mucosal abrasions and pulmonary changes, caused by the foreign body, its complications or manipulations during removal, are indications for a course of antibiotics. The earlier the diagnosis and treatment, the less the likelihood of residual pulmonary or mucosal damage.

FOREIGN BODIES IN THE EAR, NOSE AND PHARYNX

In the ear

Unless there is a definite history, children with a foreign body in the ear present with a blood-stained discharge, irritation or deafness. The requirements for the removal include sedation, local anaesthesia, good illumination and the correct instrument. Forceps are not the best instrument to remove most foreign bodies; they tend to push them further in. Some, such as insects, tend to break up. Most are best removed with a fine probe with the terminal 2 to 4 mm bent to a right angle. This hook is passed beyond the foreign body and then rotated to withdraw and remove it. A head light and viewing system is essential. If these techniques are used, few objects need to be removed under general anaesthesia.

In the nose

The child, usually between 2 and 4 years of age, presents with nasal irritation and obstruction, or a

site of lodgement and the time elapsed since the object was inhaled. Large objects in the larynx or trachea produce obstruction that may be complete if they impact in the narrow glottis. Inspiratory stridor and retraction of the supraclavicular, substernal or intercostal areas indicate that the object is in the larynx or subglottic area.

Foreign bodies in the trachea or a bronchus cause a wheeze and clinical and radiographic evidence of a ball-valve type of obstruction during expiration resulting in emphysema. Objects impacted more distally may present with symptoms of chronic chest infection from lobar or segmental consolidation.

X-rays may show an opaque object, or the segmental pulmonary collapse and lobar emphysema that occurs with small radiolucent purulent discharge. The object can often be seen after the local application of an anaesthetic with adrenaline, but X-rays are sometimes necessary. Before the removal of a nasal foreign body is attempted, topical anaesthesia and vasoconstriction is induced. Five centimetre lengths of 8 mm ($\frac{1}{2}''$) ribbon gauze are dampened with cocaine and adrenaline. These are introduced 1 or 2 cm into the nose in a non-frightening way with fingers, rather than instruments. Suction is safe and effective for smooth, round objects, such as a bead or button.

In the pharynx

The commonest object to get lodged in the tonsil, the piriform fossa or the back of the tongue is a fish bone. Subjective localisation is poor and pain may be constant or felt only during swallowing.

After spraying the fauces and the pharynx with a local anaesthetic the usual sites are examined with the aid of a spatula or a laryngeal mirror and proper illumination, and the object is removed with forceps.

FOREIGN BODIES IN THE URINARY TRACT

These are rare but most frequently involve the bladder — in girls in the preschool age-group during play, or in boys during puberty, when objects may be introduced to seek erotic stimulation. Sometimes a fragment of a ureteric catheter may break off and remain after surgery to the urinary tract. Any of these objects may cause infection, haematuria or pain, and may act as a nidus for the formation of a calculus.

Foreign bodies in the urinary or genital tract are removed by endoscopy.

OTHER FOREIGN BODIES

In the hand

Apart from superficial splinters a small fragment of metal or wood may be driven into the palm, and if it is unrecognised, a painless cystic swelling within a fibrous capsule may develop around the object. Exploration and removal under general anaesthesia are required, with tourniquet control. Unrecognised foreign bodies in the palm may cause deep web space infections similar to those seen in adult practice.

In the lower limb

Nails, pins or needles driven into the foot or knee can be shown radiographically. When they are not visible through the skin, they are most easily removed under general anaesthesia by a pair of fine artery forceps inserted through a tiny incision and guided by an image intensifier.

FURTHER READING

Brown T.C.K. & Clark C.M. (1983) Inhaled foreign bodies in children. *Med. J. Aust.* **2**: 322

Geddes N.K. & Raine P.A.M. (1994) Respiratory obstruction, thoracic trauma and ingestion of foreign body. In: *Surgical Emergencies in Children: A Practical Guide*, Raine P.A.M. & Azmy A.A.F (eds). Butterworth Heinemann, Oxford. pp. 193–219.

Jones P.G. (1963) Swallowed foreign bodies in childhood. *Med. J. Aust.* **1**: 236.

Stringer M.D. & Capps S.N.J. (1991) Rationalising the management of swallowed coins in children. *B.M.J.* **302**: 1321–2.

— 40 —

The Ingestion of Corrosives

CASE

Chamel drank from an unlabelled soft drink bottle that she found in her father's garage. She immediately developed severe mouth, throat and epigastric pain and had difficulty swallowing. The fluid ingested was identified as caustic soda.

Q. 1.1   *What should be your initial first aid?*

Q. 1.2   *What investigation should be performed in hospital? What major complication of this injury do you wish to prevent?*

In children, swallowing corrosive fluids or solids nearly always is accidental, and the exploring toddler aged between 1 and 3 years is most often the victim. Symptoms of caustic ingestion include cervical and epigastric pain, irritability, excessive drooling, dysphagia and respiratory distress. However, about 20 per cent present with no symptoms; in some, this is despite significant oesophageal injury.

PREVENTION

The most effective way to prevent such accidents is to keep all chemicals used in the home and garden out of reach of small children and in their proper containers. They should not be stored under the kitchen sink or in unlabelled containers.

PATHOLOGY

The oesophagus is the most common organ seriously injured by corrosive ingestion. Extensive or circumferential oesophageal burns may lead to severe strictures that cause dysphagia within weeks of injury.

Burns of the buccal mucosa, soft palate or tongue suggest that the oesophagus has been damaged as well.

Mucosal injury and oedema of the larynx occurs in 15 per cent of cases and can be life-threatening, requiring intubation or tracheostomy.

FIRST AID

(1) If ingestion has just occurred, wash off any excess corrosive material from the lips and skin, using plenty of water.

(2) Immediately dilute any corrosive in the mouth, oesophagus or stomach by giving cold water or milk to drink. Do not attempt to use an 'antidote' acid or alkali because the corrosive may have been identified incorrectly, and the chemical antidotes themselves may cause damage.

(3) If ingestion of the corrosive was not witnessed or confirmed by an adult, always assume it has occurred if the lips or mouth are blistered or if the toddler is drooling excessively and unable to swallow saliva.

(4) Where the nature or composition of the corrosive is uncertain, consult the Poisons

Information Service or equivalent by telephone. Induce vomiting with ipecac syrup only if directed by a poisons service.

(5) Send a sample of the corrosive agent with the child when transferring him or her to hospital if identification has not been made with certainty.

(6) After caustic ingestion the child should be referred urgently to a paediatric surgical centre.

DEFINITIVE MANAGEMENT

An oesophagoscopy at 24 hours is necessary in corrosive ingestion whenever injury to the oesophagus is suspected. This will determine the severity of oesophageal injury, and hence the need for prophylactic treatment to reduce the likelihood of subsequent oesophageal stricture formation. Where there is no damage to the oesophageal mucosa on oesophagoscopy, no treatment is required.

Patchy oedema of the intact oesophageal mucosa is regarded as the minimal degree of burn and is not likely to cause a stricture. No treatment is required and the patient may leave hospital as soon as normal feeding is re-established. A white mucosal slough or circumferential ulceration is more serious and may lead to a stricture. In these patients antibiotics are given to limit the effects of secondary infection. Steroids may diminish the extent of fibrosis, although their value is uncertain. Dilatation of the oesophagus is carried out several times a week by the passage of a mercury-filled Hurst bougie of appropriate size (for example, no. 18 with a diameter of 1 cm, for a 2-year-old). The unpleasant aspects are short-lived and the patient comes to tolerate the bouginage within a few days. Many older children can pass the bougie themselves.

This regimen is conducted initially in hospital, where the child's swallowing and the ease of bouginage can be assessed. Later the procedure can be performed at home. Oesophagoscopy is repeated 1 to 3 weeks after the injury, and if the mucosa has healed and there is no evidence of narrowing, treatment is discontinued. If there are abnormal findings at 3 weeks, treatment is continued for a further 6 weeks. Where there is worsening dysphagia and the stricture cannot be dilated effectively by bouginage, segmental resection and anastomosis may be required. Occasionally, an extensive resection and replacement of the oesophagus is unavoidable, but in the long term the best oesophagus is the patient's own, and prolonged bouginage is justified to avoid an extensive oesophagectomy.

FURTHER READING

De Peppo F., Zaccara A., Dall' Oglio L., Federici di Abriola G., Ponticelli A., Marchetti P., Lucchetti M.C. & Rivosecchi M. (1998) Stenting for caustic strictures: esophageal replacement replaced. *J. Pediatr. Surg.* **33**: 54–7.

Fyfe A.H.B & Auldist A.W. (1984) Corrosive ingestion in children. *Z. Kinderchir.* **39**: 229–33.

Gorman R.L., Khin-Maung-Gyi M.T., Klein-Schwartz W. *et al.* (1992) Initial symptoms as predictors of esophageal injury in corrosive ingestions. *Am. J. Emerg. Med.* **10**: 189.

Millar A.J.W. & Cywes S. (1998) Caustic strictures of the oesophagus. In: O'Neill J.A., Rowe M.I., Grosfeld J.L., Fonkalsrud E.W. & Coran A.G. (eds) *Pediatric Surgery*, 5th edn, pp. 969–80, Mosby, St. Louis.

Vergauwen P., Mouin D., Buts J.P. *et al.* (1991) Caustic burns of the upper digestive and respiratory tracts. *Eur. J. Pediatr.* **150**: 700.

— 41 —

Burns

CASE 1

During your intern year, you are rotated to a rural base hospital. At 5 p.m. an 18-month-old boy is rushed into the emergency department after tipping hot tea on to himself 10 minutes earlier. The tea was just boiled and no milk had been added. The area of scald estimated with a Lund–Browder chart is 15 per cent.

> *Q. 1.1*   *What are the management principles prior to transfer to the regional burns unit next morning?*

CASE 2

Jeremy is a 6-month-old infant who has been brought to your clinic with red, weeping lower legs and feet after being scalded by a hot bath.

> *Q. 2.1*   *What is the likely mechanism of injury?*

CASE 3

William and Ali are brought to the emergency department after they poured petrol on a campfire. Their faces are blackened and their hair and eyebrows are singed.

> *Q. 3.1*   *Why might the oximeter show falling oxygen saturation?*

The severity of a burn injury depends on the size and depth of the burn and its anatomical site. A burn may be caused by heat, electricity, radiation, chemical agents or friction. Burns caused by heat may be due to hot liquids, commonly referred to as scald injury. Dry thermal injury can occur from flames or contact with hot surfaces. The care of a burned child requires the services of a multidisciplinary team and may extend over many years. A burned child has a rapidly progressive illness: within a short time a healthy, alert, adventurous youngster may be in danger of losing his life. He will suffer pain and anxiety and may develop lifelong physical and psychological scars.

PREVENTION

Most burns in children are due to scalds; are self-inflicted; are twice as common in boys (usually toddlers); and occur at home, mostly in the kitchen or bathroom. The child at greatest risk therefore is the male toddler, in the kitchen and while under the care of a parent preparing or drinking a hot beverage. Flame burns occur mainly in boys playing with fire, most commonly matches and flammable fluids.

Prevention of burns rests on three main approaches:

(1) *Education*, of both children and adults, concerning potential dangers and the need for continual vigilance. Current government programs stress to the public that injuries to children can be prevented by (i) supervising them, (ii) separating them from the hazard, (iii) reducing the hazard or access to it and (iv) removing the hazard. It is hoped that by introducing such programs the incidence of burn injury will be reduced; in the last 25 years the frequency of burns has declined by 50 per cent in the State of Victoria.

(2) *Design*, for example, improvements in clothes, heating appliances, guards on stoves and temperature regulators in hot water systems.

(3) *Legislation*, for example, government (legal) control of fireworks, nightwear materials and design regulations.

When visiting a home the family doctor is in a unique position to prevent burning accidents by warning the parents of specific hazards. These include the ability of young children to reach table-tops and over-hanging saucepan handles on stoves, hot water in bathrooms, old model radiators and unguarded fires, loose cotton nightwear, and access to flammable liquids.

TREATMENT

Early, competent assessment of the burn is essential. The child should be admitted to a burns unit when there is:

(1) full-thickness skin-loss, > 5 per cent of the total body-surface area

(2) more than 10 per cent of the total body surface burned

(3) a sustained inhalation injury

(4) an important area(s) involved; for example, face, hands, buttocks and genitalia

(5) a poor social circumstance and probable non-accidental injury.

Treatment requires a team approach involving a surgeon, anaesthetist, social worker, school teacher, dietitian, physiotherapist and other paramedical therapists, all of whom confer and

> ### Box 41.1 The management of burns in children
>
> (1) first aid
>
> (2) transportation
>
> (3) assessment
>
> (4) resuscitation
>
> (5) prevention and control of infection
>
> (6) adequate nutrition
>
> (7) wound care
>
> (8) early excision of dead tissue with grafting
>
> (9) minimisation of scars and contractures, pressure garments, splints, etc.
>
> (10) psychological support and rehabilitation
>
> (11) reconstructive surgery, if necessary

work together to ensure that the child is healed and back at home as soon as possible. The phases of treatment are summarized in Box 41.1

First aid

First aid involves limiting the extent and severity of the burn. The child must be removed quickly from the source of injury; flames are smothered, by water if at hand; clothing should be removed immediately, especially with a scald; and the whole body or limb immersed in cold water for 10 minutes. Iced water is dangerous because it may cause general hypothermia or local ischaemia, and thus is contra-indicated in children.

Transportation

In major burns, transport is arranged to a hospital and intravenous fluids (for example, Hartmann's solution) should be commenced early if a delay

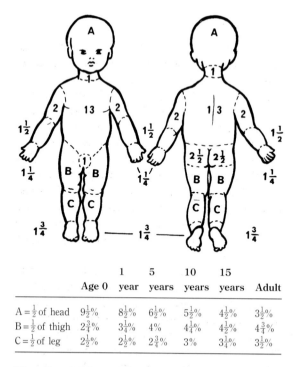

	Age 0	1 year	5 years	10 years	15 years	Adult
A = $\frac{1}{2}$ of head	$9\frac{1}{2}\%$	$8\frac{1}{2}\%$	$6\frac{1}{2}\%$	$5\frac{1}{2}\%$	$4\frac{1}{2}\%$	$3\frac{1}{2}\%$
B = $\frac{1}{2}$ of thigh	$2\frac{3}{4}\%$	$3\frac{1}{4}\%$	4%	$4\frac{1}{4}\%$	$4\frac{1}{2}\%$	$4\frac{3}{4}\%$
C = $\frac{1}{2}$ of leg	$2\frac{1}{2}\%$	$2\frac{1}{2}\%$	$2\frac{3}{4}\%$	3%	$3\frac{1}{4}\%$	$3\frac{1}{2}\%$

Fig. 41.1 Method of estimating the extent of burned surfaces, allowing for differences according to age (after Lund and Browder).

in transportation is likely. If intravenous fluids are not available a saline solution can be given orally, in small amounts at first and later in an increased volume, if tolerated. Intravenous morphine is administered and the child wrapped in a clean sheet and covered with a blanket to prevent hypothermia.

Assessment

The severity of the burn depends on the burn surface area, the depth of damage and the anatomical site involved; in particular, the face, hands, feet or perineum. In children the area and depth of the burn are mapped on a figure chart (Fig. 41.1), which allows an accurate estimation of the area involved, according to age. Unless this estimate is charted carefully, the area of the burn may be over-estimated and excessive fluids given.

A full-thickness skin burn (white, charred and painless) is usually obvious early, but partial skin loss may be superficial (erythematous, blistering and painful white slough) or deep (mottled, red and painless). The depth of partial skin loss may not be evident for several days, even to the trained eye.

Resuscitation

If shock is present or the burn area exceeds 15 per cent of the body surface (10 per cent in a young child), intravenous fluids are required, along with morphine (0.05 to 0.1 mg/kg) given slowly over 3 to 5 minutes.

Fluids required during the first 24 hours after the burn include:

(1) *Maintenance fluids*: in most children, burn injury maintenance fluids can be given orally and should initially be milk or a milk substitute. If oral intake is impossible, early nasogastric or nasojejunal feeding should be considered. If either of these methods fail, intravenous maintenance fluid should be given (N/2 saline in 5 per cent dextrose according to weight). One-third of the estimated daily requirement is given every 8 hours.

(2) *Resuscitation fluids*: 2 to 3 mL/kg body weight/1 per cent burn surface are given, with one-half of the volume as colloid; for example, 5 per cent normal serum albumin and the remainder as Hartmann's solution. Half of the estimated volume is administered in the first 8 hours and a quarter in each of the next two 8-hour periods. The volume required in the second 24 hours is approximately half that of the first 24 hours.

The rate of intravenous fluid administration depends on the general condition of the child and an expected urine flow of 0.75 mL/kg/hr, obtained via a catheter in the bladder. If the expected urine flow is not reached the intravenous fluid rate is increased. Once shock has been controlled and urine output established the rate can be decreased. After approximately 3 days, a diuresis will occur and the serum electrolytes, urine osmolality and specific gravity will indicate the further requirements.

Blood transfusion rarely is required in the first few days after the burn, but is necessary when anaemia develops and when the burn is to be excised surgically and grafted.

The pH of the gastric juice is estimated regularly in severe burns, and antacids or sucralfate are prescribed to prevent the development of stress ulcers.

Infection

Infection is the major cause of death following the initial burn injury. On admission, swabs are taken from the nose, throat, faeces and burned areas, but antibiotics are given only if there are specific indications. The major aim in treating burns patients now is to prevent infection, and it is thought that early enteral nutrition, which prevents translocation of gastro-intestinal bacteria into the bloodstream, combined with early excision of the burned escar and the uses of silver sulfadiazine (SSD) with chlorhexidine cream, have reduced the risk of both local wound infection and septicaemia.

Tetanus toxoid is given routinely.

Nutrition

Appropriate nutritional management of the severely burned patient is necessary to ensure optimal outcome. Initiation of early enteral feeding within 6 to 18 hours post-burn improves nitrogen balance, reduces the hypermetabolic response and also reduces immunological complications. Young children with major burn injuries often require nasogastric feedings as they have difficulty meeting their nutritional goals with oral intake alone. The hypermetabolic response associated with severe burn injury results in high caloric and protein requirements to ensure optimal healing and outcome. The addition of trace elements and vitamins is also important in ensuring optimal healing of both injury and skin-graft donor sites.

Wound care

After cleaning the wound with an antiseptic, loose skin is removed and gross blisters punctured, leaving removal of blistered skin to a later date. Very superficial burns, for example, sunburn, can be left exposed or covered with a bland ointment, allowing a fine eschar to form — this lifts when the underlying epithelium has healed. Erythematous weeping burns do well with a closed dressing (vaseline tulle, or a plastic covering; for example, Opsite® or Tegaderm®) that is left undisturbed beneath gauze and a firm crepe bandage for 5 days. The inner dressing can be left to separate spontaneously, the outer dressings being changed as necessary.

When there is a burn slough, or a full thickness burn, the area is washed daily with a mild soap, and SSD applied, along with a non-Px adherent plastic dressing (for example, Melolin) until healing has occurred or surgical intervention becomes necessary. Burns on the face or buttocks are left exposed, but other areas usually are treated by the closed method, which allows some freedom of movement and close contact with parents.

Surgical treatment

The aim of surgery is to excise dead skin and apply split-skin grafts as early as possible. Early skin coverage prevents many problems, including infection, long hospitalization, scar formation and psychological disturbances.

Full-thickness burns are treated as soon as the child has recovered from the shock phase. When a large area has been burned, the child is taken to the theatre twice a week for staged excision and grafting. If there is a lack of patient's skin, allograft skin from the Skin Bank is used as a biological dressing, while awaiting re-epithelialisation of the donor sites.

Deep partial burns will heal in time from deeper cells remaining in the skin appendages, but may form hypertrophic scars. As soon as the depth of such a burn becomes evident (this may take up to 1 week) the area is submitted to 'tangential' excision, down to a living base of skin matrix, and then grafted.

Scars and contractures

Burn injuries, particularly deep dermal burns, are notorious for becoming hypertrophic and creating unsightly scars. These will improve spontaneously but long-term pressure garments will accelerate their resolution and are very worthwhile. Application of silicon and Hypafix are valuable also.

Physiotherapy is employed from the time of admission, to assist movements of the chest, joints and muscles to achieve the recovery of full function. Splints and pressure garments are tailored and may be needed for 6 to 12 months to prevent contractures and scars.

Psychological support and rehabilitation

Psychological support (ideally from parents, siblings and friends) is important during hospitalisation and rehabilitation, and may be required for some years. Guilt feelings in the child and parents are common. Discussion groups for parents, and burn support groups, should be available to help the child return to a normal life.

Reconstructive surgery

Contractures and scars can lead to functional disabilities and leave cosmetic blemishes. Surgical excision, inlay grafts and corticosteroid injections may be required until adolescence is reached and active growth has ceased.

FURTHER READING

British Burn Association Recommended First Aid for Burns Scalds. *Burns* 1987, 13.

Herndon D.N. (1994) Accepting the challenge. *J. Burn. Care Rehab.* **15**: 463–9

Herndon D.N. & Pierre E.J. (1998) Treatment of burns. In: O'Neill J.A., Rowe M.I., Grosfeld J.L. Fonkalsrud E.W. & Coran A.G. (eds) *Pediatric Surgery*, 5th edn, Mosby, St. Louis, pp. 343–58.

Monafo W.W. (1996) Initial management of burns. *New Engl. J. Med.* **335**: 1581–4.

— 42 —

Neonatal Orthopaedics

CASE 1

A 1-day-old baby, weighing 3.75 kg and born by a 'difficult' delivery, was not moving his right arm soon after birth. Examination revealed no deformities, but the baby cried when the arm was moved, or when lifted. Two weeks later a painless swelling was noted in the middle third of the right humerus.

Q. 1.1   What is the swelling?

Q. 1.2   What is the natural history?

CASE 2

A newborn baby was unable to leave the neonatal nursery because of being generally unwell with signs of sepsis. On the tenth day a lack of normal kicking movements were noted in the left lower limb. There was a low grade pyrexia and the white cell count and ESR were elevated.

Q. 2.1   What might be seen on hip ultrasonography?

CASE 3

A baby boy weighing 4.65 kg was born by a shoulder presentation to a diabetic mother. There were no left shoulder or elbow movements but normal grasp reflex and finger movements.

Q. 3.1   What is the likely diagnosis?

Q. 3.2   What is the likeliest outcome?

CASE 4

A newborn baby was noted to have both feet turned in to face each other immediately after birth. The father had had multiple operations for 'club feet' in childhood. On examination the feet could be corrected to the normal position with gentle pressure from one finger.

Q. 4.1   What is the likely diagnosis?

Q. 4.2   What is the prognosis?

CASE 5

In a country hospital a newborn was noted to have both feet pointing upwards, lying along the lower tibia. The child was referred for an orthopaedic opinion, but the position improved before the consultation took place and then resolved without treatment.

Q. 5.1   Is there a risk of other anomalies?

CASE 6

A male infant was born with the right foot turned down and inwards. The foot felt stiff and could not be placed in a normal alignment. There was a strong family history of club foot.

Q. 6.1   What is the treatment and likely outcome?

Parents may bring their child to an orthopaedic surgeon in the first month of life because something looks wrong (club foot or bowed tibia) or because something is not moving or working properly (brachial plexus palsy or birth fracture). Alternatively, the paediatrician or orthopaedic surgeon may find something on examination of which the parent was not aware of (congenital dislocation of the hip).

Newborn children have limited ways in which to respond to pain, be it from a birth fracture, osteomyelitis or a tumour. They often reduce or stop moving the limb: a condition known as 'pseudoparalysis'. The limb is not paralysed, but is held still because pain can be relieved by reducing or abolishing movements. The most common causes of 'pseudoparalysis' are fractures or infection.

BIRTH FRACTURES

Birth fractures are quite common. They have an incidence of 1 to 5 per 1000 live births and they are usually found in large, healthy babies after a difficult delivery, especially by the breech. The most common sites are the clavicle, the humerus and femur. Fractures of the clavicle may not be diagnosed until a painless swelling is noted because of callus formation. Not all birth injuries are fractures; separations of the humeral and femoral epiphyses also occur and can be difficult to diagnose without a high index of suspicion and special imaging techniques. Most birth injuries heal quickly with simple splinting and recover fully. Multiple fractures in a newborn suggest a bone fragility syndrome, such as osteogenesis imperfecta, or a generalised problem such as arthrogryposis multiplex congenita.

NEONATAL MUSCULOSKELETAL INFECTION

Osteomyelitis and septic arthritis are difficult to distinguish in the neonatal period. The infection usually affects the end of the bone and the joint, and a better term is 'osteoarticular sepsis'. Infection in the neonate is the result of bacteraemia or septicaemia, and presents with non-specific signs of generalised infection rather than signs of a localised bone and joint infection. Diagnosis may be delayed, during which time the growth plate or joint may be destroyed, with resulting lifelong disability. A high index of suspicion is required in the neonate with reduced limb movements and signs of sepsis.

The most common organism is Staph. aureus, but a wide range of Gram positive and Gram negative organisms are recovered. Some are acquired from the birth canal. Identification of the organism from blood culture or joint aspirate is very important to direct antibiotic therapy appropriately.

The most important factor in prognosis is the interval between onset and intervention. Growth plates and joints can be destroyed quickly and quietly in the neonate. Joint aspiration is a diagnostic procedure, but once pus is identified the affected joint must be drained by arthrotomy and splinted for comfort. For the hip, abduction splintage is used to treat septic dislocation.

BIRTH BRACHIAL PLEXUS PALSY ('OBSTETRIC PALSY')

A true paralysis of the upper limb may occur — usually in a large baby and as the result of a difficult delivery. Injuries to the spinal cord are rare, and present as a partial or complete quadriplegia or paraplegia. A partial palsy of the upper limb is usually caused by a traction injury to the brachial plexus. The majority of injuries are neuropraxias, the nerve trunks are in continuity and 80 per cent recover fully. As a general rule, a child who recovers elbow flexion by the age of 3 months will make a full recovery. These babies require careful evaluation at intervals to document recovery and to prevent secondary contractures and deformities by a simple program of stretching exercises. Internal rotation contracture of the shoulder can be prevented more effectively by physiotherapy than by splinting.

Microsurgical repair may be helpful for those infants with complete tears to the roots of the brachial plexus, where there is little or no recovery.

NEONATAL FOOT DEFORMITIES

Most parents have a good idea of what a baby's foot should look like, and are anxious and distressed when they see a deformity. The majority of deformities are postural variations or 'packaging defects'. In the womb the foot has been compressed in an abnormal position, either because the baby is large, the womb is crowded (twin pregnancy) or

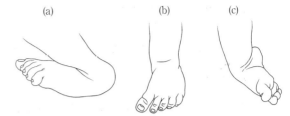

Fig. 42.1 (a) Congenital talipes calcaneovalgus. The foot has been folded back against the front of the tibia, but there is no fixed deformity. (b) Metatarsus adductus. (c) Congenital talipes equinovarus (club foot): this can be postural (mobile) or structural (stiff).

lacking in amniotic fluid (oligohydramnios). Soon after birth, when the baby has room to move, the posture improves and the appearance becomes normal. Occasionally, this process is sped up by a short period of stretching in a splint or cast, but surgery is not required. Postural club foot, metatarsus adductus and talipes calcaneovalgus, are good examples of packaging disorders (Fig. 42.1).

In metatarsus adductus the foot curves inwards, especially the great toe, so that the sole of the foot has a 'bean' shape, but the hind foot is normal. The deformity is flexible and resolves rapidly, either with a short period of casting or spontaneously (Fig. 42.1b).

The foot in talipes calcaneovalgus (Fig. 42.1a) has been lying along the tibia in the womb, the heel in a downward position referred to as calcaneus, in comparison to the heel in an upward position of club foot, referred to as equinus. The deformity is flexible and corrects rapidly.

Postural club foot looks just like structural club foot, hence parental anxiety (Fig. 42.1c). However, the two conditions do not feel in the least like each other. Postural club feet are soft and supple. Gentle pressure from an examiner's finger can place the foot in a normal position.

By contrast, 'manufacturing defects' are structural and require surgical correction. Club foot (talipes equinovarus) is a good example and is easily recognised because of the stiffness of the deformity when the examiner attempts to place the foot in the correct position (Fig. 42.2).

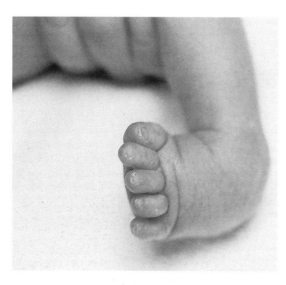

Fig. 42.2 Congenital talipes equinovarus. The foot lies in a typical position and is rigid.

The incidence of club foot is about 1 per 1000 live births in white people, 0.5 per 1000 in Asians but 5 per 1000 in Polynesians. It is more common in males, and is bilateral in about 40 per cent of cases. A family history is present, but both genetic and environmental factors are implicated. Club foot may be an isolated deformity, associated with conditions such as congenital hip dislocation, part of a syndrome or acquired because of neuromuscular disease. A long period of conservative treatment and operative treatment are often required. The affected foot is usually smaller and the leg on the affected side shorter in unilateral cases.

Another important 'manufacturing defect' is congenital dislocation of the hip. This rarely presents in the neonate because the parents have noted something; rather, it is found thanks to a screening program.

DEVELOPMENTAL DYSPLASIA OF THE HIP (DDH OR CDH)

The preferred term is Developmental Dysplasia of the Hip (DDH) rather than 'Congenital Dislocation of the Hip' (CDH). This reflects two important features of the natural history of the condition:

- Not all cases are found at birth; some develop during the first year of life.
- Not all hips are dislocated; some have only a shallow or dysplastic acetabulum.

DDH covers a spectrum of hip dysplasia and instability, presenting from birth to early childhood. It is the result of both genetic and environmental factors, so that family history is a risk factor but so also is breech birth. According to diagnostic criteria it affects 1 to 2 per 1000 live births, and is at least 5 times more common in females than males. Dysplasia usually refers to a shallowness or malformation of the acetabulum; subluxation to a partial displacement of the head of the femur from the acetabulum; and dislocation, to displacement of the head of the femur completely outside the acetabulum.

The condition is best diagnosed soon after birth through the tests of neonatal hip instability (Fig. 42.3), supplemented by the selective use of ultrasonography examination. Hip X-rays (Fig. 42.3) are of little value in the neonatal period because the femoral head is cartilaginous and hence invisible until the age of 4 to 8 months, when the ossification centre develops.

Ideally, the examination should be performed by an experienced examiner. In practice, DDH is uncommon and not every paediatrician or GP is able to gain the necessary experience. The baby should be undressed, warm, relaxed and placed on a firm but comfortable surface. Offering a bottle, finger or dummy to suck can help.

The examiner holds the leg to be examined in the hand with the hip and knee flexed, the thumb on the inner side of the thigh over the lesser trochanter and the middle finger over the great trochanter. The right hand is used to examine the baby's left hip and the left hand to examine the right hip.

The pelvis is steadied by the other hand and the flexed thigh is abducted and adducted, carefully felt for any 'clunk' or jerk that may denote the hip entering or leaving the acetabulum (Ortolani test). Then, with the hip adducted, gentle down-

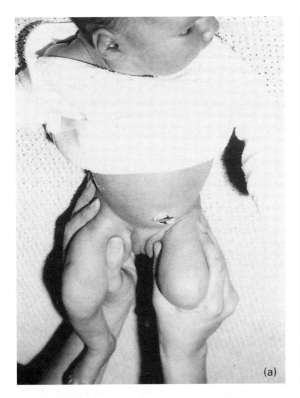

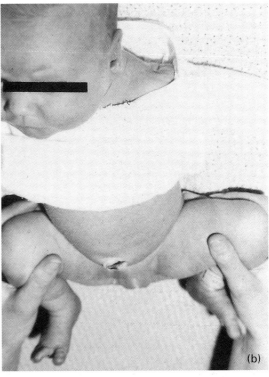

(a)

(b)

Fig. 42.3 Congenital dislocation of the hips. Ortolani's test: the thumbs are placed over the front of the hip joints as both are fully abducted with the knees and hips flexed.

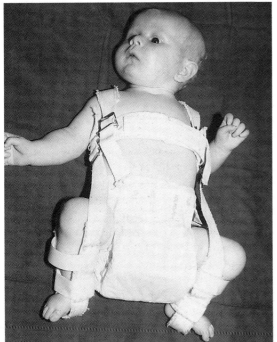

wards pressure is exerted to determine if the head of the femur is stable, or whether it may slip posteriorly out of the acetabulum (Barlow test).

A fine 'click' is not evidence of dislocation or instability, but the baby should be examined again. A 'clunk' as the hip enters the socket from a dislocated position is the most important finding and is an indication for immediate treatment. The unstable neonatal hip tends to dislocate in adduction and extension, and to reduce in flexion and abduction. Treatment is directed towards gently placing the hips in a position of abduction and flexion while allowing movement within a safe arc of motion. This is most efficiently and safely achieved by using a Pavlik harness (Fig. 42.4).

Fig. 42.4 Pavlik harness. In the flexed and abducted position, the dislocated hip is held in the reduced position.

The progress of treatment is best monitored by careful repeated hip examinations, supplemented by ultrasonography, which can be performed while the harness is in place. Most hips will stabilise quickly and become normal. If the golden opportunity for early diagnosis and treatment is missed, operative treatment and a less satisfactory result are much more likely.

FURTHER READING

Green N.E. & Mencio G.A. (1998) Major congenital orthopedic deformities. In: O'Neill J.A., Rowe M.I., Grosfeld J.L., Fonkalsrud E.W. & Coran A.G. (eds) *Pediatric Surgery*, 5th edn, Mosby, St. Louis, pp. 1859–78.

— 43 —

Orthopaedics in the Infant and Toddler

CASE 1

A mother brought her 12-month-old child to her GP because he had just started to pull to stand, and she was worried that he had flat feet and bow legs. Examination revealed a healthy toddler with symmetric bowing of the lower limbs: the gap between the knees when standing was 4 cm. There was no medial arch in the feet in the standing position.

> *Q. 1.1   What is the likely outcome for this child?*

CASE 2

Jessica, an 18-month-old, presented because she was walking with in-toeing. She had a normal birth and developmental history but walked with both feet facing inwards and sometimes tripped. Examination revealed mild bowing and medial tibial torsion.

> *Q. 2.1   What is the natural history and management?*

CASE 3

Susan, a 14-month-old, presented with a limp. She was the first born to a young mother who walked with a severe limp because of an arthritic hip. Susan had been born by breech delivery and was referred for an X-ray of her hips.

> *Q. 3.1   What is the diagnosis?*
>
> *Q. 3.2   Could the problem be diagnosed earlier?*

CASE 4

John, an 18-month-old, was brought to his paediatrician because he limped on his right leg and when he ran, his right arm was held stiffly with the elbow flexed. On examination, the muscles of the right arm and leg felt stiff when compared with the left, and the deep tendon reflexes were brisk.

> *Q. 4.1   What is the likely problem?*

CASE 5

Bruce, a 22-month-old, was collected from child care by his mother who was told that he had been limping on his right leg. He was put to bed but next morning refused to walk. He had a fever and was sore when his nappy was changed. His mother took him to his GP, who arranged admission to hospital.

Q. 5.1   *What might be wrong?*

Q. 5.2   *What would a bone scan show?*

CASE 6

Mary, a 4-month-old, presented to her GP because of persistent crying and a swollen left thigh. She was a 'difficult' baby with feeding and sleeping problems. There were several bruises and abrasions.

Q. 6.1   *What is the diagnosis?*

Q. 6.2   *What would X-rays show?*

CASE 7

Toby was well known at the Emergency Department of his local hospital. At the age of 20 months he had been seen three times for fractures to both his upper and lower limbs. On this occasion his blue sclerae were noted.

Q. 7.1   *What is the diagnosis?*

Limp, or abnormal gait, are the most common reasons for orthopaedic referral in the infant and toddler. As children grow there are rapid changes in the appearance and alignment of the lower limbs, such that the bow-legged toddler becomes a knock-kneed child, and eventually an adult with straight legs. Many toddlers who are referred to orthopaedic clinics are normal and have no specific disease or deformity. They are referred with a variation of normality, such as flexible flat foot, in-toeing, out-toeing, knock knees or bow legs. It is essential to recognise that there can be just as much parental anxiety in these circumstances as there is about a child with a definable pathological condition.

The general principles of the management of these children are as follows:

(1) These conditions are common because they are normal variations.

(2) A reasonable description of normal is the mean value of the measurement plus or minus 2 standard deviations. This is of value to surgeons, but not to parents.

(3) These conditions generally resolve spontaneously and there is little evidence that intervention changes the natural history.

(4) Over-investigation of these children should be resisted.

(5) Over-treatment should be resisted.

(6) Within the large group of normal children with physiological variants there are a small number with specific pathology. These children should be identified, investigated, diagnosed and treated appropriately.

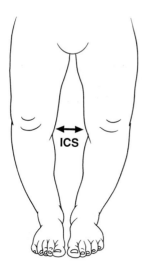

Fig. 43.1 Bow legs: the tibia has an outward curve and an inward twist (internal torsion), both of which accentuate the normal 'flat' appearance of the feet.

THE TODDLER WITH A SYMMETRICALLY ABNORMAL GAIT

Bow legs

When the toddler first begins to walk the appearance of bowing is very common. It is frequently accompanied by some degree of internal tibial torsion and the one deformity accentuates the other. Bowing seems to be pronounced in overweight children.

Physiological bowing is symmetrical, not excessively severe, and improves with time. Measurement of the distance between the knees (the intercondylar separation (ICS)) in the standing child provides a simple means of follow-up to assess whether the condition is improving or not (Fig. 43.1). Often this is all that parents require for reassurance. Night splints have been abandoned with the recognition that they do not influence the natural resolution of the condition.

Pathological bowing may be asymmetrical, it is often more severe and it deteriorates with time. Causes of pathological bowing include Blount's disease, rickets, trauma and skeletal dysplasia.

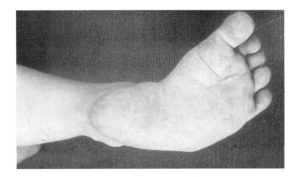

Fig. 43.2 Metatarsus adductus. The midfoot and forefoot are adducted, but the heel is normal.

In-toeing

This is one of the commonest presenting symptoms at paediatric orthopaedic clinics because of its appearance and parental concern about long-term sequelae (Fig. 43.2). Sometimes the concern is from the grandparents or a kindergarten teacher. There may also be a complaint that the child is clumsy or trips frequently. There is often a marked contrast between parent and child. The parent is anxious about the 'deformity', whereas the child runs around the consulting room in a carefree fashion, frequently not demonstrating nearly as much in-toeing as the parents claim is the case at home.

Internal tibial torsion

Internal or medial tibial torsion is very common in toddlers, and usually presents as in-toeing between 1 and 3 years of age. It is probably a 'packaging defect'; the result of intrauterine positioning. It frequently coexists, and may be confused, with bowing of the tibia, physiological genu varum.

The natural history is for spontaneous resolution. A number of orthotic devices have been used; principally boots on a curved metal bar with the feet turned outwards (Denis Browne splint). This is used as a night splint and is a potent cause of disturbed sleep and family distress. It may speed resolution of the deformity, but this has never been proven. Surgery is almost never required in normal children. In pathological conditions such as spina bifida it can be treated by derotation tibial osteotomy at the supramalleolar level.

THE TODDLER WITH A PAINLESS, CHRONIC LIMP

Developmental dysplasia of the hip (DDH)

DDH may present at walking age because of an asymmetric gait (Fig. 43.3). At this age the hip is not painful and does not cause an undue delay in walking. Bilateral hip dislocations may present even later than a unilateral dislocation because the deformity is symmetrical. The risk factors are the first-born female child, breech delivery, and having a positive family history. In addition to the usual neonatal clinical examination of the hips, an infant with many risk factors should have ultrasonography examination of the hips in the neonatal period and an X-ray of the hips at 6

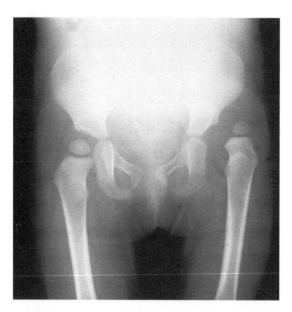

Fig. 43.3 Congenital dislocation of the hip. An X-ray showing a permanently dislocated hip and poor acetabular development in an infant where the diagnosis was missed at birth.

months. Delayed presentation leads to a high risk of arthritis in young adults.

Hemiplegia

The typical hemiplegic gait is a limp with a stiff, ipsilateral arm with a flexed elbow. Most children with hemiplegia have a brain lesion acquired in the perinatal period, but the mildly involved may not present until walking age. Walking and running may unmask or accentuate the posturing in the upper limb.

Cerebral palsy (CP) is the most common cause of physical disability in developed countries. It is classified according to the type of movement disorder (spastic, athetoid, ataxic or mixed) and the distribution in the limbs (hemiplegia, diplegia or quadriplegia).

Toe-walking

When children are learning to walk a short period of intermittent toe-walking is very common. It is then followed by a period of 'flat foot' strike before the gait matures to the adult pattern, in which a heel strike is normal. In some children the period of toe-walking is prolonged and pronounced, causing parental concern and referral to the orthopaedic surgeon.

Differential diagnosis

The majority of these children are otherwise normal and are called 'idiopathic toe-walkers'. The pathological causes of 'toe-walking' are diplegic CP, muscular dystrophy, Charcot Marie Tooth disease and spinal dysraphism. Unilateral toe-walking is almost always pathological and the most common causes are hemiplegic CP and unilateral DDH.

ACUTE ONSET LIMPING IN THE TODDLER

This is a common age for the presentation of acute haematogenous osteomyelitis (AHO). Over

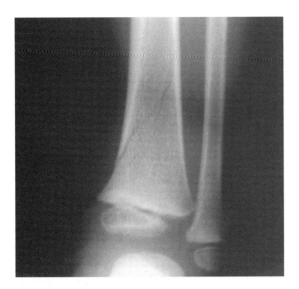

Fig. 43.4 The 'toddler's fracture'. A spiral fracture of the distal tibia often presenting as a limp of unknown cause, which is difficult to see on X-ray.

a period of 12 to 48 hours the child develops fever, a limp and then refuses to walk. A toddler's fracture of the tibia may present in a similar manner because the fall or injury is not observed and the fracture may be difficult to see on X-ray (Fig. 43.4).

FRACTURES IN THE INFANT AND TODDLER

It is difficult for a normal infant to sustain a femoral fracture. Infants cannot climb, they have limited mobility and most accidental falls in this age group do not result in a fracture. The younger the child with any fracture, especially a femoral fracture, the higher the incidence of child abuse. As many as 40 per cent of femoral fractures in the under 12 month age-group are caused by child abuse. A bone scan will detect any occult fractures (Fig. 43.5).

Most infants and children with fractures and an unconvincing history have been abused. However, a number may have fragile bones because of osteogenesis imperfecta, and a premature

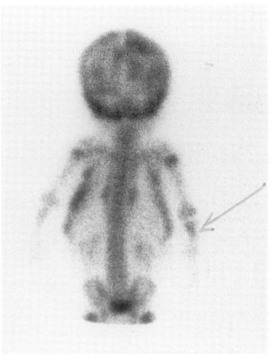

Fig. 43.5 A Technetium bone scan is a sensitive means to detect occult fractures in child abuse.

diagnosis of child abuse may cause irreparable harm (Fig. 43.6).

FURTHER READING

Baxter A. & Dulberg C. (1988) Growing pains in children *J. Pediatr. Orthop.* **8**: 402–6.

Benson M.K.D., Fixsen J.A. & Macnicol M.F. (ed.) (1994) *Children's Orthopaedics and Fractures*, Churchill Livingstone, Edinburgh.

Fraser R.K., Menelaus M.B., Williams P.F. & Cole W.G. (1995) The Miller procedure for flexible flat feet. *J. Bone Joint Surg.* **77B**: 396–9.

Glasgow J.F.T. & Graham H.K. (1997) *Management of Injuries in Children*, BMJ Publishing group, London.

Griffin P.P., Wheelhouse W.W., Shiavi R. & Bass W. (1997) Habitual toe walkers. A clinical and EMG gait analysis. *J. Bone Joint Surg.* **59-A**: 97–101.

Hensinger R.N. (1986) *Standards in Pediatric Orthopedics*. Raven Press, New York.

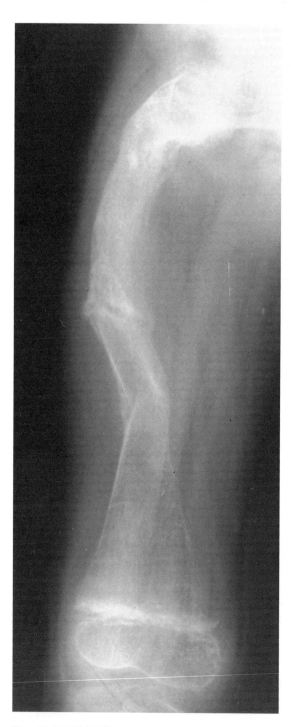

Fig. 43.6 Multiple fractures and deformity of the femur in osteogenesis imperfecta.

Kling T.F. & Hensinger R.N. (1983) Angular and torsional deformities of the limbs in children. *Clin. Orthop. Rel. Research,* **186**: 136–42.

McCoy F.G., Graham H.K. & Piggot J. (1987) Non-union of fractures of the carpal scaphoid in a child. *Ulster Medical Journal,* **56 (1)**: 66.

Piggot J., Graham H.K. & McCoy F.G. (1986) Supracondylar fracture of the humerus in children: Treatment by straight lateral traction. *J. Bone Joint Surg.* **68-B**: 577–83.

Pirone A.M., Graham H.K. & Krajbich J.I. (1988) The management of displaced extension type supracondylar fractures of the humerus in children. *J. Bone Joint Surg.* **70(A)**: 541–650.

Rang M. (1983) *Children's Fractures,* 2nd edn, J.B. Lippincott Co., Philadelphia.

Staheli L. (1990) Lower positional deformity in infants and children: a review. *J. Pediatr. Orthop.* **10**: 559–63.

Steele J.A. & Graham H.K. (1992) Angulated radial neck fractures in children, a prospective study of percutaneous reduction. *J. Bone Joint Surg.* **74-B**: 760–4.

Svenningsen S., Terjesen T., Apalset K. & Anda S. (1990) Osteotomy for femoral anteversion. *Acta Orthop. Scand.* **61**: 360–3.

Wenger D., Maudlin D., Speck G., Morgan D. & Leiber R. (1989) Corrective shoes and inserts as treatment for flexible flat feet in infants and children. *J. Bone Joint Surg.* **71-A**: 800–10.

Wenger D.R. & Rang M. (1993) *The Art and Practice of Children's Orthopaedics,* Raven Press, New York.

Williams P.F. & Cole W.G. (eds) (1991) *Orthopaedic Management in Childhood,* 2nd edn, Chapman & Hall, London.

— 44 —

Orthopaedics in the Child

CASE 1

Mary, a 4-year-old, was brought to her GP because of in-toeing. Examination revealed that she walked with both feet and knees facing inwards by 20 degrees. Her mother commented that she had been described as 'double jointed' as a child. Both had signs of generalised joint laxity.

> *Q. 1.1   What is the diagnosis?*

CASE 2

Jacky, a 5-year-old, was brought to see an orthopaedic surgeon because of knock knees. Examination revealed symmetric genu valgum with 6 cm between the ankles in the standing position.

> *Q. 2.1   Is treatment required?*

CASE 3

Sara, a 6-year-old, was a keen gymnast and was noted to have 'flat feet'. Expensive orthotics were prescribed.

> *Q. 3.1   Are these necessary?*

CASE 4

A 7-year-old boy falls out of a tree on to his outstretched hand. He presents shortly after with a very swollen, painful elbow and decreased radial pulse.

> *Q. 4.1   Why is this important?*

As children become older, parental anxiety about the appearance of their feet, legs and walking continues. As in the younger age groups, the majority of these children are also normal, but a different spectrum of problems are seen from those seen in the toddler. It may be rare to see CDH or cerebral palsy presenting for the first time in the child, but irritable hip, Perthes' disease (Fig. 44.1), osteomyelitis and septic arthritis are all seen.

As children become more adventurous in play and participate in sport, an increasing number and variety of fractures and epiphyseal injuries are seen.

INTERNAL FEMORAL TORSION (INSET HIPS)

This is frequently seen in children between the ages of 3 and 10 years. The in-toeing is symmetrical. Parents complain that their children look awkward and trip frequently, but the degree of disability is not great. The child often has signs of generalised joint laxity and may have associated features, such as flexible flat feet.

Examination reveals a characteristic shift of the arc of hip rotation inwards, hence the synonym 'inset hips'. A typical finding would be internal rotation of 80 to 90 degrees and external rotation

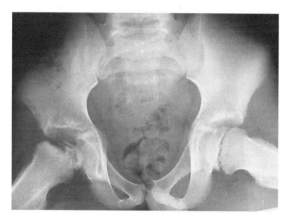

Fig. 44.1 Typical X-ray appearance of Perthes' disease.

of 0 to 10 degrees. This is the reason why the children can sit comfortably in the 'W' position (Fig. 44.2). It is doubtful if sitting in this position causes the condition, but there is some evidence that habitually sitting in this posture slows down the natural tendency to spontaneous recovery.

In some children the correction of in-toeing is accomplished by a compensatory tibial torsion. In these children the feet no longer turn in, but in standing and walking the patellae are facing inwards or 'squinting'. This combination of deformities can look unattractive and give the appearance of bow-legs.

Management

The natural history of the condition is for spontaneous resolution during the growing years. There is no evidence that any form of exercises or orthotic devices influences the resolution. The condition can be treated surgically by means of external rotation osteotomy of the femur, but the vast majority of children improve spontaneously and do not require intervention.

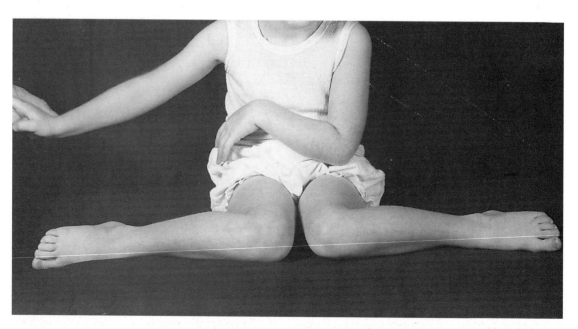

Fig. 44.2 Internal femoral torsion (inset hips): the child can sit on the floor in the 'W' position.

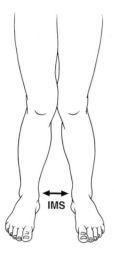

Fig. 44.3 Knock knees (genu valgum).

Perthes' disease (Legge–Calvé–Perthes; pseudocoxalgia)

This is a form of osteochondritis juvenilis affecting the head of the femur, mainly in boys (80 per cent) between 3 and 10 years of age. The cause is unknown, though trauma is partly responsible.

The symptoms include intermittent painless limp, or less commonly, severe, painful limp. Patients with a good prognosis need no treatment, although admission to hospital may be needed to rest the leg in Pugh's traction.

KNOCK KNEES

Physiological genu valgum, or knock knee deformity, is often seen in children between the ages of 3 and 8 years (Fig. 44.3). The majority of children straighten spontaneously. The deformity is symmetrical, not excessive (for example, the gap [intermalleolar separation (IMS)] between the ankles on standing is < 10 cm) and improves with time. Pathological genu valgum is usually more severe, asymmetrical and increases with time. Causes include trauma (proximal metaphyseal greenstick

fracture of the tibia or growth plate injury) rickets, skeletal dysplasias and congenital limb deficiencies.

Management

There is no evidence that the natural history of the condition is affected by exercises, shoe inserts or night splints.

A small number of children with physiological genu valgum do not correct completely. The reasons to consider surgery are discomfort from 'knee-swishing' while running, concern about the appearance, and progression of the deformity in the pathological cases. In order to assess the degree and site of deformity a standing X-ray of the lower limb should be obtained. Correction can be achieved by restricting growth in the distal femoral or proximal tibial growth plates on the medial side of the knee. When the growth plates are fused, osteotomy of the distal femur or proximal tibia is required.

FLAT FEET

Almost all infants have 'flat feet' and in the majority an arch will develop by the age of 6 years. The clinical findings of a flexible flat foot include absence of the medial longitudinal arch and a variable degree of hind foot valgus. When the child stands 'at ease', the only support to the medial arch is the interosseus ligaments and intrinsic muscles of the foot, which are not continuously active. When the child stands on tip-toe, the long flexor and extensor muscles are recruited into continuous activity. In the correctable flat foot the medial longitudinal arch usually appears and the heel tilts into neutral or varus. This 'tip toe test' can be used to explain the nature of the condition to parents and to reassure them that the internal structure of the foot is normal. In the flexible flat foot the medial arch is also reformed on weight bearing when the hallux is passively dorsiflexed. This is referred to as the 'toe-raising test of Jack'.

Pathological causes of flat foot include hypermobility syndromes and cerebral palsy.

Management

Most of the enthusiasm for 'treating' flat foot has probably been based on the observation that through the use of any of the popular forms of treatment, the majority of children are noted to get 'better'.

Although shoe modifications and inserts do not change the shape of the foot in the long term, there is some evidence that orthotics may prolong the life of the shoe by decreasing deformation and wear. If excessive shoe wear and the cost of replacements are important to the parents, or pain is a problem, the 'Helfet' heel cup or a simple medial arch support may be helpful. Expensive, custom made orthotics are rarely, if ever, required.

In children with normal flexible flat foot, surgery is very rarely required.

GROWING PAINS AND NIGHT CRAMPS

About 15 per cent of children go through a period where they wake at night, crying because of pains in their legs. The child goes to sleep after an energetic day only to wake in misery, but the following day all is well. Presentation is often delayed until there have been many disturbed nights.

Clinical features

The child has no day-time pain and no limp. The pain at night is relieved by rubbing, heat and simple analgesics. Examination reveals no abnormalities.

Differential diagnosis

Night pains are a feature of osteoid osteoma, but this is always unilateral and often reasonably well localised. One cause of bilateral leg pains is leukaemia, which can be excluded in most children by a full-blood count. There are usually other features in leukaemia or an atypical story, so investigation is not necessary in all children with bilateral nocturnal leg pain.

Management

Full history-taking and thorough examination excludes pathological causes and allays parental anxiety. Reassurance is very important and fortunately most parents can accept the situation. There may be a role for a program of stretching exercises.

FRACTURES AND EPIPHYSEAL INJURIES IN THE CHILD

As the child becomes more adventurous in play, and then active in organised sport, the incidence of musculoskeletal injuries increases dramatically. The weak link in the child's skeleton is the growth plate or physis. In children, epiphyseal separations are common, as are fractures of the long bones.

Specific soft tissue injuries, such as collateral ligament tears, are rare and the diagnosis of a 'sprain' in the child is frequently incorrect. A valgus force at the knee, which would result in a tear of the medial collateral ligament in an adult, is more likely to cause a separation of the distal femoral epiphysis in the child (Fig. 44.4). The equivalent of an anterior cruciate tear in a child is avulsion of the tibial spine.

Non-specific, minor soft tissue injury is common in the child, including abrasions and bruising.

FRACTURES IN CHILDREN

Fractures are caused by forces applied to the skeleton that result in failure of the bone under the applied load. Because children's bones have different biomechanical qualities from adult bones, the patterns of failure are different. Children's bones may bend and buckle rather than break cleanly (Fig. 44.5). Plastic bowing, buckle fractures and greenstick fractures are all incomplete fractures frequently seen in children but not in adults. Children's fractures heal more quickly than adult fractures, and recovery of function is also faster and generally more complete. Children's fractures

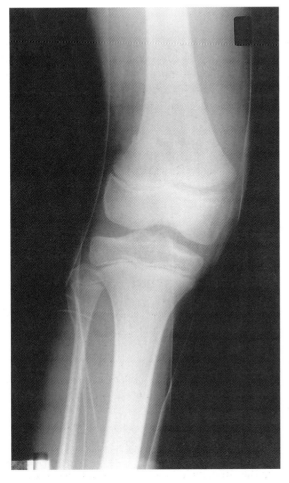

Fig. 44.4 Valgus injury to the knee. In an adult, a tear of the medial ligament would be likely, whereas in this child the result is a Harris–Salter type 2 separation of the distal femoral plate.

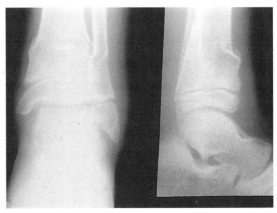

Fig. 44.5 Children's bones may bend and buckle, as in this fracture of the distal tibia and fistula.

than 12 months, the hyperaemia results in faster growth of the injured limb compared with the uninjured limb. During the first year after fracture, this may amount to between 0.5 and 1.5 cm. With this in mind, femoral fractures in this age group may be allowed to heal with up to 1 cm of overlap or shortening, in the expectation that overgrowth will tend to make up the deficit and equalise the length of the lower limbs (Fig. 44.6).

In children, most fractures are isolated injuries caused by indirect forces:

- in the upper limb, a fall on the outstretched hand
- in the lower limb, a twisting injury; for example, roller-skating.

These are usually closed injuries, with a good prognosis.

A small percentage of injuries are caused by direct violence, usually road trauma. These injuries are more likely to be multiple, severely displaced, open or compound, and have associated injuries to the head, spinal cord or abdomen.

Fractures in children are treated in many ways including cast immobilisation, traction, internal fixation and external fixation. The choice of management is based on an understanding of the risks and benefits of each type of treatment, with safety, efficacy and convenience being the most important factors.

are subject to a process of remodelling during further growth by which residual deformity may correct and function improve. Remodelling is faster and more complete in younger children and for fractures close to an active growth plate. Hence, residual angulation or displacement of distal radial fractures in younger children is well tolerated and there are few poor results in the long term. Fractures of the femur in children aged between 4 and 10 years are subject to 'overgrowth'. During the remodelling phase, which may last for more

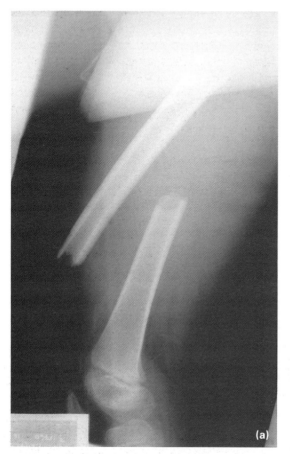
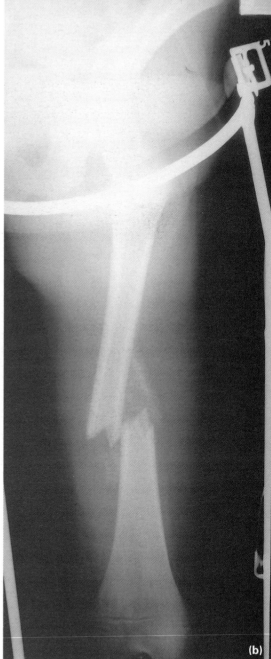

Fig. 44.6 (a) Open fracture of the femur as a result of a fall from a tree. Note the gross displacement and shortening; (b) after wound care, reduction and traction, the fracture is healing in good position. Up to 1 cm of overlap is acceptable because of anticipated overgrowth.

UPPER LIMB FRACTURES

Fractures occur most frequently at the ends of the long bones but may be seen in the midshaft. The

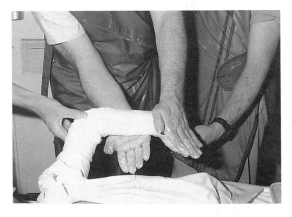

Fig. 44.7 Treating fractures in children: moulding a plaster for a distal radial fracture.

area next to the growth plate, the metaphysis, is especially vulnerable. In the upper limb the most common injuries are fractures of the distal radial metaphysis, the diaphyses of the radius and ulna, and fractures around the elbow. Most fractures of the radius and ulna are managed by closed reduction and cast immobilisation for about 6 weeks (Fig. 44.7).

Elbow fractures in children are common; there are many types and a variety of management strategies are required. An accurate diagnosis is required that in turn requires good quality anterior–posterior (AP) and lateral X-rays, and a knowledge of the normal growth patterns of the elbow.

The most common of the more serious injuries is the supracondylar fracture of the distal humerus. This is a transverse fracture of the distal humerus, just above the growth plate, and is usually displaced backwards as the result of a fall on the outstretched hand (Fig. 44.8a). The

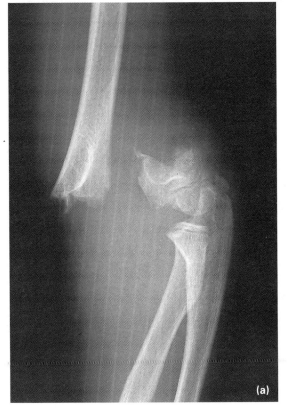

(a)

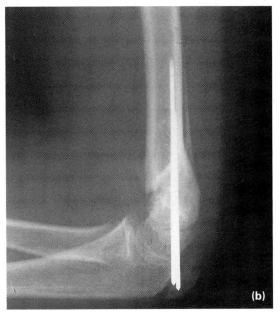

(b)

Fig. 44.8 (a) Supracondylar fracture of the humerus with gross displacement: the neurovascular structures are at risk; (b) the appearance after closed reduction and Kirschner wire fixation.

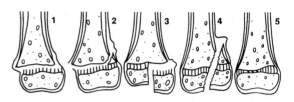

Fig. 44.9 The types of growth-plate injury, as classified by Salter & Harris.

fracture displacement or subsequent swelling may result in vascular problems in the forearm and hand and Volkman's ischaemia (Box 44.1). Nerve palsies are also common. In the past these fractures were usually managed by reduction and casting with the elbow flexed, but this increases the risk of Volkman's ischaemia. The preferred management for displaced supracondylar fractures is now closed reduction and percutaneous fixation with Kirschner wires (Fig. 44.8b).

Displaced fractures of the lateral condylar physis are Harris–Salter type 4 injuries and require open reduction and internal fixation. Fractures of the radial neck can usually be managed by closed reduction or an indirect percutaneous reduction with a Kirschner wire.

THE HARRIS–SALTER CLASSIFICATION OF GROWTH PLATE INJURIES

There are many classifications of growth plate injuries, but that by Harris and Salter is the most popular and useful (Fig. 44.9). The line of separation of the growth plate is identified on good quality AP and lateral X-rays, looking for both horizontal and vertical components. Most injuries can be readily classified in 1 of the 5 groups. Some complex injuries require further imaging including CT scans or MRI.

Type 1 and 2 injuries are the most common and are usually managed by closed reduction and cast immobilisation. Epiphyseal injuries heal very quickly and in type 1 and 2 injuries the prognosis is usually good. In type 3 and 4 injuries the growth cartilage and articular cartilage are both disrupted. Precise reduction is required (this usually means an open reduction) but growth disturbance is still a possibility. Partial growth arrest may cause a progressive angular deformity in the limb; a complete arrest results in progressive shortening.

LOWER LIMB FRACTURES

Fractures of the femur and tibia are common and are usually classified according to the position of the fracture in the diaphysis; for example, the upper, lower or middle third. Femoral fractures can be managed by a wide variety of methods including traction, hip spica casts, internal fixation and external fixation (Fig. 44.6). The method is chosen according to the age of the child, the fracture type and displacement, and the experience and preference of the surgeon. Younger children tolerate traction and casts very well. Open fractures and those associated with head injuries, tibial fractures and multiple injuries are better managed by internal fixation. The time to healing is closely related to age: 2 to 3 weeks in the first year of life, 6 to 12 weeks in children, and 8 to 16 weeks in teenagers. Remodelling and overgrowth have been referred to above.

Tibial fractures are very common but are usually more easily managed than femoral fractures. The majority are treated by closed reduction and cast immobilisation for 6 to 10 weeks. Displaced diaphyseal fractures carry a risk of compartment syndrome, and neurovascular monitoring is important for 48 hours after injury. Tibial and femoral fractures cause a prolonged period of limping in most children because of weakness, stiffness and loss of confidence. Time and reassurance of parents is of more help than physiotherapy.

FURTHER READING

Baxter A. & Dulberg C. (1988) Growing pains in children *J. Pediatr. Orthop.* **8**: 402–6.

Benson M.K.D., Fixsen J.A. & Macnicol M.F. (ed.) (1994) *Children's Orthopaedics and Fractures*, Churchill Livingstone, Edinburgh.

Fraser R.K., Menelaus M.B., Williams P.F. & Cole W.G. (1995) The Miller procedure for flexible flat feet. *J. Bone Joint Surg.* **77B**: 396–9.

Glasgow J.F.T. & Graham H.K. (1997) *Management of Injuries in Children*, BMJ Publishing Group, London.

Griffin P.P., Wheelhouse W.W., Shiavi R. & Bass W. (1997) Habitual toe walkers. A clinical and EMG gait analysis. *J. Bone Joint Surg.* **59-A**: 97–101.

Hensinger R.N. (1986) *Standards in Pediatric Orthopedics.* Raven Press, New York.

Kling T.F. & Hensinger R.N. (1983) Angular and torsional deformities of the limbs in children. *Clin. Orthop. Rel. Research,* **186**: 136–42.

McCoy F.G., Graham H.K. & Piggot J. (1987) Non-union of fractures of the carpal scaphoid in a child. *Ulster Medical Journal*, **56 (1)**: 66.

Piggot J., Graham H.K. & McCoy F.G. (1986) Supracondylar fracture of the humerus in children: treatment by straight lateral traction. *J. Bone Joint Surg.* **68-B**: 577–83.

Pirone A.M., Graham H.K. & Krajbich J.I. (1988) The management of displaced extension type supracondylar fractures of the humerus in children. *J. Bone Joint Surg.* **70(A)**: 541–650.

Rang M. (1983) *Children's Fractures,* 2nd edn, J.B. Lippincott Co., Philadelphia.

Staheli L. (1990) Lower positional deformity in infants and children: a review. *J. Pediatr. Orthop.* **10**: 559–63.

Steele J.A. & Graham H.K. (1992) Angulated radial neck fractures in children, a prospective study of percutaneous reduction. *J. Bone Joint Surg.* **74-B**: 760–4.

Svenningsen S., Terjesen T., Apalset K. & Anda S. (1990) Osteotomy for femoral anteversion. *Acta Orthop. Scand.* **61**: 360–3.

Wenger D., Maudlin D., Speck G., Morgan D. & Leiber R. (1989) Corrective shoes and inserts as treatment for flexible flat feet in infants and children. *J. Bone Joint Surg.* **71-A**: 800–10.

Wenger D.R. & Rang M. (1993) *The Art and Practice of Children's Orthopaedics*, Raven Press, New York.

Williams P.F. & Cole W.G. (eds) (1991) *Orthopaedic Management in Childhood*, 2nd edn, Chapman & Hall, London.

— 45 —

Orthopaedics in the Teenager

CASE 1

Kylie, a 12-year-old, was on holidays with her family. When she was on the beach in her swimsuit her mother noticed that her shoulders were uneven and when she bent forwards the ribs on the right side were prominent. Although Kylie had no pain she agreed to go for an X-ray of her back.

> Q. 1.1   What is the diagnosis?
>
> Q. 1.2   What did the X-ray show?
>
> Q. 1.3   What is the management?

CASE 2

A 14-year-old boy attended the Emergency Department for the third time in 6 weeks. He complained of pain in his left knee, which was associated with limping. Symptoms were worse after basketball and relieved by rest. Blood tests and X-rays of the knee were normal and a diagnosis of sprained knee ligaments had been made. He had been prescribed anti-inflammatory medication and a knee brace. On this occasion it was noted that his left hip lacked internal rotation and that the hip went into external rotation during flexion.

> Q. 2.1   What is the diagnosis?
>
> Q. 2.2   What investigations are appropriate?
>
> Q. 2.3   What is the management?

CASE 3

Sue, a 14-year-old, presents with painful knees. There has been pain in the right knee, then the left, and currently both are sore. She has been seeing a physiotherapist for over a year for similar symptoms, including pain, giving way and clicking. Many sets of X-rays had been taken and were reported as normal.

> Q. 3.1   What is the diagnosis?
>
> Q. 3.2   What investigations are appropriate?
>
> Q. 3.3   What is the management?

CASE 4

Mary, a 13-year-old, has complained of pain in her right knee for the past 8 weeks. The pain has been mild and intermittent, but has become more constant, keeping her awake at night. She had physiotherapy for a pulled muscle with some temporary benefit. She agreed to her mother's request to see her GP after she noted a lump on the inner aspect of her thigh, just above the knee.

Q. 4.1   What is the differential diagnosis?

Q. 4.2   What investigations are needed?

Q. 4.3   What is the management?

The teenage years encompass the final period of skeletal growth leading to the closure of the growth plates. The adolescent growth spurt is relatively short but intense, a time of rapid growth in the length of long bones and remodelling of the skeleton to meet the needs of the young adult.

Evaluating musculoskeletal symptoms in teenagers can be difficult. Pain that may be referred to the lower limbs from the back and hip pathology frequently presents with knee pain. Teenagers may conceal symptoms and signs from their parents. A scoliosis may reach an advanced degree of deformity before being noticed by parents.

SCOLIOSIS

Scoliosis means a lateral curvature of the spine and may be classified as structural or non-structural. Non-structural curves have a cause outside the spine, the most common being a difference in leg lengths. Structural scoliosis is a complex, 3-dimensional deformity of the spine, in which a rotational deformity is an important component (Fig. 45.1). Idiopathic adolescent scoliosis is equally common in both sexes (minor curves are found in up to 4 per cent of the population), but far more girls than boys come to surgery because their curves are more likely to progress. There is often a family history and curves may progress rapidly during the adolescent growth spurt. Scoliosis is recognised clinically by the 'forward bend test' and confirmed on X-ray. Curve progression should be monitored clinically and by measuring directly from the X-ray. Curves of less than 20 degrees are unlikely to progress, curves of between 20 degrees and 40 degrees may be controlled by bracing, and curves of more than 40 degrees may require surgical correction by spinal instrumentation and fusion.

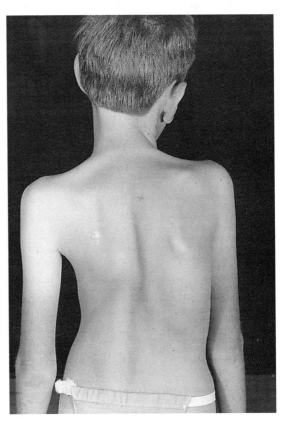

Fig. 45.1 Scoliosis. There is a right thoracic scoliosis producing prominence of the right scapula and ribs due to rotation of the vertebral bodies. The left shoulder is lowered and the left waist is increased. The deformity of the spine and chest is more apparent on forward bending.

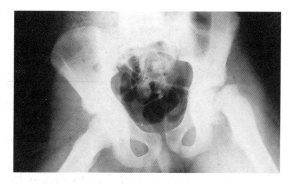

Fig. 45.2 Slipped upper femoral epiphysis on X-ray.

SLIPPED UPPER FEMORAL EPIPHYSIS

Diagnoses such as 'sprains' and 'pulled muscles' can be dangerous. They lack precision and are often incorrect, a smokescreen for fuzzy thinking, wrong diagnoses and/or incorrect treatment.

There is only one growth plate that may fail under normal physiological loads: the proximal femoral growth plate. During the last 2 years of rapid growth that lead to the closure of the growth plate, the upper femoral growth plate may slip, allowing posterior displacement of the femoral head in relation to the shaft (Fig. 45.2). This process may occur in normal teenagers, but is more likely if the loads on the growth plate are increased (for example, in obesity) or the growth plate is weakened by endocrine disorders, radiation or renal disease.

The time frame of the slipping dictates the clinical presentation. If the slip is acute, the adolescent will have severe pain in the hip, will be unable to walk and all movements of the hip will be grossly restricted. The X-ray appearances are usually easily recognised and ultrasonography of the hip will usually show a haemarthrosis, as well as the acute slip. However, if the slipping occurs gradually over a period of many weeks, the presentation can be much more difficult to recognise. The pain, which may be mild and intermittent, is often felt mainly or only in the knee. The adolescent can walk, but there may be an intermittent limp. There is usually a good range of hip motion except internal rotation, which is lost or restricted early in the slipping process, and eventually there will be a characteristic sign whereby the hip rolls into external rotation when it is flexed. Early chronic slips are often difficult to recognise on X-ray and the lateral view is the most sensitive projection. Delay in the diagnosis of chronic slips is frequent because of a failure to consider that knee pain may be referred from the hip, or because a lateral hip X-ray is not done. Delay in diagnosis may result in continued slipping and a much worse prognosis. Such delays frequently lead to litigation.

Both types of slip require immediate operation. Chronic slips are pinned *in situ* to prevent progression, and have a good outcome if the degree of slip is not severe. The management of acute slips is more controversial and the outcome is uncertain. Reduction by traction followed by pinning may be the safest option but there is a significant risk of avascular necrosis and later degenerative arthritis.

ANTERIOR KNEE PAIN

Knee pain is very common in adolescents and there are many causes. Most knee disorders are self-limiting and are managed by advice and reassurance. However, knee pain may be the presenting symptom of a limb- and life-threatening condition, such as an osteosarcoma. Not every patient with knee pain should have a bone scan or MRI. The history and examination are the primary tools to distinguish the serious from the trivial.

Anterior knee pain is a common clinical syndrome in adolescents, especially girls, with up to 20 per cent affected. Pain is usually intermittent, is located around or behind the patella, and is made worse by exercise and relieved by rest and simple analgesics. It is often bilateral, but one side may be more symptomatic than the other.

Examination is usually unremarkable, apart from patellar tenderness and crepitus. X-rays are normal but are done to exclude more serious pathology. Arthroscopic examination of the knee may reveal changes in the retropatellar cartilage, which are sometimes called chondromalacia. However, the relationship of these changes to pain is not clear. Some of the most painful knees are normal on arthroscopic examination, and the changes of chondromalacia may be present without pain. Anterior knee pain can be considered to be an overuse syndrome affecting the immature retropatellar cartilage, which is ultimately benign and self-limiting. It does not lead to arthritis or any other sequelae in later life.

Management is conservative: explanation, education and simple measures should be used to control symptoms, including analgesics, restricting activities that provoke symptoms, hamstring stretching and quadriceps strengthening. Neither arthroscopic examination nor surgery should be advised routinely.

The differential diagnosis includes osteochondritis dissecans of the tibial tuberosity (Osgood–Schlatter's disease), bipartite patella, meniscal tears, plica syndrome, patellar instability and referred pain from the hip.

BONE TUMOURS

The principal symptoms of a bone tumour are pain and the presence of a mass or lump. Slow-growing bone tumours often present as a mass, with pain as a less prominent feature. The most common bone tumour is the benign osteocartilaginous exostosis, usually abbreviated to 'exostosis' (Fig. 45.3). Exostoses are benign bone tumours that are usually solitary and are found near the ends of long bones because they originate from aberrant cartilage cells from the growth plate. Some children have multiple exostoses and this may be inherited as an autosomal dominant condition: 'hereditary multiple exostoses'. The bony lumps are noticed incidentally or after minor trauma. They grow slowly until skeletal maturity or a little later. Clinically and radiologically they are benign in behaviour, although incomplete excision may lead to local recurrence. Excision is

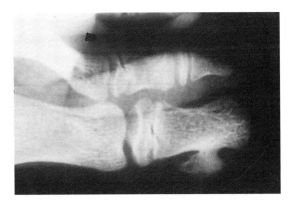

Fig. 45.3 Exostosis of the distal phalanx of the great toe.

advised if the lumps are symptomatic or the diagnosis is in doubt.

A solitary bone cyst usually presents as a patholgical fracture of the proximal humerus or femur (Fig. 45.4). Often the fracture stimulates healing of this benign lesion.

Painful benign bone tumours include osteoid osteoma and osteoblastoma. These are small tumours that present with night pain, characteristically relieved by aspirin. Diagnosis may be delayed because the tumours are small and are not always easily demonstrated on X-ray. Excision is usually performed by CT guidance using a trocar passed percutaneously into the nidus.

Malignant bone tumours usually present with well-localised pain, which is progressive, disturbs sleep and is not easily or fully relieved by rest or analgesics. The rapidly growing ends of long bones are most likely to be affected, including around the knee (the distal femur and proximal tibia) and the proximal femur and the proximal humerus. The two most common primary malignancies of bone, osteosarcoma and Ewing's sarcoma (Fig. 45.5), are most common in childhood and adolescence.

Diagnosis and staging is achieved by imaging studies that may include plain X-rays, bone scans, CT and MRI followed by biopsy — in all cases. Although there are features that suggest malignancy on X-ray (for example, bone destruction by the lesion, a large soft tissue mass and a

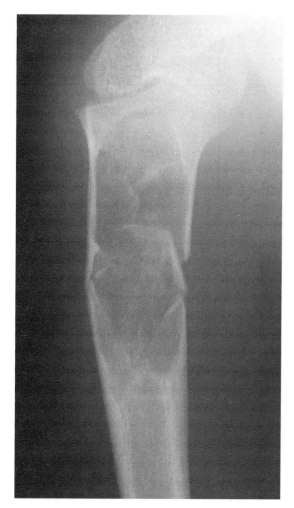

Fig. 45.4 Solitary bone cyst of the humerus. Note the fractures of the thinned cortex.

marked periosteal reaction) these features can be mimicked by benign bone tumours, bone dysplasias and infection.

The prognosis for saving both life and limb in adolescents with primary bone tumours has improved dramatically with limb salvage surgery and chemotherapy. The tumour must be completely excised with a margin of healthy tissue, and the limb reconstructed, whenever possible, using a variety of techniques including bone grafts (autografts and allografts) and endoprosthetic

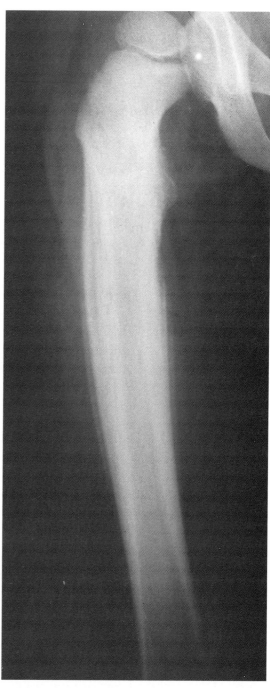

Fig. 45.5 Ewing's sarcoma involving the proximal half of the diaphysis of the femur, with layers of new bone and fusiform swelling of the soft tissue.

replacement. Chemotherapy is usually commenced after the diagnosis has been established by biopsy but before the tumour excision surgery.

FURTHER READING

Baxter A. & Dulberg C. (1988) Growing pains in children *J. Pediatr. Orthop.* **8**: 402–6.

Benson M.K.D., Fixsen J.A. & Macnicol M.F. (ed.) (1994) *Children's Orthopaedics and Fractures*, Churchill Livingstone, Edinburgh.

Fraser R.K., Menelaus M.B., Williams P.F. & Cole W.G. (1995) The Miller procedure for flexible flat feet. *J. Bone Joint Surg.* **77(B)**: 396–9.

Glasgow J.F.T. & Graham H.K. (1997) *Management of Injuries in Children*, BMJ Publishing group, London.

Hensinger R. N. (1986) *Standards in Pediatric Orthopedics*, Raven Press, New York.

Kling T.F. & Hensinger R.N. (1983) Angular and torsional deformities of the limbs in children. *Clin. Orthop. Rel. Research,* **186**: 136–42.

McCoy F.G., Graham H.K. & Piggot J. (1987) Non-union of fractures of the carpal schapoid in a child. *Ulster Medical Journal*, **56(1)**: 66.

Rang M. (1983) *Children's Fractures,* 2nd edn, J.B. Lippincott Co., Philadelphia.

Steele J.A. & Graham H.K. (1992) Angulated radial neck fractures in children, a prospective study of percutaneous reduction. *J. Bone Joint Surg.* **74(B)**: 760–4.

Svenningsen S., Terjesen T., Apalset K. & Anda S. (1990) Osteotomy for femoral anteversion. *Acta Orthop. Scand.* **61**: 360–3.

Wenger D.R. & Rang M. (1993) *The Art and Practice of Children's Orthopaedics*, Raven Press, New York.

Williams P.F. & Cole W.G. (eds) (1991) *Orthopaedic Management in Childhood,* 2nd edn, Chapman & Hall, London.

— 46 —

The Hand

CASE 1

A 3-year-old has a fixed flexion deformity of the thumb. X-rays are normal.

Q. 1.1   *What is the diagnosis?*

Q. 1.2   *Is splinting indicated?*

Q. 1.3   *Is surgery required?*

CASE 2

An 8-month-old child of a diabetic mother has a weak right arm. Hand movement has recovered since birth; however, elbow flexion and shoulder control have not yet appeared.

Q. 2.1   *What is the diagnosis, cause (aetiology, pathology and anatomy) and treatment?*

The results of reconstructive surgery of the hand in a child are much better than for similar conditions in adults. Injuries should be repaired immediately. The correction of malformations is often completed in the first year of life, or at least prior to starting school. The stiffness that adults experience after upper-limb surgery is seldom a problem. The hand needs to be protected, immobilised and maintained in an elevated position until sufficient healing has taken place to allow the child to play and use the hand without restriction. A plaster slab or cast must be applied in such a way that the child cannot easily remove it. It must be comfortable and immobilise the hand, wrist and often the elbow in a safe position. In most cases the tips of the digits should be able to be inspected to ensure that vascular compromise does not occur. Elevating the arm in a well-designed sling under the clothing is the best way of ensuring that the limb is protected. In a child, a plaster should be maintained for 2 weeks after simple suturing, 3 weeks after skin-

grafting (for example, syndactyly release) and almost 4 weeks following tendon surgery. Ongoing protective splinting may then be required.

CONGENITAL ANOMALIES

These are common and varied. A classification based on embryological aberrations is useful in describing and recording malformations (Box 46.1). Unfortunately, many unrelated conditions, such as trigger thumb, syndactyly and clinodactyly, are classified as a failure of differentiation. Anomalies may be localised to the hand or be a local manifestation of a generalised condition, such as arthrogryposis multiplex congenita. Some deformities, for example, certain forms of syndactyly, are strongly familial; others are sporadic, with no known cause.

Other associated congenital conditions are common and should be looked for. Many are potentially lethal, such as radial club hand

Box 46.1 Classification of malformations of the hand

(1) Failure of formation (transverse congenital amputations, phocomelia, radial club hand and cleft hand).

(2) Failure of differentiation (syndactyly, clinodactyly, camptylodactyly, clasp thumb).

(3) Duplication (polydactyly and triphalangeal thumb).

(4) Overgrowth (giantism and macrodactyly).

(5) Undergrowth (hypoplasia, brachydactyly and symbrachydactyly).

(6) Constriction ring syndrome (intra-uterine amputations, congenital constriction bands and acrosyndactyly).

(7) Congenital skeletal abnormalities (achondroplasia).

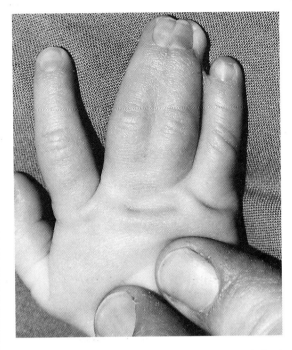

Fig. 46.1 Syndactyly, complete and complex (fused distal phalanges) between ring and middle fingers, with simple and almost complete syndactyly between the ring and little fingers.

being linked to cardiac and haemopoietic abnormalities.

Management

Children with a hand anomaly (congenital 'difference') may have functional and/or cosmetic impairment. They will, however, learn to use it with dexterity, provided certain basic anatomical elements are present. The psychological effects on the parents need to be managed.

Syndactyly

This affects 1 : 2000 births and may be incomplete or complete (to the finger-tip) and simple or complex (fused bones). It may be part of a syndrome, such as Poland or Apert's syndrome. Family history is positive in up to 40 per cent of cases; inheritance is dominant but there is reduced expression and penetrance. Early surgery (in the first 6 months) is indicated in acrosyndactyly and when border

digits, particularly the thumb, are involved, leading to growth disturbance in digits of unequal length (Fig. 46.1).

Clasp thumb

This may be due to a congenital trigger thumb caused by a swelling within the flexor pollicis longus tendon impinging on the fibrous flexor sheath. Alternatively, it may represent a weakness in the extensor muscles that can be improved by splinting initiated in the first month of life. Rarely a deficiency of skin on the palmer surface requires correction.

Trigger thumb

'Trigger thumb' is a common, and often bilateral abnormality. It is sometimes identified at birth but is usually found in children up to 5 years of age.

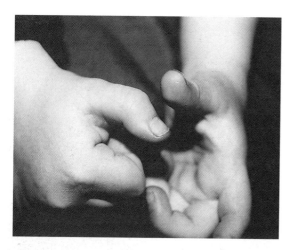

Fig. 46.2 Right trigger thumb presenting as a fixed flexion deformity.

The primary lesion is a fusiform thickening or nodule in the flexor tendon of the thumb; this is associated with a narrowing of the tendon sheath at the metacarpophalangeal joint (Fig. 46.2). Once the affected digit is flexed, extension is restricted by an impingement of the nodule proximal to the narrowing. Often children present with fixed flexion deformities of the interphalangeal joint. Clinically, the nodule in the tendon can be palpated at the level of the metacarpal head in the palm. A similar nodule can sometimes be palpated in the identical position in the opposite hand, and may give rise to symptoms. Treatment involves longitudinal incision of the tendon sheath to allow full excursion of the tendon through the area of narrowing.

Distal arthrogryposis

This condition, which may be inherited, is associated with skin deficiency, under-developed flexure creases and weakness associated with under-development of the musculature. The thumbs may be clasped and the digits ulnar deviated. An intense program of splintage, initiated in the neonatal period, produces quite dramatic improvements.

Camptylodactyly

This affects 1 in 100 hands, and causes a flexion contracture, particularly of the proximal interphalangial joint of the little finger, and is due to an imbalance of anomalous muscles.

Clinodactyly

This affects 1 in 100 hands with radial deviation, particularly of the little finger due to a delta-shaped middle phalanx associated with an anomalous C-shaped cartilage growth plate.

Polydactyly

Radial (preaxial) polydactyly involving the thumb occurs in 1 in 1000 births, particularly in Asia. This condition is sporadic and unilateral, except when 1 of the duplicated thumbs is triphalangeal. In this case the condition is often bilateral and is inherited as an autosomal dominant condition. Ulnar (post-axial) polydactyly occurs in 1 in 300 in black people, and in 1 in 3000 in white people. This condition is often bilateral, inherited in an autosomal recessive pattern and may be part of a syndrome.

Symbrachydactyly

This is a sporadic unilateral condition with hypoplasia of the digits that are short and stiff (aplasia of bones and joints). In many cases the digits are represented by soft tissue nubbins. Microsurgical transfer of toes can significantly improve function in some patients. Others may benefit from the free grafting of toe proximal phalanges into redundant soft tissues in the first 2 years of life.

Obstetric brachial plexus palsy

This is due to a traction injury associated with a difficult delivery (for example, Erb's palsy). These improve in 90 per cent of cases. If there is no recovery after 3 months, particularly if all nerve roots are involved, then exploration and reconstruction with nerve grafts should be contemplated within the first year of life. The results of reconstruction are far better than those achieved in adults.

INJURIES TO THE HAND

The repair of injuries to the hand differs little from that in adults, except that the results are generally better. Absorbable skin sutures should be used. Restoration of function is more rapid and more complete. Prolonged hand therapy is rarely necessary and re-education takes days or weeks, instead of months or years.

Failure to diagnose the extent of the injury when the child is first seen leads to unsatisfactory results and the need for later reconstruction. Subjective tests for nerve injuries are of little value and co-operation during a detailed examination is unlikely. Injuries to tendons and nerves may be overlooked until the loss of function is noted by parents, weeks or months later. Awareness of the likelihood of these injuries associated with lacerations of the hand is essential. Abnormal posture of the fingers with the hand at rest suggests possible tendon injury. Soft tissue damage rarely is severe. Most injuries are cuts or crushing injuries. Any wound in a child that cannot be adequately examined, particularly if it overlies an important structure, must be explored under general anaesthesia. Any damage to tendons and nerves can be repaired primarily under ideal conditions. No matter how minor the injury, a full plaster and sling should be used to promote uncomplicated healing.

Injuries to finger-tips

Crushing and slicing injuries with a loss of part of the finger-tip are common in childhood (Fig. 46.3). In most crush injuries the tissue remaining after judicious debridement and thorough lavage is viable. Any associated fracture of the distal phalanx

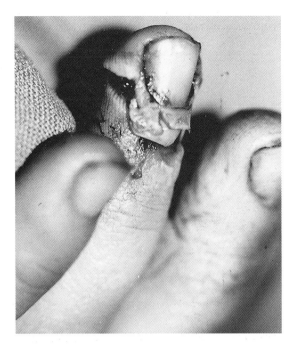

Fig. 46.3 Finger crushed in a door.

should be reduced and in some cases pinned with a fine Kirschner wire. If possible, a portion of the tip of the finger should be left exposed so that the circulation can be observed in the early postoperative period.

In slicing injuries with skin-loss, some form of primary closure with a skin-graft or local flap may be indicated. In younger children the cross-sectional area of the finger-tip is small, healing is rapid and the results of healing by second intention can be excellent. Amputations at the level of the mid-distal phalanx can often be microsurgically replanted, by anastomosis of preferably two blood vessels. More distal amputations or unreplantable crushed or avulsed parts may be, after de-fatting, replaced as a graft with moderate success.

FURTHER READING

Flatt A.E. (1994) *The care of congenital hand anomalies*, Quality Medical Publishing, St. Louis.

Johnstone B.R. & Duncan J. (1998) Hand injuries in children. In: Conolly W.B. (ed.) *Atlas of Hand Surgery,* Churchill Livingstone, New York, chapter 21, pp. 135–46.

Smith P.J. & Grobbelaar A.O. (1997) Congenital hand anomalies. In: *Grabb and Smith's Plastic Surgery,* 5th edn, Lippincott-Raven, Philadelphia, chapter 80, pp. 959–73.

Tonkin M.A. (1997) Congenital deformities. In: Conolly W.B. (ed.) *Atlas of Hand Surgery,* Churchill Livingstone, New York, chapter 33, pp. 267–77.

— 47 —

The Breast

CASE 1

An 8-year-old girl presents with a slightly tender lump behind the left areola, which has been present for 2 months. There is no growth spurt or menarche.

    Q. 1.1   *What is the problem and its natural history?*

    Q. 1.2   *When is further investigation or surgery indicated?*

CASE 2

A 2-week-old has bilateral enlargement of the breast buds with milk production. The right breast is painful, red and tender.

    Q. 2.1   *What is the diagnosis and treatment?*

    Q. 2.2   *What is the gender of the baby?*

In the paediatric age group there are no serious conditions involving the breast in either sex, but there are a number of minor conditions that may give rise to anxiety or inconvenience.

ABSENT BREASTS AND MULTIPLE NIPPLES

Absence of the breast is a rare, and usually unilateral, anomaly that is frequently part of a regional dysplasia that also affects the pectoral muscles and subjacent ribs (Poland syndrome) (Chapter 50).

Multiple nipples, which are also rare, can occur anywhere along a curved line in front of the anterior fold of the axilla. It is even rarer to have a supernumerary breast, which is usually in the axilla. These can be removed simply by surgery.

NEONATAL ENLARGEMENT

Transplacental passage of lactogenic hormones may lead to hyperplasia and the secretion of breast milk in newborn babies of either sex. The enlargement usually lasts a week if left alone, but attempts to empty the breast by massage will prolong and increase milk production. Unusually overactive secretion can be stopped within 24 hours by oral oestrogens, but this is rarely necessary. The engorgement predisposes to infection, which is not particularly common, but serious.

If an abscess forms it should be drained by a small incision placed peripherally in girls to minimise disruption of the canaliculi beneath the nipple. Since the entire breast is no larger than the areola, extreme care is required to avoid unintentional mastectomy or physical damage to the breast bud.

PRECOCIOUS PUBERTY

This is very uncommon, but may occur in girls as early as 12 to 18 months of age. Menstruation and bilateral hyperplasia of the breasts should always raise the possibility of an underlying cause; for example, an ovarian (or adrenal) tumour or an intracranial lesion, but in the constitutional type, no cause is found and the possibility of dwarfism from excess production of oestrogens should be investigated.

PREMATURE HYPERPLASIA

This is probably the commonest minor physiological aberration, and when unilateral it presents a diagnostic problem. The usual finding is the development of one breast in girls, sometimes as young as 5 years, though more commonly in those 7 to 9 years of age.

The presenting feature is a firm discoid lump 1 to 2 cm in diameter, situated symmetrically and concentrically beneath the nipple. It is initially symptomless and found accidentally, although it may become tender, possibly due to repeated palpation and to anxiety. There are no other signs of puberty that develop at the normal time. The danger is that a biopsy will be performed, for it is tantamount to a total mastectomy.

The clinical signs are so diagnostic that no confirmation by other means is required. This is not precocious puberty, for the menarche occurs at the normal age. The affected breast may return to normal, but the swelling commonly remains static and the same changes usually appear in the opposite breast within 3 to 12 months: both then remain static without further increase in size until puberty. Reassurance and explanation are all that are required. Biopsy is an avoidable disaster.

PUBERTAL 'MASTITIS'

This occurs in boys as well as girls. In girls there is some tenderness, discomfort and a granular texture on palpation; and serous fluid can be expressed from the nipple — one breast is often affected more than the other. It is a temporary phase and no treatment is required.

In boys the discoid, subareolar lesion as described in premature hyperplasia occurs in one or both breasts at about 12 to 14 years. No treatment is necessary.

GYNAECOMASTIA

This occurs in several conditions, perhaps most commonly in a spurious form in obese pre-adolescents, when it is formed of fat alone.

In thin boys the possibility of ambiguous sexual development requires elucidation by a close examination of the genitalia, chromosomal studies, the estimation of ketosteroids in the urine, urethroscopy, biopsy of the gonads, or even laparoscopy (Chapter 10).

It may arise as a side effect of oestrogen therapy for some other condition.

In most cases no cause can be found, and if the enlargement is of sufficient magnitude to cause embarrassment, simple mastectomy is justified. The standard curved submammary incisions should not be used, for the scar may simulate the contour of a breast even after it has been removed. A half-circle peri-areolar incision is preferable if the breast is not too large.

FURTHER READING

Seashore J.H. (1998) Disorders of the breast. In: O'Neill J.A., Rowe M.I., Grosfeld J.L., Fonkalsrud E.W. & Coran A.G. (eds) *Pediatric Surgery*, 5th edn, Mosby, St. Louis, pp. 779–86.

— 48 —

Chest Wall Deformities

CASE

Bruce, a 7-year-old, presents with his mother because of increasing concern about the appearance of his deformed chest, which is preventing him from playing sport. He is embarrassed about the defect and wants it repaired.

> *Q. 1.1*   *Is the deformity significantly limiting his cardiorespiratory performance?*
>
> *Q. 1.2*   *What investigations are required?*
>
> *Q. 1.3*   *What advice would you give his mother?*

Deformities of the chest wall are almost all congenital and are classified as follows:
(1) primary depression deformities of the sternum (funnel chest: pectus excavatum)
(2) primary protrusion deformities of the sternum (pigeon chest: pectus carinatum)
(3) deficiency deformities of the chest wall
(4) failure of midline sternal fusion.

AETIOLOGY

The deformity is a primary condition, except in a few of the protrusion deformities, where it may be secondary to chronic asthma, congenital heart disease, a massive lung cyst, diaphragmatic hernia or hydatid cysts of the liver. Extremely rarely, depression deformities may be seen in Marfan's syndrome, homocystinuria and congenital laryngeal stridor with inspiratory retraction.

A hereditary factor can generally be established, but it is recessive and consequently may slip one or more generations.

Abnormal action of the diaphragm may influence the nature of the anomaly whether there is protrusion or depression. It is important to realize that the type of deformity is not always the same in successive generations, or even among siblings.

DEPRESSION DEFORMITY (FUNNEL CHEST)

Clinical features

Pectus excavatum (funnel chest) is four times as common as pectus carinatum (pigeon chest). It is appreciably more frequent in males, and may be symmetrical or asymmetrical. These children are usually thin, muscular and ligamentous laxity is marked, and posture tends to be poor. The sternal depression is always maximal at the sterno-xiphisternal junction, but may extend up the sternum to any level.

When most of the sternum is affected, the depression is shallow and the deformity may be described as the 'saucer' type. A localized depression is compatible with a well-developed upper chest and the very localized 'funnel' may be referred to as the 'cup' type.

In asymmetrical lesions the sternum is rotated,

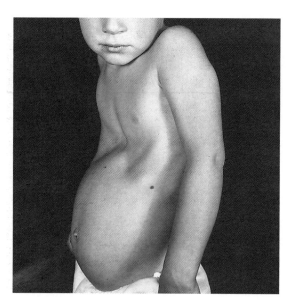

Fig. 48.1 Depression deformity. An extensive deep depression centred on the sterno-xiphisternal junction. Note the lateral sulcus, in profile, on the right side.

usually from right to left around its longitudinal axis, producing prominence of the costal cartilages on one side and recession of those on the other.

A shallow sulcus may extend laterally on each side from the sterno-xiphisternal junction, a sulcus that corresponds to the attachment of the diaphragm to the lower costal cartilages; that is, Harrison's sulcus. The costal margin on each side may become generally everted or protrude as a boss. Postural kyphosis is common and scoliosis not infrequent.

The deformity may be of any degree of severity, from being barely detectable to one in which the lower sternum almost touches the front of the vertebral column (Fig. 48.1).

A funnel chest may be present at birth, or become apparent at any age up to 16 years. There is a group of males in which it develops rapidly at about 15 years of age, when rapid growth in height is occurring.

When the deformity is severe at birth there is paradoxical retraction of the sternum on inspiration. This ceases at about the age of 4 years and is replaced by orthodox respiratory movement of subnormal amplitude. In the great majority of cases there is a tendency for the deformity to progress until growth ceases, but in others it becomes less severe.

Symptoms

These are largely related to psychological effects and to cardiac function (in severe defects).

Psychological features may become apparent from an early age. The child resents being 'different' and when undressed for examination he brings the arms together to try to conceal the shape of the chest. Older children may refuse to go swimming for fear of becoming an object of attention. Comments from schoolmates may be frequent and unkind. The psychological effects can completely alter the child's personality and his reaction to his environment.

Diminished exercise tolerance is uncommon, and confined to those with severe deformity. Pain may be mentioned but it has no organic basis. The deformity is not responsible for any supposedly increased tendency to respiratory infections.

The progression and severity of the condition, and its significance to the patient and his parents, can best be assessed by several examinations at yearly intervals, with photographs recording the deformity at each visit.

An X-ray of the chest may be undertaken to demonstrate the position of the heart and to establish the distance of the sternum from the vertebral column.

Treatment

The deformity cannot be improved by any form of exercises or retaining apparatus. Encouragement of participation in physical activity helps some children to become less self-conscious about lesser degrees of depression deformity. In selecting patients for surgical correction of the deformity it is important that the patient wants to have the correction. Only in very severe cases is surgery indicated in the first decade of life.

At operation, which is usually performed at puberty, the chest cage is exposed through a transverse incision, with elevation of muscle flaps. The sternum is mobilized and the costal cartilages divided to correct the deformity. The corrected position of the sternum is maintained by struts (usually of steel) placed transversely behind the sternum.

PROTRUSION DEFORMITIES (PIGEON CHEST)

A high protrusion

This may be associated with a deficiency deformity and is never an acquired lesion. The sternum is angulated forwards at the level of the third sternochondral junction, and below this point it recedes as a depression. There may be 'pinching-in' of the lower costal cartilages.

The radiological findings are unique, for there is osseous fusion of all the synchondroses of the sternum, which probably occurs before the age of 1 year.

The symptoms produced are purely the result of cosmetic defect. The deformity tends to increase with age, and never regresses spontaneously.

Surgical treatment is for cosmetic reasons and achieves excellent results. In less severe cases in girls the decision to operate may be deferred until after puberty, for breast development may help to mask the deformity.

Low protrusion

These may be secondary, particularly to chronic asthma. In a few of those in whom it is a primary condition there is a tendency towards spontaneous improvement, which is usually apparent by the age of 8 years; otherwise, there is a general tendency for the deformity to increase until growth ceases.

The maximal protrusion is at the sterno-xiphisternal junction or a little higher, and there is usually some pinching-in of the lower costal

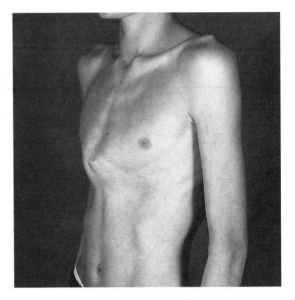

Fig. 48.2 Low protrusion deformity maximal just above the sterno-xiphisternal junction.

cartilages (Fig. 48.2). Prominence of the costal cartilages on each side near their junction with the sternum may be present, forming a median trough which, though locally depressed, is still part of the sternal protrusion. Rotation of the sternum producing an asymmetrical deformity is not uncommon.

Radiography is necessary to confirm the degree of protrusion and to exclude the presence of any intrathoracic condition that might be contributory. The symptoms are related entirely to the cosmetic defect.

Treatment

Secondary deformities usually resolve spontaneously after elimination of the underlying cause.

Primary lesions may also show a tendency to spontaneous improvement. In the first decade of life, repeated observation will indicate the trend. Many patients present for the first time after puberty.

Operation is indicated in the patient with severe and/or progressive cosmetic deformity.

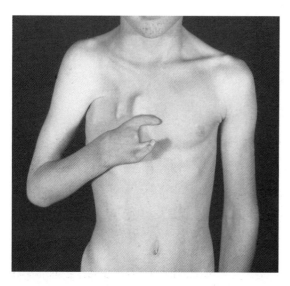

Fig. 48.3 Deficiency deformity. Poland syndrome; absent nipple, areola and pectoral muscles with hypoplasia of the chest wall and syndactyly.

DEFICIENCY DEFORMITIES

In the usual type the pectoral muscles are absent on one side and there is a variable degree of hypoplasia of the underlying ribs and costal cartilages.

The third and fourth cartilages may be deficient anteriorly, with some paradoxical respiratory movement visible through the chest wall. (This is rarely of any clinical significance.) All elements of the breast may be absent, but usually the nipple and areola are present. Hypoplasia of the upper limb on the affected side and syndactyly may occur (Poland syndrome; Fig. 48.3). The sternum in these patients may show a high protrusion deformity of cosmetic significance. The dominant problem, however, is the soft tissue deficiency.

Treatment

Surgery is only rarely indicated for filling in the bony chest wall deficiency or for the correction of sternal protrusion. Muscular flaps, utilizing the *latissimus dorsi*, can be used to provide soft tissue bulk, to be followed in girls by augmentation mammoplasty. It is more difficult to replace absent tissues than it is to reorganize disordered tissues; despite this, much can be done to improve the appearance in these children.

FURTHER READING

Bax N.M.A., Ottenschot T., Gil D. & Vismeer H. (1990) Does early subperichondral removal of several costal cartilages interfere with chest wall growth? An experimental study in kittens. *Pediatr. Surg. Int.* **5**: 165–9.

Chetcuti P., Dickens D.R.V. & Phelan P.D. (1989) Spinal deformity in patients with oesophageal atresia. *Arch. Dis. Child.* **64**: 1427–30.

Kandel J. & Haller J.A. (1998) Chest wall and breast. In: Oldham K.T., Colombani P.M. & Foglia R.P. (eds) *Surgery of Infants and Children: scientific principles and practice*, Lippincott-Raven, Philadelphia, pp. 871–82.

Martinez D., Juamne J., Stein T. & Pena A. (1990) The effect of costal cartilage resection on chest wall development. *Pediatr. Surg. Int.* **5**: 156–64.

von der Oelsnitz G. (1990) Operative correction of pectus excavatum. Experience at the Children's Hospital of Bremen. *Pediatr. Surg. Int.* **5**: 150–5.

— 49 —

Lungs, Pleura and Mediastinum

CASE 1

Jemma, a 3-year-old, became unwell with a viral upper respiratory infection. Forty-eight hours later she became very sick with high fever, lethargy, cough and shortness of breath, eventually becoming cyanotic.

Q. 1.1   *What could be the problem?*

Q. 1.2   *How is it best treated?*

CASE 2

Adrian is 16 and tall for his age. He developed sudden severe chest pain and shortness of breath, not relieved at all by his usual asthma medication.

Q. 2.1   *What is the diagnosis and its management?*

While the principles of diagnosis and treatment of pulmonary disease in children are similar to those of adults, there are additional aspects that need to be considered:

(1) The respiratory passages are small and encroachment on the lumen by exudate or oedema may cause obstruction of the airways.

(2) The cough reflex is relatively ineffectual in infancy and retention of secretions may have serious consequences.

(3) Obstruction may cause superimposed infection and patchy or lobar collapse.

(4) Hypoxia develops rapidly in neonates and increased respiratory effort increases the consumption of oxygen; the vicious circle may culminate in respiratory failure.

(5) Disturbances of intrathoracic pressure relationships are tolerated poorly and a tension pneumothorax may cause irreversible cardio-respiratory failure, particularly if there is pre-existing lung disease.

With few exceptions, for example, hydatid disease, operations on the lungs and pleura in childhood are of two kinds: the resection of pulmonary tissue and the provision of pleural drainage.

Resection, usually lobectomy, is required for a variety of developmental anomalies, including lobar emphysema, hamartoma, sequestrated lobe, and for carefully selected cases of bronchiectasis. Metastases from osteosarcoma or Wilms' tumour may also warrant resection.

Inhaled foreign bodies sometimes produce few symptoms. The final diagnosis of an intrabronchial foreign body occasionally is made after resection of a diseased segment of lung.

Pleural drainage may be necessary in three conditions:

(1) pneumothorax, for example, neonatal pneumothorax (Chapter 4); traumatic pneumothorax (Chapter 38)

(2) empyema (see below)

(3) haemothorax, an unusual condition because of the rarity of major thoracic injuries in childhood.

Aspiration of the pleural cavity may be used diagnostically to obtain pleural fluid for microscopy and culture, or as a preliminary step in providing immediate continuous drainage of an empyema by means of an intercostal catheter.

STAPHYLOCOCCAL PNEUMONIA

This occurs usually as a complication of a viral infection of the upper respiratory tract (Fig. 49.1).

Diagnosis

Although X-rays enable the diagnosis to have a high degree of certainty, identification of the organism responsible is the absolute criterion. When *Staphylococcus aureus* is isolated from a throat swab or sputum, and typical changes are present in lung radiographs, the diagnosis is at least presumptive. The development of a pleural

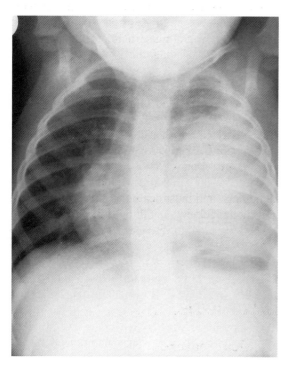

Fig. 49.1 Staphylococcal pneumonia involving the left hemithorax.

complication and culture of staphylococcus from a specimen of pus from the pleural cavity confirm the diagnosis.

The diagnosis may be delayed at presentation because the clinical signs suggest upper respiratory tract infection, and the pathological changes initially are confined to this area. When the condition progresses to pneumonia, this may not be recognized immediately. The baby or young child may become worse rapidly for the following reasons:

(1) Septicaemia and a shock-like state of collapse.
(2) An air leak under tension at one or more of three sites: (i) intrapleural-pneumothorax; (ii) intrapulmonary-pneumatocele; (iii) in the mediastinum-pneumomediastinum.
(3) A collection of pus: (i) intrapleural-empyema, or pyopneumothorax, when both pus and air are present; (ii) intrapulmonary-single or multiple lung abscess.
(4) Obstruction of the airways.

Treatment

Intravenous antibiotics are given, and until the results of culture and sensitivity tests are known, an effective combination is flucloxacillin and gentamicin. Serial X-rays are obtained because of the rapid evolution of the pathological changes on radiology.

Complications and sequelae

Suppurative pericarditis, meningitis, septicaemia and osteomyelitis may complicate staphylococcal pneumonia, but are uncommon when appropriate antibiotics are given early and in adequate dosage.

EMPYEMA

Spread of infection from the lower respiratory tract may cause a fibrinous or serofibrinous pleurisy, a pyopneumothorax or an empyema.

An empyema may be unilateral or bilateral, generalised or loculated, and the rate of resolution is variable. These factors determine the clinical course and the type of treatment required.

Staphylococcus aureus is the predominant organism and 80 per cent are resistant to penicillin. Other Gram-positive cocci, for example, pneumococci and streptococci, and Gram-negative bacilli, for example, *Escherichia coli*, are encountered less commonly. In 75 per cent of patients an acute viral respiratory infection is the precipitating factor. The exanthems (particularly measles), focal staphylococcal infections or an underlying pulmonary disease are responsible in the other 25 per cent of cases.

Those with underlying disease form a heterogeneous group that includes developmental anomalies, prematurity, birth injury, degenerative diseases of the CNS, anaemia, skin diseases and malabsorption syndromes.

Clinical features

The onset of staphylococcal pneumonia is marked by acute toxaemia associated with cough, dyspnoea and grunting respirations, but initially without localising signs in the chest. As toxic signs become less severe, the clinical features of an empyema can be recognised: diminution in the movement of the chest, dullness to percussion and diminished air entry. In others the illness remains static or progresses more slowly. In either type the clinical picture may become suddenly worse with the occurrence of an 'air leak' caused by a bronchopleural fistula and leading to a pneumothorax or pyopneumothorax. These may occur in any type of infection, but they are particularly typical of staphylococcal pneumonia (Fig. 49.1).

In staphylococcal empyema, cyanosis is a variable feature, and peripheral circulatory failure may develop. The interpretation of the clinical signs is difficult without concomitant X-rays because similar clinical signs can be caused by a pneumothorax with tension, which demands urgent relief.

The symptoms and signs of an empyema, other than staphylococcal, vary widely according to the underlying disease, the duration of illness and the age of the patient. As in other infections the picture in the neonatal period is frequently quite different, and there may be little fever or toxaemia, even when there is extensive intrathoracic suppuration.

Investigation

Bacteriological investigation will determine the organisms present in the nasopharynx, in focal areas of sepsis and in the empyema.

The radiographic findings are a composite of those in the underlying lung and in the pleura. The course of the disease and the response to treatment are closely followed by serial X-rays.

Treatment

Treatment is directed to the underlying condition and drainage of the empyema. Intermittent paracentesis has as limited place, and in most cases continuous drainage is required. Open thoracotomy and drainage is the method of choice when paracentesis has failed, the pus is thick or there is evidence of loculation.

Drainage is needed in most cases and surgical consultation is desirable. The paediatric surgeon should observe the early stages of a disease, to give advice on whether and when thoracotomy is appropriate. Chronic empyemas are rare in childhood and decortication is practically never required.

In previously healthy children the mortality is minimal and most deaths occur early when the infection is fulminant and the child is septicaemic. The highest mortality is in the newborn, in bilateral empyemas and in those with serious pre-existing pulmonary disease.

PNEUMOTHORAX

Clinical features

The clinical picture is determined by the age of the patient, the size of the pneumothorax, the

Box 49.1 Causes of pneumothorax

(1) Spontaneous; often in a teenager, from an apical bleb.

(2) Rupture of subpleural abscess in staphylococcal pneumonia.

(3) Neonatal pulmonary disease; for example, hyaline membrane disease.

(4) Rupture of subpleural emphysematous bulla; for example, asthma, cystic fibrosis.

(5) Traumatic; following chest wall injury (Chapter 38).

(6) Perforation of oesophagus by an ingested foreign body or during oesophagoscopy.

(7) Iatrogenic; for example, after paracentesis.

(8) Rupture of the hydatid cyst.

(9) Postoperative, after thoracotomy.

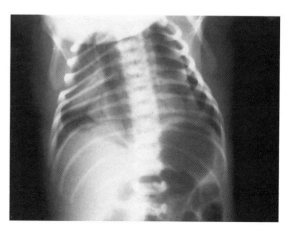

Fig. 49.2 Neonatal pneumothorax. The tension pneumothorax has caused displacement of the mediastinum to the right with a collapse of the right lung.

Box 49.2 Causes of pleural effusions

(1) Pulmonary infection: acute (staph. pneumonia), chronic (TB).

(2) Disturbed haemodynamics: cardiac failure, hypoproteinaemia.

(3) Malignancy: lung, pleura, mediastinum.

(4) Chylothorax: damaged obstructed thoracic duct.

presence or absence of tension and the nature of any underlying pulmonary disease (Box 49.1). Symptoms include pain in the chest, dyspnoea and those of the underlying disease.

Signs include displacement of the trachea and the apex beat, diminished movement of the chest wall, a hyper-resonant percussion note and diminished air entry.

X-rays are usually diagnostic (Fig. 49.2) but occasionally a huge cyst or unusual types of diaphragmatic hernia may look similar radiologically.

Treatment

Urgent relief of tension by needling or intercostal drainage with an intercostal chest tube is required. The underlying cause may require further investigation and treatment.

PLEURAL EFFUSION

The accumulation of fluids (pus, serofibrinous exudate, blood, chyle or transudate) in the pleural cavity occurs in a variety of conditions (Box 49.2).

The physical signs are usually unmistakable, but radiographs are necessary and may require careful interpretation to distinguish a pleural 'collection' from such conditions as hydatid cyst or neuroblastoma.

Paracentesis provides information on the nature of the fluid and material for cytological and bacteriologic examination, and indicates the necessity for further drainage.

Chylothorax may occur spontaneously, and after thoracic operations; some cases require aspiration or even thoracotomy. Replacing the fat content of the diet with medium-chain triglycerides that are absorbed via the portal vascular system may control, or even cure, the condition: long-chain fats enter the lacteals and travel via the thoracic duct.

BRONCHIECTASIS

Recurrent or chronic bronchitis is the most common precursor of bronchiectasis. This type of bronchiectasis tends to be widespread, although the disease is usually most marked in one area. Bronchiectasis may complicate an exanthem.

Infection associated with permanent collapse of one or more lobes of one lung may be the cause, but the bronchiectasis may remain 'dry'; that is, structural changes can be demonstrated by bronchography but symptoms and signs are minimal or absent if the affected area remains free of infection.

Other causes include pulmonary tuberculosis, hydatid disease, congenital weakness of the bronchial wall (bronchomalacia), cystic fibrosis and the inhalation of a foreign body. In healed tuberculosis the bronchiectasis is usually 'dry', while in bronchomalacia and cystic fibrosis, dilatation of the bronchi is usually wide-spread and associated with copious sputum.

Clinical features

Physical signs may be diffuse, localised or even absent, according to the aetiology and the extent of the disease. Clinical assessment of the nature and amount of sputum, any interference with normal life and school attendance, and the frequency of acute toxic episodes of pneumonitis, should precede any investigations.

Bronchoscopy and bronchography aim to confirm the diagnosis and determine the distribution

and severity. A CT scan of the chest confirms its location. Culture of the sputum is a useful guide to chemotherapy, particularly during exacerbations of infection.

Treatment

Conservative treatment, with physiotherapy, postural drainage and antibiotics, is usually effective. The co-operation of fully informed patients is all-important in the success of this program.

Lobectomy and/or segmental resection is required occasionally and in localised disease it is curative. As a general rule, resection should be deferred until late childhood in case progressive disease in the remaining lobes of the lungs develops. When the bronchiectasis is more widespread, resection of a particularly diseased area may considerably improve the patient's well-being and reduce the amount of sputum produced, although some coughing may persist.

CONGENITAL MALFORMATIONS

Congenital lobar emphysema and congenital cystic lung (Chapter 4) may present in older children, and there is no typical clinical pattern. Often recurrent respiratory infections lead to an X-ray examination of the chest and the diagnosis.

Bronchography may provide additional information and fluoroscopy may demonstrate 'trapped air' in the lobe concerned; that is, movement of the mediastinum towards the affected side during inspiration and away from it during expiration.

Treatment involves removal of the affected portion of the lung.

PULMONARY SEQUESTRATION

A sequestrated lobe is pulmonary tissue that does not communicate with the bronchial tree by an anatomically normal bronchus and receives its blood supply from an anomalous systemic artery, usually the aorta. It does not participate in the normal function of the lung and is prone to infection. Two types are recognised: extralobar and intralobar.

In extralobar sequestration there is complete anatomical and physiological separation from the normal lung and the sequestrated portion may be above or below the diaphragm. This is sometimes seen in association with congenital diaphragmatic hernia. The arterial supply is from the aorta (above or below the diaphragm) or one of its branches.

In intralobar sequestration the abnormal tissue is contiguous with the related lung that partially surrounds it. This type is almost always in the posterolateral portion of the right or left lower lobe. The blood supply comes from large direct branches of the aorta (75 per cent) or other thoracic or abdominal vessels (25 per cent), and the venous drainage is through the pulmonary veins.

The sequestrated lobe may consist of a large cyst, multiple cysts, branching bronchi without cysts, or all three of these.

Clinical features

The usual history is of repeated episodes of pulmonary infection with signs confined to one area. Although the infection commonly subsides, acute suppuration may supervene. Subsidence of the acute phase leaves in its wake chronic suppuration with poor health, a persistent cough and sometimes low grade pleural pain. Haemoptysis occasionally occurs.

Chest X-rays show an opacity in the posteromedial part of one of the lower lobes or cystic spaces with or without fluid levels in a lower lobe. In the acute phase the opacity increases in size and may produce mediastinal displacement.

Aortography or Doppler ultrasonography demonstrates the anomalous arterial supply, confirms the diagnosis and is useful in planning the surgical approach (Fig. 4.3).

Treatment

Resection is indicated because of the susceptibility

to infection, but preliminary evacuation and drainage of pus may be required. More often the acute infection subsides with antibiotics and the patient can be investigated, and operated on, in a quiescent phase.

THE CHILD WITH A MEDIASTINAL MASS

A child may present with a mediastinal mass in one of two ways:

(1) a symptomless mass demonstrated in a chest X-ray; or
(2) symptoms caused by compression of mediastinal structures.

A symptomless mass

The thymus is large in infancy, and determining whether its appearance on chest X-ray is normal requires experience. Some radiographic techniques cause apparent enlargement.

A symptomless mediastinal mass may develop in the course of a generalised disease; for example, from enlarged hilar lymph nodes in leukaemia or Hodgkin's disease, or as metastases from a known malignant disease. Paravertebral and para-aortic masses of neuroblastoma may involve the mediastinum, often as the primary site but also as metastases from a tumour elsewhere; for example, in the abdomen (Chapter 25).

Compression of mediastinal structures

In childhood this is nearly always the result of a malignant mass, of which lymphosarcoma is the commonest. Congestion of the veins of the head, neck and upper limbs from obstruction of the superior vena cava, wheezing respirations, an unproductive or reverberating brassy cough and increasing dyspnoea are all ominous signs.

Lymphosarcomas usually arise in the anterior mediastinum in the region of the thymus, and X-rays usually show a large mass that extends

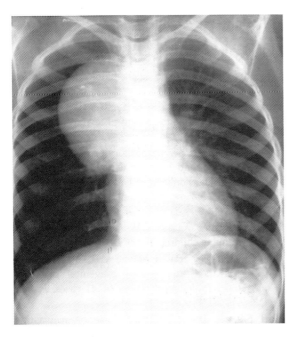

Fig. 49.3 A mediastinal mass: in this case a neuroblastoma with calcification in the posterior mediastinum.

laterally. The edges are irregular, rounded or ill-defined; the tumour may extend into the pleura and cause a pleural effusion. The histological diagnosis can be made from cytology of the cells in the pleural effusion.

A neural crest tumour (neuroblastoma or ganglioneuroma) is the usual cause of a paravertebral mass: areas of both neuroblastoma and ganglioneuroma may be present in a single tumour (Fig. 49.3). Erosion of the ribs and extension into a vertebral foramen causing spinal symptoms are seen with infiltrating mediastinal neuroblastomas.

A ganglioneuroma is a benign tumour arising in a paravertebral gutter. It often grows through a vertebral foramen into the spinal canal, resulting in two solid elements connected by a narrow isthmus in the intervertebral foramen, a 'dumb-bell' tumour.

Thymomas are much less common and are difficult to distinguish from lymphosarcomas. They tend to grow slowly, to reach an even larger size and to have a more distinct margin in X-rays of the chest.

Teratomas in the anterior mediastinum are very rare. They are cystic or solid, only occasionally malignant and may extend laterally into one or other pleural cavity.

Bronchogenic cysts arise close to the trachea or the hilum of the lung; they usually contain air and many show a fluid level in X-rays. There may be a history suggestive of intermittent partial obstruction of one of the larger bronchi and surgical excision is curative.

Management

Compression of the trachea and/or bronchi may cause severe respiratory distress, sometimes precipitated by a supervening virus infection. Nasotracheal intubation may be necessary as an emergency.

When a chest X-ray shows a mediastinal mass, tracheostomy is usually of no assistance for the obstruction is below the level of the suprasternal notch. This situation is most commonly caused by a lymphosarcoma, and this presumptive diagnosis should be confirmed quickly by examination of the peripheral blood, the bone marrow or an accessible enlarged lymph node (or occasionally the mass itself). As with other malignancies the stage of the disease will determine treatment. However, use of cytotoxic agents, even without a histological diagnosis, is justified in an emergency and brings dramatic relief. The prognosis for most types of lymphosarcoma is good.

Incidental chest X-ray presentation

Sometimes a mass is found incidentally on chest X-ray. Initial investigations should include:
(1) Examination of the peripheral blood for evidence of leukaemia.
(2) Examination of the bone marrow for metastatic neuroblastoma.

lesions represent malformations of various parts of the lymphatic system, from capillary lymphatics to ducts and sacs, and may also have an element of venous ectasia. Lymphangiomas have a propensity to infection that must be treated with antibiotics. Well-defined lesions should be excised if possible. Cystic hygromas are usually located deep in the cervical and upper thoracic area, and they may be associated with inflammatory and infectious complications. These should also be excised as completely as possible. However, they are not encapsulated or confined by tissue planes (Fig. 16.2).

PIGMENTED NAEVI

True pigmented naevi are melanocytic in origin.

Junctional naevus

Histologically, these naevi show clusters of melanocytes in the basal layers of the skin. They are flat brown or black spots clinically, and normally persist throughout childhood. Junctional activity after puberty is a very slight risk for malignant melanoma. Malignant change is so rare that excision of these in childhood should be avoided unless they have particularly worrying features or if they are a significant cosmetic blemish.

Compound and intradermal naevi

A compound naevus has both junctional and intradermal components. Naevus cells bud off into the dermis where they proliferate and form a cluster of cells resulting in a raised palpable lesion. In later years the junctional activity ceases and the lesions become mature intradermal naevi. They are felt to be benign with no risk of malignant transformation. Surgical excision is for cosmetic reasons.

Spitz naevi

The juvenile or Spitz naevus is usually reddish in colour, as melanin is less prominent. There is considerable junctional activity and spindle cells are present in the dermis. The presence of mitotic figures and atypical cells sometimes leads to confusion with malignant melanoma.

Congenital naevi

Congenital naevi are found in 1 per cent of babies. They may be small (< 1.5 cm), medium or large (> 20 cm). These are histologically similar to acquired compound naevi and the cells form nests deep within the dermis in association with hair follicles and sebaceous glands. The giant naevus occurs in 1 : 20 000 babies and covers a major segment of the body; for example, 'bathing-trunk' naevus (Fig 50.5a). Multiple smaller naevi may also be present in other areas and there may be meningeal involvement. The giant naevus is largely intradermal but it may have a junctional component. The risk of malignant melanoma, mainly after puberty, is about 4 per cent over a lifetime in large naevi and may be higher in giant naevi. With adolescents the lesions tend to become more nodular and hairy.

Treatment is performed mainly for cosmetic reasons by excision and direct closure where possible, or reconstruction with flaps, with or without tissue expansion. In many instances, complete removal is impossible. In giant naevi, extensive skin-grafting is best avoided. Early referral is essential, as many giant naevi can be dramatically improved by curettage in the first few months of life (Fig. 50.5b).

Halo naevi

A halo naevus occurs when melanocytes disappear from the periphery of a pigmented naevus. This is felt to be an immunological phenomenon, and lymphocytes are seen on histological examination. The naevus may disappear completely, leaving a pale patch of skin that later re-pigments.

Ephilis

An ephilis or freckle is a localised increase in

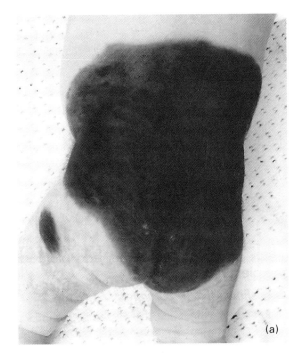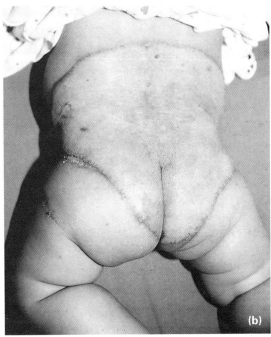

Fig. 50.5 Giant hairy naevus: (a) at 3 weeks of age; (b) following healing after removal using a sharp curette (and excision of the rim that failed to cleave off with the curette).

epidermal pigmentation only. The melanocytes are normal in number.

Lentigo

A lentigo is a patch of increased numbers of melanocytes occupying the basal layer of the epidermis.

Blue naevi

A blue naevus consists of spindle-shaped melanocytes with large amounts of pigment in the deeper dermal layers. The presence of the dark pigment beneath the translucent epidermis produces the characteristic blue-grey colour. The 'Mongolian spot' found on the back and buttock of Asian and black infants, which fades with age, is a classic example.

FURTHER READING

Lorentzen M., Pers, M. & Bretteville–Jensen A.L. (1997) The incidence of malignant transformation in giant pigmented nevi. *Scand. J. Plast. Reconstr. Surg.* **11**: 163–7.

Mulliken J.B. (1990) Cutaneous vascular anomalies. In: McCarthy, J.G. (ed.) *Plastic Surgery*, W.B. Saunders, Philadelphia, pp. 3191–274.

Mulliken J.B. (1997) Vascular anomalies. In: *Grabb and Smith's Plastic Surgery*, 5th edn, Lippincott-Raven, Philadelphia, pp. 191–203.

Orlow S.J. (1997) Congenital melanocytic nevi. In: *Grabb and Smith's Plastic Surgery*, 5th edn, Lippincott-Raven, Philadelphia, pp. 127–30.

Swerdlow A.J., English J.S.C. & Qiao Z. (1995) The risk of melanoma in patients with congenital nevi: a cohort study, *J. Am. Acad. Dermatol.* **32**: 595–9.

Zarem H.A. & Lowe N.J. (1997) Benign growths and generalized skin disorders. In: *Grabb and Smith's Plastic Surgery*, 5th edn, Lippincott-Raven, Philadelphia, pp. 141–60.

Q. 3.2 Craniofacial surgery for synostosis; repair of fingers; genetic counselling.

Q. 3.3 IQ may be impaired if craniosynostosis is not corrected early; but if so, should be normal.

Chapter 16

Q. 1.1 Cervical lymphadenitis; abscess; sialectasis.

Q. 1.2 Once proven/suspected to contain pus: incision and drainage.

Q. 2.1 External angular dermoid; excision.

Q. 3.1 Thyroglossal cyst ± infection; ectopic thyroid; dermoid cyst; submental lymph node; rarely: goitre.

Q. 3.2 Sistrunk operation (removal of cyst, track including middle 1/3 of hyoid bone).

Chapter 17

Q. 1.1 No; spontaneous closure in > 90 per cent by 2 years of age.

Q. 1.2 If not closed by 2 to 3 years because of increasing risk of incarceration.

Q. 1.3 Normal gap in abdominal wall of fetus for placental vessels (umbilical arteries × 2, umbilical vein × 1).

Q. 2.1 Residual necrotic tissue from cord stump colonised by skin organisms. Granulation tissue ('granuloma') is produced in response to subacute inflammation. Silver nitrate cauterisation or excision.

Q. 3.1 Patent vitello-intestinal duct or urachus; ectopic bowel mucosa.

Q. 3.2 By urinary, faecal or mucus only discharge. Excision.

Q. 4.1 Extraperitoneal fat.

Q. 4.2 No.

Q. 4.3 Yes, if symptoms are troublesome.

Chapter 18

Q. 1.1 Observe visible peristalsis and palpate pyloric tumour.

Q. 1.2 Refer to paediatric surgeon.

Q. 1.3 Serum electrolytes and acid-base looking for metabolic alkalosis.

Q. 2.1 Malrotation with volvulus.

Q. 2.2 Barium meal.

Q. 2.3 Ladd's operation (laparotomy and detorsion of bowel) — extremely urgent.

Q. 3.1 Gastro-oesophageal reflux.

Q. 3.2 Reduce handling after feeds, thickening feeds.

Chapter 19

Q. 1.1 Intussusception.

Q. 1.2 Per rectum, plain abdominal X-ray and gas enema.

Q. 1.3 Seven per cent recurrence rate.

Q. 2.1 Bowel obstruction secondary to intussusception (or other causes).

Q. 2.2 Resuscitation with I.V. fluids, nasogastric tube decompression, cross-match blood.

Q. 2.3 Operative reduction ± resection.

Chapter 20

Q. 1.1 Mesenteric adenitis, but should exclude urinary infection.

Q. 1.2 Urine micro and culture, rectal examination.

Q. 2.1 Appendicitis (retrocaecal/retroileal).

Q. 2.2 No, as you have already made a diagnosis.

Chapter 21

Q. 1.1 Fear of serious underlying dissorders, particularly cancer.

Q. 1.2 Frequent short-lived pains, referred to the periumbilical region, perhaps associated with stress in the child's life. Physical examination rarely shows anything other than constipation.

Q. 1.3 The surgeons' role is to exclude serious disease after a careful history and physical examination, and then to reassure.

Chapter 22

Q. 1.1 Needs diet (fluid and fibre increase) and laxative treatment. Rule out (rare) organic causes.

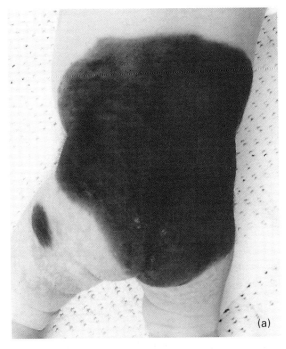 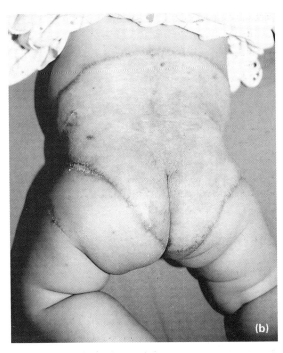

Fig. 50.5 Giant hairy naevus: (a) at 3 weeks of age; (b) following healing after removal using a sharp curette (and excision of the rim that failed to cleave off with the curette).

epidermal pigmentation only. The melanocytes are normal in number.

Lentigo

A lentigo is a patch of increased numbers of melanocytes occupying the basal layer of the epidermis.

Blue naevi

A blue naevus consists of spindle-shaped melanocytes with large amounts of pigment in the deeper dermal layers. The presence of the dark pigment beneath the translucent epidermis produces the characteristic blue-grey colour. The 'Mongolian spot' found on the back and buttock of Asian and black infants, which fades with age, is a classic example.

FURTHER READING

Lorentzen M., Pers, M. & Bretteville–Jensen A.L. (1997) The incidence of malignant transformation in giant pigmented nevi. *Scand. J. Plast. Reconstr. Surg.* **11**: 163–7.

Mulliken J.B. (1990) Cutaneous vascular anomalies. In: McCarthy, J.G. (ed.) *Plastic Surgery*, W.B. Saunders, Philadelphia, pp. 3191–274.

Mulliken J.B. (1997) Vascular anomalies. In: *Grabb and Smith's Plastic Surgery*, 5th edn, Lippincott-Raven, Philadelphia, pp. 191–203.

Orlow S.J. (1997) Congenital melanocytic nevi. In: *Grabb and Smith's Plastic Surgery*, 5th edn, Lippincott-Raven, Philadelphia, pp. 127–30.

Swerdlow A.J., English J.S.C. & Qiao Z. (1995) The risk of melanoma in patients with congenital nevi: a cohort study, *J. Am. Acad. Dermatol.* **32**: 595–9.

Zarem H.A. & Lowe N.J. (1997) Benign growths and generalized skin disorders. In: *Grabb and Smith's Plastic Surgery*, 5th edn, Lippincott-Raven, Philadelphia, pp. 141 60.

— 51 —

Soft Tissue Lumps

CASE 1

A 1-year-old has a non–hair-bearing patch of yellow, slightly raised and irregular skin measuring 2 × 3 cm on the scalp.

    Q. 1.1   *How and when should this be treated?*

    Q. 1.2   *What may happen if it is not treated?*

CASE 2

A year ago a 13-year-old girl who's parents are Pakistani had her ears pierced. She now has 1 cm lumps at the sites of the piercing.

    Q. 2.1   *What is the diagnosis and how should this be managed?*

There are many cutaneous and subcutaneous lesions in childhood. Some of the more common are covered in this chapter. Vascular and pigmented lesions of the skin are discussed in Chapter 50.

WARTS

These are small epidermal tumours produced in response to papilloma virus infections of the skin. They are contagious to a limited degree. Those on the soles of the feet can cause discomfort on weight-bearing. Treatment involves destruction of the lesion by topical application of liquid nitrogen, salicylic acid or podophyllin paint, or curettage.

MOLLUSCUM CONTAGIOSUM

This is caused by a pox virus that produces clusters of pink papules with a central plug that can be squeezed out. They usually resolve after 2 months or may be treated like warts.

EPIDERMAL AND PILAR CYSTS

These are common cysts of epidermal and pilar (hair follicle = tricholemmal) origin respectively. Although they are most often seen in adults, these cysts are not uncommon in children. Treatment is by complete surgical excision.

DERMOID CYSTS

These are most commonly found in the head and neck. Dermoid cysts contain epithelium and adnexal structures, such as sweat glands or hair follicles of varying degrees of differentiation. Nasal dermoids may have a small pit or sinus with associated hair growth. External angular dermoids appear in the lateral eyebrow region (Fig. 16.7). They are sometimes located under the pericranium and appear hard and fixed. Treatment is by complete surgical excision; however, for deep nasal dermoids possible intra-cranial extension should be excluded.

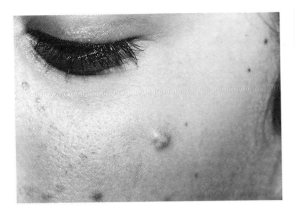

Fig. 51.1 Pilomatrixoma.

PILOMATRIXOMA

This relatively common skin appendage tumour occurs on the face, neck and upper extremities of young children. It is a hard, non-tender and irregular intradermal or subcutaneous lesion, which may appear white or yellow in colour through the skin (Fig. 51.1). It is characterised histologically by areas of calcification and 'ghost cells'. Excision is recommended. Multiple lesions should arouse suspicion of Gardner's syndrome, with multiple polyposis.

NAEVUS SEBACEOUS

Naevus sebaceous is present at birth and appears as a yellowish, slightly raised lesion, usually on the scalp or face. There is a 15 to 20 per cent incidence of basal cell carcinoma developing during adulthood if it is left untreated. These lesions are best excised electively during early childhood.

HYPERTROPHIC SCARS AND KELOIDS

Children tend to produce thick red scars that take 1 to 2 years to involute to become acceptably pale and flat. This is more common on the earlobes, sternum and deltoid regions, particularly in

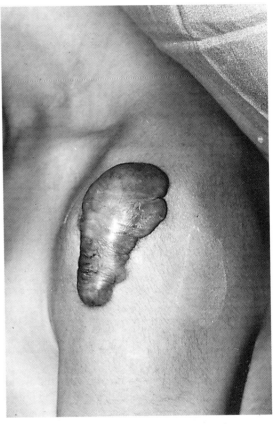

Fig. 51.2 Keloid scar in an adolescent Asian male following a BCG vaccination.

African and Asian people. A keloid continues to grow beyond the margins of the original wound (Fig. 51.2). The appearance is often very unsatisfactory, they are itchy and sometimes cause contractures. Management can be difficult and involves counselling parents (about the time course and expected outcome), intralesional corticosteroid injections, pressure (often applied through specially designed lycra garments) and the use of silicon gel sheeting.

GANGLIA

Ganglia contain gelatinous synovial fluid and frequently arise from joints: particularly the wrist and principally from the scapholunate ligament. They also arise from tendon sheaths. They may be uncomfortable and can be treated with aspiration and corticosteroid injections followed by splintage or by excision.

NEUROFIBROMATOSIS

This autosomal dominant condition affects 1 in 3000 children, and may present as café-au-lait pigmented spots or soft tissue tumours. These consist of fibroblasts, Schwann cells and nerve fibres. Large plexiform lesions of the nerve trunks may be quite disfiguring. Neurofibrosarcoma occurs in approximately 5 per cent of patients later in adulthood.

FIBROMATOSIS

This is an idiopathic, self-limiting fibroblastic proliferation that infiltrates and tends to recur but never metastasises. This often affects the digits or palm, and may be aggressive (extra-abdominal desmoid).

SOFT-TISSUE SARCOMAS

These make up 6 to 8 per cent of all malignancies in childhood, with rhabdomyosarcoma and un-differentiated sarcoma being the most common. After diagnostic biopsy and complete staging, combined treatment with chemotherapy, wide excision, and sometimes radiotherapy, is planned. Sophisticated reconstruction, often with micro-surgically transferred tissues, may be required.

FURTHER READING

Cohen I.K. & Peacock E.E. (1990) Keloids and hypertrophic scars. In: McCarthy, J.G. (ed.) *Plastic Surgery*, Vol. 1, W.B. Saunders, Philadelphia, pp. 732–47.

Zarem, H.A. & Lowe, N.J. (1997) Benign growths and generalized skin disorders. In: *Grabb and Smith's Plastic Surgery*, 5th edn, Lippincott-Raven, Philadelphia, pp. 141–60.

— 52 —

Answers to Case Questions

Chapter 1

Q. 1.1 Regular ultrasonography to monitor progress; ongoing discussion with and counselling by a paediatric surgeon.

Q. 1.2 Yes; antenatal ultrasonography allows antibiotic prophylaxis and early postnatal investigation to be initiated before the kidney becomes further damaged by infection and/or obstruction.

Q. 2.1 Chromosomal analysis and search for other major anomalies.

Q. 2.2 No, only rarely is the time or mode of delivery important.

Chapter 2

Q. 1.1 Wrap the exposed viscera and abdomen in plastic wrap (be careful not to twist the bowel); insert I.V. line for 4 per cent dextrose and 1/5 (0.18 per cent) normal saline; nil orally; nasogastric tube with aspiration; put the baby in the incubator; check for other anomalies; talk to parents about surgery and prognosis (good); obtain consent for transport and surgery; take a photograph for the parents.

Chapter 3

Q. 1.1 No. General anaesthetic is required to prevent fear and to keep the patient still during surgery. A local anaesthetic is used for postoperative analgesia.

Q. 1.2 Removal of sutures (with blade or scissors) is frightening to children because they assume it will be painful (which it is).

Q. 2.1 Fear of pain; staying overnight away from home and parents; unknown technology; unfamiliar people.

Chapter 4

Q. 1.1 Cystic lung disease (sequestration; cystic adenomatoid malformation; congenital tumour — for example, teratoma).

Q. 1.2 Excision.

Q. 2.1 Pneumothorax ± tension.

Q. 2.2 Intercostal drainage: formal catheter (fourth IC space, mid-axillary line) or needle (second IC space, mid-clavicular line) if urgent.

Chapter 5

Q. 1.1 Diaphragmatic hernia.

Q. 1.2 X-ray of chest and abdomen (± insertion of NG tube to determine the position of the stomach).

Q. 1.3 Pulmonary hypoplasia and pulmonary hypertension are main intrinsic factors. Iatrogenic factors include excessive ventilation with pneumothorax and rough handling or premature surgical intervention prior to stabilisation.

Q. 2.1 No.

Q. 2.2 Insert a nasogastric tube and apply gentle suction to keep the bowel decompressed.

Q. 2.3 Tension pneumothorax.

Chapter 6

Q. 1.1 Pass a stiff 10F catheter gently via the mouth: arrested at 9 to 11 cm from gums confirms the diagnosis.

Q. 1.2 Yes, look for VATER/CHARGE and others.

Q. 1.3 Standard neonatal pre-operative 'first aid' plus 10 minutely suction of the oesophagus.

Q. 2.1 VATER: clinical examination and imaging.

Q. 2.2 Renal and cardiac ultrasonography, as well as a pre-operative work-up.

Chapter 7

Q. 1.1 Hirschsprung's disease; small bowel atresia; volvulus neonatorum; meconium ileus.

Q. 1.2 Call the Neonatal Emergency Transport Service.

Q. 1.3 See under General Treatment.

Q. 2.1 Rectal biopsy for histochemical tests and an examination for ganglion cells.

Q. 2.2 Colostomy above the transition zone in the newborn period and a pull-through operation at 3 to 6 months of age.

Q. 2.3 Initial prognosis is good and surgery is life-saving, but there are problems with long-term morbidity (see Prognosis).

Q. 3.1 Duodenal atresia; volvulus neonatorum; high jejunal atresia.

Q. 3.2 Plain X-ray and barium meal.

Q. 3.3 Volvulus neonatorum is one of the most urgent conditions seen by paediatric surgeons.

Chapter 8

Q. 1.1 Exomphalos.

Q. 1.2 Failure of the formation of the umbilical ring with embryonic folding.

Q. 1.3 Wrap defect and abdomen in plastic wrap (avoid kinking contents of sac); incubator; I.V. fluids ± extra glucose if the baby is large; nasogastric tube to keep bowel empty; nil orally; examination for other anomalies; talk to parents.

Q. 1.4 Aim to excise the sac and umbilical cord and close the defect primarily. A prognosis is reasonable if no other anomalies are present.

Q. 2.1 Yes, if 'first aid' is good.

Q. 2.2 Heat- and water-loss cause rapid hypothermia and dehydration.

Q. 2.3 Yes, but it is not very common, except for secondary atresia of the bowel compressed at the level of defect in the abdominal wall.

Q. 3.1 Bladder exstrophy.

Q. 3.2 Yes, but a prognosis for urinary continence is guarded.

Q. 3.3 Each corpus cavernosum forms separately. Sexual function should be fair, but not normal (penis bent and short).

Chapter 9

Q. 1.1 Level and appearance at birth; motor and sensory levels; any secondary deformities; other abnormalities (for example, hydrocephalus).

Q. 1.2 There is a high risk of Arnold–Chiari malformation and associated hydrocephalus.

Q. 1.3 The intellect should be reasonable, as long as hydrocephalus is controlled; walking is unlikely although hip flexion and adduction may be preserved.

Q. 2.1 Incontinence ± partial outlet obstruction; infection; stone; renal failure.

Q. 2.2 Clean intermittent catheter for urine (± reconstruction procedures); diet and wash outs/laxatives for faeces.

Chapter 10

Q. 1.1 Any child with an: (i) apparently enlarged clitoris; (ii) apparent hypospadias with bifid scrotum and/or undescended testes; (iii) truly ambiguous genitalia.

Q. 1.2 As much as possible, so they understand and can participate in decision-making.

Q. 1.3 Genital anomaly is a medical and social emergency requiring urgent referral to a tertiary centre.

Q. 1.4 (i) Potential for adult fertility; (ii) relative degree of development of male versus female organs.

Q. 2.1 No.

Q. 2.2 Bifid 'scrotum' and/or bilateral or unilateral 'cryptorchidism'.

Chapter 11

Q. 1.1 Same as for Case 1, Chapter 2.

Q. 1.2 Either definitive surgery if low anomaly, or colostomy if high anomaly, then pull-through at about 3 months

Q. 1.3 Outcome for faecal continence is poor for high anomalies: bowel wash outs ± diet and laxative treatment required. Low anomalies with better outlook, but soiling or constipation is still common.

Q. 2.1 MRI.

Q. 2.2 Diet and laxatives or regular wash outs (via the anus or appendicostomy).

Chapter 12

Q. 1.1 Head circumference crosses the percentiles (hydrocephalus); abnormal shape.

Q. 2.1 Headaches are frequent/'different'; significant child/parental anxiety; other symptoms of raised ICP or epilepsy; focal signs.

Q. 2.2 Some are benign (pilocytic astrocytoma, craniopharyngioma, pineocytoma) and may be cured with surgery. Germinoma and medulloblastoma are malignant but prognosis is good with treatment. The rest do badly (for example, brain stem glioma, pineoblastoma, disseminated medulloblastoma or ependymoma).

Q. 3.1 Sometimes; slow refill may indicate blockage. Clinical diagnosis.

Q. 4.1 Surgery is possible but the prognosis varies (occipital is worse than sincipital because of blindness/hydrocephalus/ataxia). Genetic counselling needed.

Q. 5.1 Plagiocephaly secondary to 'sticky' lamboid suture. Often improves but strip craniectomy is needed sometimes. Definitive synostosis needs operation.

Chapter 13

Q. 1.1 Amblyopia may develop if squint ± poor vision untreated.

Q. 1.2 Eye examination, including cover test and check of vision.

Q. 2.1 Yes: there is nystagmus which may be secondary to poor vision.

Q. 2.2 Vision and eye examination; referral to ophthalmologist.

Q. 3.1 Cause is nasolacrimal duct obstruction, which resolves in 95 per cent by 1 year. Probing (under GA) reserved for persisting symptoms only.

Q. 3.2 Antibiotic drops only needed if secondary infection with conjunctivitis occurs.

Q. 4.1 History and examination should reveal cause; for example, a foreign body.

Chapter 14

Q. 1.1 The infant has otitis media with effusion (± acute suppuration). The fluid in the middle ear reduces hearing. A pale, opaque membrane occurs with fluid behind the membrane and inflammatory thickening.

Q. 1.2 Amoxicillin 40 mg/kg/day: 3 doses for 5 days.

Q. 1.3 Yes.

Q. 2.1 Tonsillectomy plus adenoidectomy is recommended if attacks of tonsillitis are very frequent.

Q. 3.1 Physical examination to determine the site of stridor plus the degree of airway obstruction, followed by flexible laryngoscopy.

Q. 3.2 Nose blocked, stenosis, choanal atresia; glossoptosis; laryngomalacia; vocal cord lesions; subglottic stenosis; tracheomalacia.

Chapter 15

Q. 1.1 Pierre Robin syndrome with mandibular hypoplasia and secondary cleft palate.

Q. 1.2 Nurse prone ± airway for first few days. Long-term spontaneous resolution with growth.

Q. 2.1 Four per cent if no parents affected.

Q. 2.2 Sixteen per cent if parent affected.

Q. 3.1 Apert syndrome.

Q. 3.2 Craniofacial surgery for synostosis; repair of fingers; genetic counselling.

Q. 3.3 IQ may be impaired if craniosynostosis is not corrected early; but if so, should be normal.

Chapter 16

Q. 1.1 Cervical lymphadenitis; abscess; sialectasis.

Q. 1.2 Once proven/suspected to contain pus: incision and drainage.

Q. 2.1 External angular dermoid; excision.

Q. 3.1 Thyroglossal cyst ± infection; ectopic thyroid; dermoid cyst; submental lymph node; rarely: goitre.

Q. 3.2 Sistrunk operation (removal of cyst, track including middle 1/3 of hyoid bone).

Chapter 17

Q. 1.1 No; spontaneous closure in > 90 per cent by 2 years of age.

Q. 1.2 If not closed by 2 to 3 years because of increasing risk of incarceration.

Q. 1.3 Normal gap in abdominal wall of fetus for placental vessels (umbilical arteries × 2, umbilical vein × 1).

Q. 2.1 Residual necrotic tissue from cord stump colonised by skin organisms. Granulation tissue ('granuloma') is produced in response to subacute inflammation. Silver nitrate cauterisation or excision.

Q. 3.1 Patent vitello-intestinal duct or urachus; ectopic bowel mucosa.

Q. 3.2 By urinary, faecal or mucus only discharge. Excision.

Q. 4.1 Extraperitoneal fat.

Q. 4.2 No.

Q. 4.3 Yes, if symptoms are troublesome.

Chapter 18

Q. 1.1 Observe visible peristalsis and palpate pyloric tumour.

Q. 1.2 Refer to paediatric surgeon.

Q. 1.3 Serum electrolytes and acid-base looking for metabolic alkalosis.

Q. 2.1 Malrotation with volvulus.

Q. 2.2 Barium meal.

Q. 2.3 Ladd's operation (laparotomy and detorsion of bowel) — extremely urgent.

Q. 3.1 Gastro-oesophageal reflux.

Q. 3.2 Reduce handling after feeds, thickening feeds.

Chapter 19

Q. 1.1 Intussusception.

Q. 1.2 Per rectum, plain abdominal X-ray and gas enema.

Q. 1.3 Seven per cent recurrence rate.

Q. 2.1 Bowel obstruction secondary to intussusception (or other causes).

Q. 2.2 Resuscitation with I.V. fluids, nasogastric tube decompression, cross-match blood.

Q. 2.3 Operative reduction ± resection.

Chapter 20

Q. 1.1 Mesenteric adenitis, but should exclude urinary infection.

Q. 1.2 Urine micro and culture, rectal examination.

Q. 2.1 Appendicitis (retrocaecal/retroileal).

Q. 2.2 No, as you have already made a diagnosis.

Chapter 21

Q. 1.1 Fear of serious underlying dissorders, particularly cancer.

Q. 1.2 Frequent short-lived pains, referred to the periumbilical region, perhaps associated with stress in the child's life. Physical examination rarely shows anything other than constipation.

Q. 1.3 The surgeons' role is to exclude serious disease after a careful history and physical examination, and then to reassure.

Chapter 22

Q. 1.1 Needs diet (fluid and fibre increase) and laxative treatment. Rule out (rare) organic causes.

Q. 2.1 Needs exclusion of organic causes, especially Hirschsprung's disease and intestinal neuronal dysplasia. Initial management includes enemas ± faecal disimplaction (under GA).

Chapter 23

Q. 1.1 See Box 23.2.
Q. 1.2 Anal fissure, secondary to constipation.
Q. 1.3 Correct the constipation with diet and laxatives.
Q. 2.1 Meckel's diverticulum; duplication; peptic ulcer; varices.

Chapter 24

Q. 1.1 Ulcerative colitis; barium enema, colonoscopy with biopsy, full blood examination and bacteriological cultures.
Q. 2.1 'Top-and-tail' endoscopy with biopsies; barium meal and follow-through; full blood examination; liver function tests; stool cultures.
Q. 2.2 Extent of disease; extra-intestinal signs and symptoms; histology.

Chapter 25

Q. 1.1 Hydronephrosis.
Q. 1.2 Renal ultrasonography; DTPA scan ± cystoscopy with retrograde pyelogram to distinguish pelvi-ureteric junction obstruction from vesico-ureteric junction obstruction.
Q. 2.1 Wilms' tumour or neuroblastoma, once ultrasonography confirms the lesion is solid.
Q. 2.2 Biopsy/excision, chemotherapy ± radiotherapy.
Q. 3.1 Catecholamine measurements (VMA, MHMA) in urine, CT scan, bone scan, bone marrow, FBE; neuroblastoma.
Q. 3.2 Prognosis is poor, but some are still curable with chemotherapy and surgery.

Chapter 26

Q. 1.1 Trauma (handle-bar, child abuse, MCA); bile duct stone; idiopathic.
Q. 1.2 Serum lipase level; epigastric peritonism and ileus; ultrasonography/CT scan shows swollen gland.
Q. 1.3 A cystic cavity secondary to leakage of enzymes from the pancreatic duct.
Q. 2.1 Liver function tests; ultrasonography; HIDA scan.
Q. 2.2 Stone is removed by laparotomy, laparoscopy or ERCP. Biliary atresia requires Kasai portoenterostomy.

Chapter 27

Q. 1.1 Perianal abscess with fistula *in ano*; incision of abscess and tract.
Q. 2.1 Labial adhesions.
Q. 2.2 Separation with thermometer, paper clip or gentle pressure (± anaesthetic jelly). Regular application of vaseline and general measures to prevent nappy rash.

Chapter 28

Q. 1.1 Risk of subsequent ascent at 5 to 10 years of age.
Q. 1.2 If ascent occurs orchidopexy is recommended once the testis no longer can reside spontaneously in the scrotum.
Q. 2.1 Ambiguous genitalia; bilateral intra abdominal testes; bilateral perinatal torsion/agenesis.
Q. 2.2 Hormone/chromosome tests; laparoscopy ± orchidopexy/orchidectomy.
Q. 3.1 Six months.
Q. 3.2 Not known for certain but expected to be normal or near normal in most boys with early treatment.

Chapter 29

Q. 1.1 Indirect inguinal hernia.
Q. 1.2 Bilateral inguinal herniotomy.

Q. 2.1 Torsion of testis or appendage; epididymitis; idiopathic scrotal oedema.

Q. 2.2 No.

Q. 2.3 Exploration of the scrotum, R/O appendage or detorsion and fixation of testes (both).

Chapter 30

Q. 1.1 No, not necessary; normal washing (externally) is sufficient.

Q. 1.2 After 5 years in the majority of boys; partial adherence is still normal until adolescence.

Q. 2.1 Urethral meatus and glans visible in normal child on retraction or traction.

Q. 2.2 Topical corticosteroid cream or circumcision.

Q. 3.1 Neonatal circumcision is not necessary for hygiene and the procedure is dangerous.

Q. 3.2 The acceptable standard is a general anaesthetic (after 6 months); full surgical technique; adequate postoperative analgesia.

Q. 3.3 Bleeding; infection; penile deformity; glanular/meatal ulceration; acute retention (pain).

Q. 4.1 Six months.

Q. 4.2 Fix chordee; put urethra on top of the glans; satisfactory cosmetic appearance; minimum complications.

Q. 4.3 Extensive mobilisation to fix chordee; foreskin advance to ventral surface; neourethra constructed; ± postoperative stenting/urinary diversion, 1 or 2 stages.

Chapter 31

Q. 1.1 Urine micro and culture to confirm UTI, then renal ultrasonography. Further tests only if ultrasonography is abnormal.

Q. 1.2 Low risk of anomaly but still possible.

Q. 1.3 Perineal contamination is secondary to poor perineal hygiene ± constipation with soiling.

Q. 2.1 Suprapubic aspirate.

Q. 2.2 Renal and bladder ultrasonography, MCU ± DTPA or DMSA scan.

Chapter 32

Q. 1.1 Renal ultrasonography; MCU ± DMSA scan.

Q. 1.2 Unpleasant and invasive, but gold standard for VUR, urethral and bladder anomalies.

Q. 1.3 Indirect MCU.

Q. 2.1 Both.

Q. 2.2 It should not (although scars become visible very slowly and may appear to be occurring later).

Q. 2.3 Failed medical treatment; anatomical anomalies; persisting VUR in prepubertal girls.

Chapter 33

Q. 1.1 Spontaneous resolution is common, especially in the less severe cases. Severe dilatation suggests progressive obstruction requiring treatment.

Q. 1.2 Pelvi-ureteric junction obstruction; vesico-ureteric junction obstruction; vesico-ureteric reflux; urethral obstruction.

Q. 1.3 Antibiotic prophylaxis, early ultrasonography and MCU (< 1 to 2 weeks), and MAG3/DTPA scan (2 to 6 weeks).

Q. 2.1 Vesico-ureteric obstruction; vesico-ureteric reflux; urethral obstruction.

Q. 2.2 MCU and renal ultrasonography, especially in infants and preschool children. MCU less useful in older children.

Chapter 34

Q. 1.1 Each predisposes to the other.

Q. 1.2 Renal and bladder ultrasonography; X-ray ± MCU; ± cystoscopy to document bladder anatomy; CMG for bladder function.

Q. 1.3 Correct VU reflux surgically if still present; bladder training; antibiotics ± anticholinergics.

Q. 2.1 Ectopic ureter in the perineum.

Q. 2.2 Patch test; renal ultrasonography; DTPA scan.

Q. 2.3 Heminephroureterectomy.

Q. 3.1 Occult spina bifida: hairy/pigmented patch, lipoma, sinus, palpable defect in vertebral spines. Absent sacral segments.

Q. 3.2 Secondary spinal and meningeal infection may occur.

Q. 3.3 Clean intermittent catheterisation is the mainstay of treatment.

Chapter 35

Q. 1.1 Meatal ulcer.

Q. 1.2 Soak off scabs; apply vaseline; leave off nappy; treat nappy rash.

Q. 2.1 Ruptured kidney; Wilms' tumour; hydronephrosis.

Q. 2.2 Renal ultrasonography: if minor renal trauma, then treat conservatively unless there is a significant urine leak. For tumour and hydronephrosis: treat condition.

Chapter 36

Q. 1.1 Airway, breathing, circulation; resuscitation; secondary (head-to-toe) survey; continued resuscitation; definitive care.

Q. 1.2 Detailed examination of all body systems to identify all injuries.

Q. 1.3 Airway obstruction (from tongue or blood) may depress conscious state.

Q. 2.1 Surgical debridement under anaesthetic.

Q. 2.2 Tetanus management; excision of devitalised tissue.

Chapter 37

Q. 1.1 See Box 37.1.

Q. 1.2 See Box 37.3.

Q. 1.3 See Box 37.2.

Q. 2.1 See Box 37.4.

Q. 3.1 Acute left extradural haemorrhage.

Q. 3.2 Extremely urgent.

Q. 3.3 Determine the GCS. Urgent resuscitation and x-match, CT, then craniotomy and R/O collection. If delay before surgery give

Mannitol. **N.B.**: Urgent problem with risk of death.

Q. 4.1 See Box 37.5.

Q. 5.1 Transient/prolonged amnesia after HI. No pathology with minor concussion; severe concussion with diffuse axonal injury (swelling on CT with haemorrhage in corpus callosum/dorsal brain stem) — may cause a persisting vegetative state.

Chapter 38

Q. 1.1 Ruptured spleen.

Q. 1.2 ABC; correction of hypovolaemia; CT or U/S to confirm rupture; conservative treatment (unless uncontrollable haemorrhage, which is very rare).

Q. 2.1 The girl has a fractured femur and possible intra-abdominal bleeding (possible liver or splenic rupture). The leg needs an air-splint and traction/fixation. After airway control and oxygen, the girl needs resuscitation with fluids and urgent transfusion. A CT scan will demonstrate the injury; however, conservative treatment is likely unless there is bowel perforation.

Chapter 39

Q. 1.1 No.

Q. 1.2 No.

Q. 2.1 Under general anaesthesia with a mosquito forcep inserted via a small incision guided with an image intensifier.

Chapter 40

Q. 1.1 Immediate copious irrigation of face and mouth with water, and drinking copious water/milk.

Q. 1.2 Observation to see if drooling/dysphagia is present, and if so, oesophagoscopy is needed to diagnose the full-thickness oesophageal burn that needs treatment to prevent stricture.

Chapter 41

Q. 1.1 Remove clothing and immerse the affected parts in cold water for 10 minutes. Commence IV (Hartmann's solution). Give I.V. morphine: 0.05 to 0.1 mg/kg over 5 minutes. Wrap the child in a clean sheet and blanket. Take swabs of the nose, throat, faeces and burn. Insert urinary catheter. Give maintenance fluids orally. Start I.V. rate at $(\frac{1}{2} \times 2$ to 3 ml/kg/1 per cent burn area over the first 8 hours, giving $\frac{1}{2}$ the estimated volume as 5 per cent serum albumin and $\frac{1}{2}$ Hartmann's solution. Call the Burns Unit for advice and to arrange a transfer.

Q. 2.1 Possible child abuse by deliberate immersion.

Q. 3.1 Possible inhalation injury with airway burn.

Chapter 42

Q. 1.1 Callus of healing fracture of humerus secondary to birth injury.

Q. 1.2 Spontaneous healing with full recovery.

Q. 2.1 Dislocated hip with soft tissue oedema around the capsule. Aspiration of joint revealed pus, consistent with diagnosis of septic dislocation of hip. Even with drainage, I.V. antibiotics and abduction bracing, there is a risk of proximal femoral growth arrest and short limb.

Q. 3.1 Birth injury to brachial plexus.

Q. 3.2 Spontaneous recovery with elbow movements at 6 weeks and shoulder movements normal by 3 months. Failure to recover by 3 months suggests microsurgical repair is needed.

Q. 4.1 'Postural' club foot.

Q. 4.2 Normal function after a few weeks of stretching exercises.

Q. 5.1 Talipes calcaneovalgus may be associated with a developmental dislocation of the hip.

Q. 6.1 Serial plaster casts to commence immediately. Surgical release of contracted tendons may be required at 6 months if there is residual deformity.

Chapter 43

Q. 1.1 The child has bow legs, which resolves over 6 to 12 months. Monitoring the deformity in the standing position with serial Polaroid photographs is useful.

Q. 2.1 Internal tibial torsion is common with mild bowing. Six-monthly reviews should demonstrate resolution by 3 years of age.

Q. 3.1 Development dislocation of the hip.

Q. 3.2 Ortolani's test with confirmation by hip ultrasonography should have been done at birth, as she had all the risk factors for DDH.

Q. 4.1 Cerebral palsy with hemiparesis.

Q. 5.1 Osteomyelitis of proximal femur.

Q. 5.2 A hot area in right upper femur.

Q. 6.1 Child abuse.

Q. 6.2 Fracture of the femoral shaft and a strong likelihood of other healing fractures, such as rib, skull, collarbone.

Q. 7.1 Osteogenesis imperfecta (Type 1); a skull X-ray would show multiple Wormian bones.

Chapter 44

Q. 1.1 Internal femoral torsion.

Q. 2.1 The gap is not excessive and spontaneous resolution is expected without surgery.

Q. 3.1 Simple orthotics may prolong shoe life, but makes little difference to the condition itself.

Q. 4.1 This is likely to be a supracondylar fracture with brachial artery compromise. There is a high risk of Volkman's ischaemia unless treatment is rapid and appropriate.

Chapter 45

Q. 1.1 Scoliosis.

Q. 1.2 Likely to show an intrinsic curvature ± rotational deformity.

Q. 1.3 < 20°: observe; 20 to 40°: brace; > 40°: spinal fusion.

Q. 2.1 Slipped upper femoral epiphysis.

Q. 2.2 AP and lateral X-ray; ultrasonography may help to diagnose secondary haemarthrosis.

Q.2.3 Pinning of epiphysis *in situ* to prevent further chronic slippage.

Q.3.1 Overuse syndrome affecting immature retropatellar cartilage.

Q.3.2 No further tests needed if the X-ray is normal. Arthroscopy is indicated occasionally.

Q.3.3 Conservative; analgesics, restriction of provocative activities and gentle exercises.

Q.4.1 Osteosarcoma or Ewing's tumour.

Q.4.2 Imaging (plain X-ray, bone scan, CT/MRI) and biopsy.

Q.4.3 Chemotherapy followed by tumour excision ± limb salvage.

Chapter 46

Q.1.1 Trigger thumb.

Q.1.2 No.

Q.1.3 Yes.

Q.2.1 Erb's palsy; traction on brachial plexus during difficult delivery; surgery if not resolved after 3 months.

Chapter 47

Q.1.1 Premature thelarche; remains static or resolves over 6 to 12 months.

Q.1.2 Only if mastitis occurs, surgery for drainage of abscess (rare at this age).

Q.2.1 Neonatal hypertrophy; clean skin with antiseptic, do not squeeze breast (milk production ceases spontaneously).

Q.2.2 Either male or female (female hormones from mother).

Chapter 48

Q.1.1 Chestwall deformities only cause *subtle* changes in the cardiorespiratory function, except in severe deformity.

Q.1.2 A chest X-ray, especially if there is a low protrusion.

Q.1.3 Reassure her that there is no major functional limitation, and cosmetic surgery can be done if required (often delayed until adolescence).

Chapter 49

Q.1.1 Staph. pneumonia, and may be developing Staph. empyema.

Q.1.2 Flucloxacillin and gentamicin I.V. until cultures confirm sensitivity; regular X-ray review; ± surgical drainage of empyema.

Q.2.1 Spontaneous pneumothorax; confirm with X-ray, needle or intercostal catheter if under tension; if no tension, observe in ward; diagnose and treat cause.

Chapter 50

Q.1.1 No risk of melanoma.

Q.1.2 Cosmetic treatment if needed.

Q.2.1 Amblyopia of eye; deformity of face throughout preschool years; some residual scar.

Q.2.2 Surgical excision or laser treatment. Occasionally, intra-lesion steroid injection or interferon treatment is needed.

Chapter 51

Q.1.1 Naevus sebaceous: needs excision in childhood.

Q.1.2 Fifteen to 20 per cent risk of basal cell carcinoma in adulthood, if untreated.

Q.2.1 Keloid; counselling, intralesional steroid injections, pressure via lycra or silicon gel sheeting.

Index

Jones' Clinical
Paediatric Surgery
Diagnosis and management